THE DOCTOR, HIS PATIENT
AND THE ILLNESS

THE DOCTOR, HIS PATIENT AND THE ILLNESS

MICHAEL BALINT, M.D.

Second Edition

PITMAN

PITMAN PUBLISHING LIMITED
128 Long Acre, London WC2E 9AN

Associated Companies
Pitman Publishing Pty Ltd, Melbourne
Pitman Publishing New Zealand Ltd, Wellington

Distributed in the United States of America and Canada
by Urban & Schwarzenberg Inc.,
F East Redwood Street, Baltimore, MD 21202

© Michael Balint, 1957, 1964

First Published 1957
Second Edition 1964
Reprinted 1966, 1968, 1971, 1973, 1974, 1977, 1983, 1984

ISBN 0 272 79206 3

Printed in U.S.A. at
Whitehall Company, Wheeling, Illinois

To my wife and colleague

By the same Author

PRIMARY LOVE AND PSYCHO-ANALYTIC TECHNIQUE
First Edition London and New York 1952
Second Revised and Enlarged Edition
London and New York, 1964

PROBLEMS OF HUMAN PLEASURE AND BEHAVIOUR
London and New York, 1957

THRILLS AND REGRESSIONS
London and New York, 1959

In collaboration with Enid Balint
PSYCHOTHERAPEUTIC TECHNIQUES IN MEDICINE
London and New York, 1961

Preface

THIS book represents part of the results of a research project by a team of fourteen general practitioners and a psychiatrist. Although the theoretical conclusions are mine and the book was written by me, the work on which it is based was done entirely by my fourteen colleagues: Drs. D. Arning, G. Barasi, N. Chisholm, M. B. Clyne, A. J. Hawes, B. Hermann, P. Hopkins, J. Horder, L. Hornung, A. Lask, P. R. Saville, G. Szabo, G. Tintner and A. L. Zweig. It is with great pleasure that I acknowledge my indebtedness to them for their unselfish co-operation. Theirs was by no means a simple or easy task. The special nature of the research not only required frank disclosure by them of many intimate personal details of their daily work, details which by general tacit consent are hardly ever made public; it also required acceptance of thorough and searching criticism of such details. Anybody reading this book cannot but be impressed by the amount and severity of criticism that was given and taken in good spirit during the research; all irritation, hurt personal feelings, vexation were either disregarded or tolerated to enable the research work to proceed.

The training scheme on which the research was based was developed jointly by Enid Balint and myself. In addition she supervised a number of the cases treated and took a considerable part in the case conferences; but perhaps her most important contribution was the benevolent but unsparing comments and criticisms with which she followed the development of the atmosphere in the group discussions. On more than one occasion it was her correct and sound evaluation of the real difficulty that helped me to overcome it.

Next I wish to express my gratitude to Dr. John D. Sutherland, Medical Director of the Tavistock Clinic, who from the outset followed our venture with warm interest and put at our disposal all the services of the Clinic. Without his understanding support our research would not have been possible. He contributed Appendix IV, in which he discusses an important additional rôle for the psychological clinic. We are equally indebted to the members of the consultant staff of the Adult Department of the Clinic for supervising cases treated by participants.

We were allowed to call upon the help of the psychologists of the Adult Department whenever a patient was referred for diagnosis. Our understanding of the patient's problems profited greatly by the results of the projection tests used. I wish to mention in particular Mr. H. Phillipson and Mr. John Boreham, who did most of the work for us.

Dr. John Kelnar and Dr. R. D. Markillie gave several theoretical courses to the various groups of doctors, which were much appreciated and were found to be most helpful.

That our research was able to proceed as smoothly as it did was mainly due to our secretary, Miss Doris Young. She looked after everybody and everything; all the administrative arrangements worked without a hitch; the right people, the right papers and the right case notes appeared at the right moment as if by magic. It was she who took down in shorthand the proceedings of the case seminars, which means that a large part of this book was literally written by her. Her greatest contribution, however, was her talent for effacing herself; although she was physically always present at our seminars, we could discuss the most intimate and awkward matters confidently feeling that we were alone.

Mr. Eric Mosbacher, who read the whole manuscript, proved to be a sympathetic but inexorable critic of my English and helped considerably in making this book as readable as it is. But, as I did not always accept his amendments, the final responsibility for the text is entirely mine.

Dr. R. H. Gosling undertook the compilation of the Index and I wish to express my sincere thanks for his conscientious work. I am also indebted to Dr. Philip Hopkins who not only read the proofs but also called my attention to some unclear or ambiguous passages in the text.

And lastly, my thanks are due to my patient and long-suffering secretary, Mrs. I. Lloyd-Williams, who typed this book several times over and pointed out several badly worded passages.

* * *

I wish to acknowledge the courtesy of the Editors of the *British Medical Journal, The Lancet,* and *The British Journal of Medical Psychology* for allowing me to use previously published material.

July 1956   MICHAEL BALINT

Preface to the Second Edition

THE request to prepare a revised edition, however gratifying, caused a number of problems for which it was not easy to find satisfactory answers.

The publication of this book, eight years ago, did not coincide with a halt in our research; quite the contrary, it happened during a period of expansion. This expansion compelled us to test and retest our results and led to some considerable development of our ideas about medical practice, about psychotherapy in general, and especially about psychotherapy by general practitioners. Part of the results of this development has already been published in the Mind and Medicine Monographs, chiefly in two books: Michael and Enid Balint: *Psychotherapeutic Techniques in Medicine* (1961) and David Malan: *A Study of Brief Psychotherapy* (1963); while other results, those about training, will be published shortly in books now under preparation.

The most important aspect of this development for the field covered by the present book is a somewhat changed appreciation of the general practitioner's rôle during treatment. Whereas in this book I was mainly concerned with the demonstration of the importance of "listening," as distinct from the traditional medical history taking, recent research, especially by my wife and myself, led us to isolate and define two more aspects of the psychotherapist's tasks, which are—of course—no new discoveries. These are "understanding" and "using the understanding so that it should have a therapeutic effect." These three aspects are subsequent phases of the same process; "listening" provides the material which is then ordered into "understanding," and evidently understanding must be achieved before it can be used. The phrase: "using the understanding so that it should have a therapeutic effect," is tantamount to a demand for a more exacting form of diagnosis; the therapist is expected to predict with a fair amount of accuracy what sort of effect his envisaged intervention will have.

To embody these new ideas into the existing text would have meant rewriting a very large part of the book. This would have

ix

destroyed the simplicity of the presentation; in fact it would have meant writing another book. After some hesitation I decided against this plan and restricted my work to a careful revision of the text, to ironing out some ambiguities, and to pointing out here and there the direction of our new ideas.

One part of the book, however, had to be completely rewritten and this is Appendix III, Follow-Up Reports. I used the opportunity offered by a revised edition to ask my colleagues who took part in the original research, to follow up all their patients whose case histories were included in this book. For the sake of easier presentation the whole of Appendix III had to be rearranged. Under each case we have printed first the result of the first period of follow-up, taken over unchanged from the first edition, followed immediately by the result of the second period of follow-up.

And lastly, a very pleasant task indeed, I wish to express my great indebtedness to my fourteen colleagues who, after so many years of separation, responded without fail to my request. I am sorry to have to qualify this last sentence; one of them gave up his practice and left London; his name, however, must not be mentioned, otherwise it would give away not only his anonymity but possibly also his patients'. Next, I wish to thank Dr. John D. Sutherland, Medical Director of the Tavistock Clinic, for his continued interest in this research and for revising Appendix IV, which he kindly contributed to the first edition. Dr. Philip Hopkins has again undertaken the arduous task of proof reading, for which he has my sincere thanks. And, last but not least, my thanks are due to my secretary Miss Joan Morris for her unsparing and conscientious help during the preparation of the revised edition.

MICHAEL BALINT

October 1963

Contents

CHAPTER I

Introductory

FOR a number of years research seminars have been organized at the Tavistock Clinic to study the psychological implications in general medical practice. The first topic chosen for discussion at one of these seminars happened to be the drugs usually prescribed by practitioners. The discussion quickly revealed—certainly not for the first time in the history of medicine —that by far the most frequently used drug in general practice was the doctor himself, i.e. that it was not only the bottle of medicine or the box of pills that mattered, but the way the doctor gave them to his patient—in fact, the whole atmosphere in which the drug was given and taken.

This seemed to us at the time a very elevating discovery, and we all felt rather proud and important about it. The seminar, however, soon went on to discover that no pharmacology of this important drug exists yet. To put this second discovery in terms familiar to doctors, no guidance whatever is contained in any text-book as to the dosage in which the doctor should prescribe himself, in what form, how frequently, what his curative and his maintenance doses should be, and so on. Still more disquieting is the lack of any literature on the possible hazards of this kind of medication, on the various allergic conditions met in individual patients which ought to be watched carefully, or on the undesirable side-effects of the drug. In fact, the paucity of information about this most frequently used drug is appalling and frightening, especially when one considers the wealth of information available about other medicaments, even those most recently introduced into practice. The usual answer is that experience and common sense will help the doctor to acquire the necessary skill in prescribing himself. The shallowness of this self-reassuring advice becomes apparent when it is compared with the detailed instructions based on carefully controlled experiments with which every new drug is introduced into general practice.

When the seminar realized this disquieting state of affairs, our mood changed, and we decided forthwith that one of the aims, perhaps the chief aim, of our research should be to start devising this new pharmacology.

The importance of a study of this kind is perhaps much greater nowadays than ever before; but the reason is only partly inherent in medicine. Particularly as a result of urbanization, a great number of people have lost their roots and connexions, large families with their complicated and intimate interrelations tend to disappear, and the individual becomes more and more solitary, even lonely. If in trouble, he has hardly anyone to whom to go for advice, consolation, or perhaps only for an opportunity to unburden himself. He is more and more thrown back on his own devices. We know that in many people, perhaps in all of us, any mental or emotional stress or strain is either accompanied by, or tantamount to, various bodily sensations. In such troubled states, especially if the strain increases, a possible and in fact frequently used outlet is to drop in to one's doctor and complain. I have deliberately left the verb without an object, because at this initial stage we do not know which is the more important, the act of complaining or the complaints that are complained of. It is here, in this initial, still "unorganized" phase of an illness, that the doctor's skill in prescribing himself is decisive. We shall discuss presently the unexpected consequences that may be brought about by the doctor's response to his patient's complaints. Before doing so I propose to say something about our methods and the general set-up of our research.

Our work has been carried out exclusively in the form of discussion groups, consisting of about eight to ten general practitioners and one or two psychiatrists. The groups met once a week for two to three years, though some went on longer. The meetings were held on the early afternoon of the free half-day usually taken by general practitioners. This enabled them to attend without serious interference with their practice; in fact, this arrangement worked so well that even in the busiest months of general practice, from December to March, the attendance was very good—averaging for the whole year from ninety to ninety-five per cent of the possible total.

Our venture was a mixture of research and training. At the outset I had some idea that, psychologically, much more happens in general practice between patient and doctor than is discussed in the traditional text-books. If my ideas were correct, the events that I wanted to get hold of could be observed only by the doctor himself; the presence of a third person, however tactful and objective, would inevitably destroy the ease and intimacy of the atmosphere. Such a third person would see only an imitation, perhaps a very good imitation, but never the real thing.

Thus, the research could be conducted only by general practitioners while doing their everyday work, undisturbed and unhampered, sovereign masters of their own surgeries. But general practitioners are entirely untrained for this task; this is a matter to which we shall have several occasions to return in the following pages. Moreover, when we started, no established method was in existence, so far as I am aware, for training general practitioners in psycho-diagnosis and psychotherapy. Thus we were faced with three different though interlinked tasks. The first was to study the psychological implications in general practice; the second to train general practitioners for this job; and the third to devise a method for such training.

The chief emphasis in this book is on the research aspect of our venture. The training system is briefly described in Appendices I and II. Some of the discussions that followed the doctors' reports on their patients give some idea how our research-cum-training worked. (See especially cases Nos. 10, 15, 17, 19, 21, 23 and 24.)

The uncertainty caused by the complex structure of our venture is reflected in our terminology. The mainstay of our research-cum-training will be referred to in this book as group discussion, case conference, research seminar, discussion seminar, discussion group, etc.; all meaning the same but describing it from different angles.

As will be seen, the doctors tried hard to entice the psychiatrists into a teacher–pupil relationship, but for many reasons it was thought advisable to resist this. What we aimed at was a free, give-and-take atmosphere, in which everyone could bring up his problems in the hope of getting some light on them from the experience of the others. The material for our discussions was almost invariably provided by recent experiences with patients reported by the doctor in charge. The continuity of the course enabled us to follow the development of the patients' problems for two or three years—occasionally even longer—and thereby to examine how far our ideas, diagnoses, predictions, therapeutic attempts, etc., were correct and useful or otherwise. (Appendix III.)

Our chief aim was a reasonably thorough examination of the ever-changing doctor–patient relationship, i.e. the study of the pharmacology of the drug "doctor." In order to obtain reliable data for this study we tried to restrict to a minimum the use of written material in our discussion groups. There was no reading of prepared reports or manuscripts; the doctors were asked to report freely on their experiences with their patients. They were allowed to use their clinical notes, but only as an *aide-mémoire* and not as a *précis*. From the beginning our intention was that a doctor's report should include as full an account as possible of his emotional responses to his patient, or even his emotional involvement in his patient's problems. A frank account of this, the emotional, aspect of the doctor–patient relationship can be obtained only if the atmosphere of the discussion is free enough to enable the doctor to speak spontaneously. Any prepared manuscript or written report would of necessity involve a good deal of secondary elaboration of this spontaneous material, which was exactly what we wished to avoid. The following chapters will testify to the extent to which we were able to achieve our aim.

Let me confess at the outset that our contribution to the solution of the many problems involved in the close study of the doctor–patient relationship is meagre enough, although the general direction in which medicine, in our opinion, ought to develop will become fairly clear. But, even if it is impossible to indicate a rational therapy for an illness, a commendable step has been taken if it has become possible to describe the pathological processes involved and give a reliable diagnosis. This, then, is the chief aim of this book: to describe certain processes in the doctor–patient relationship (the undesirable and unwanted side-effects of the drug "doctor") which cause both the patient and his doctor unnecessary suffering, irritation and fruitless efforts. Hitherto these processes have certainly not been fully observed, or, if they have been observed, their importance has not been properly evaluated. Then we shall try to describe diagnostic signs to enable the doctor to recognize these pathological processes in good time. It will be only in the third instance—and only to a very modest extent—that we shall be able to indicate what sort of therapy might be applied in this most complicated field.

My first task, therefore, is to state the problem that we are to investigate. Briefly, the problem is this: why does it happen so often that, in spite of earnest efforts on both sides, the relationship between patient and doctor is unsatisfactory and even unhappy? Or in other words, why does it happen that the drug "doctor," despite apparently conscientious prescription, does not work as intended? What are the causes of this undesirable development and how can it be avoided?

I shall base all my deductions on concrete clinical observations of individual patients. None of the cases were, however, observed by me. As mentioned above, courses were arranged at the Tavistock Clinic at which general practitioners discussed the psychological implications of their everyday practice. All the cases quoted in this book were taken from this source, and they are normally reported in the practitioner's own words. Summaries made by me in some cases for the sake of brevity were submitted to the practitioners concerned for approval before inclusion.

The draft of the book was sent in instalments to each doctor taking part in the research, and we devoted a number of meetings to discussing it. Every objection was discussed, and if a considerable number of the participants identified themselves with it the passage in question was altered or omitted. Thus the final version is the result of true teamwork. Although each of us had his share in this book, the responsibility for the printed text is entirely mine.

To preserve the doctors' anonymity, only the masculine pronoun is used throughout this book, except in two case histories, Nos. 22 and 24, where the sex of the doctor was of importance in the development of the doctor–patient relationship. Each doctor, however, has been identified by a letter, in order to enable the reader to study the various individual atmospheres created by them. One of the unexpected results of our research was the realization of how greatly these atmospheres can differ. What is entirely impossible in one surgery happens as a matter of course in another. (See Chapters XIII and XVII.) The drug "doctor" is evidently far from being standardized. What is still more interesting is that patients can benefit by all these varieties of the drug. This does not mean, however, that each variety is equally beneficial. On the contrary, each has its own side-effects, and the identification by a letter of the alphabet of our anonymous doctors will help the reader to become aware of both the desirable main effects and the undesirable side-effects of each variety.

To preserve the patients' anonymity turned out to be a much more difficult task. We have done our best to make the patients quoted in this book unrecognizable. No names are mentioned, and wherever possible external circumstances have been disguised. Unfortunately there is a limit to such attempts at disguise. If one goes too far in that direction the case history differs so greatly from the original that it may amount to falsification. In order to avoid this pitfall, all the essential features, above all the psychological details, of the individual patient were left unchanged. But this means that a patient may recognize himself in the description of his case. This highly undesirable hazard is unfortunately inevitable and, so far as I can see, nothing can be done to avoid it with certainty. To minimize this risk we confined our selection to case histories of patients who were thought unlikely to read this book. But in spite of all our precautions I am aware that by some ill-luck this publication may cause inconvenience, some discomfort, or even pain to one or the other patient. Should this occur, all I can do is to express my deep and sincere regret, and to give an assurance that it is highly improbable that the individual concerned will be identifiable by anyone but himself.

The case reports are rather novelistic and some of them even long-winded. It would not have been difficult to prune them and to print only what the pruner considered essential and relevant. After some consideration I decided not to do this, but to print the reports in the form in which they were presented, unprepared, to our discussion seminars.* A carefully pruned report represents what we psychoanalysts call the results of secondary elaboration, i.e. of weeding out most of the remnants of the emotional processes in the mind of the reporter, or of his critics, thereby giving disproportionate emphasis to intellectual processes. Leaving the reports as they were presented will, I hope, enable the reader to see to some extent both the emotional and the intellectual involvement of the reporter and of his audience.

---

*As a rule an experienced shorthand-typist, Miss Doris Young, was present and took down what was said practically verbatim. The reports printed here are based on her notes.

The cases reported in this book are mostly of the simple, every-day type that occur in the surgery of every doctor from Land's End to John o' Groats'. I greatly hope that in reading them doctors will recognize one or the other of their own only too familiar patients. This was exactly our purpose; to enable doctors to take a fresh look at their everyday experience and see that there are problems which, because medicine has tried to ignore them, cause them a great deal of unnecessary work and their patients a great deal of unnecessary suffering and irritation. As I have mentioned, I am able to offer solutions for only a fraction of the problems thrown up by this book. The rest must await further research. But I hope that our findings may enable doctors to notice developing problems before they spoil their relationship with certain patients, and that better knowledge and better insight will enable them to prevent some undesirable developments.

The book is divided into three parts. The first part, Chapters II–IX on Diagnosis, is mainly critical, at times severely so. We hope that it will be clear that our criticism does not imply that the whole of medicine is in urgent need of reform. On the contrary, our aim is to demonstrate which aspects of medical thought and practice are in need of revision. In our view, these aspects may be summed up as *the pathology of the whole person.*

The second part of the book—Chapters X–XV—is concerned with Psychotherapy by General Practitioners. Only cases treated by general practitioners have been included. This part is, inevitably, somewhat patchy. The chief reason is our scanty knowledge, which does not permit us to deal with the subject systematically.

The third part—General Conclusions—consists of six somewhat disconnected chapters. In them I have tried to sum up the positive results of our research. As mentioned, on most occasions, instead of solutions, we see only problems, but also possibilities for future research.

In Appendix I the present state of our training system is described, followed by an Appendix on selection; in a third Appendix all the cases reported are followed up at least until December 31, 1955; and lastly, in a fourth appendix John D. Sutherland describes an important additional function of the psychological clinic.

At the outset I must warn the reader that he will not find in this book any references to literature. The chief reason is personal.

I am an erratic and unsystematic reader. Although I am aware that authors may have written about this or that part of our field of research, my knowledge of the literature is unreliable. To overcome this shortcoming I could either have drawn up a spurious bibliography or sat down to several months' hard library work. I should have hated either.

In consequence, I have to accept the uncertainties and limitations caused by my ignorance. It is perfectly possible that in a number of our findings we may have been anticipated by others, who may even have described them in a more accurate or more helpful form. If so, I apologize and disclaim priority.

I have one more excuse for the lack of references. Our research was deliberately kept self-contained. We wanted to see how far we—a team of general practitioners and psychiatrists—could go on our own, each of us using what he had, a condition only too well known to doctors. Thus, this book is based on what we used to call the "courage of our own stupidity" (see Appendix I); and references to other authors would have been rather out of place.

PART I

Diagnosis

CHAPTER II

The General Problem

AS stated in the introductory chapter, it happens not so infrequently that the relationship between the patient and his doctor is strained, unhappy, or even unpleasant. It is in these cases that the drug "doctor" does not work as it is intended to do. These situations are quite often truly tragic; the patient is in real need of help, the doctor honestly tries his hardest—and still, despite sincere efforts on both sides, things tend obstinately to go wrong. Our first four cases will illustrate this sort of situation.

CASE I* (*reported by Dr. M.*)

Mrs. C., aged 32 years; married, childless. This patient has been on my partner's list since early 1946. She complained then of epigastric and chest pains. My partner sent her for investigation to an eminent physician in April 1946, who reported, "You will be glad to hear that this patient's chest X-ray is quite normal. She seems very pleased at this and I think most of her symptoms are functional, and hope that the reassurance I have given her may be of some help."

A short while after, the patient was unhappy about the condition of the chest as the pain returned, and she was sent for chest X-ray to a chest clinic. The physician to the chest clinic reported in May 1946, "You will be pleased to learn that there is no evidence of pulmonary or pleural tuberculosis. I think the epigastric pain originates in the abdominal wall, that is, it is probably muscular or fibrous in origin. Massage might now be tried." Massage was accordingly tried, but with little success. She was a frequent visitor to the surgery and was seen by me first in October 1946. I thought then that her symptoms might be due to "chronic appendicitis." I referred her to a gynaecologist first, who wrote in 1947, "This lady is rather puzzling. She has been under Dr. L., who had her completely investigated and found nothing, and I must admit I can find nothing abnormal, and from the gynaecological point of view I have drawn a blank. Whether

* This case history was published in the *British Medical Journal* (1954), Vol. I., p. 115.

in view of her constant pain in the right side and her chronic constipation there is the possibility of an appendix, it is difficult to say, but if you wish I will ask one of our surgeons . . ." A surgeon was accordingly asked, and he said in October 1947, ". . . I have advised her to come into hospital for the removal of her appendix." Appendicectomy was carried out in December 1947. She came to see me then practically every week with a variety of pains, sometimes in the right iliac fossa, sometimes in the back, and drove me frantic with seemingly irrelevant chatter and unwillingness to leave me during a busy surgery. I sent her to see a well-known orthopaedic surgeon on account of her persistent backache. He said in January 1948, "She has a supple back, although there is some slight tenderness in her lumbar muscles. I am arranging for her to have some treatment in the physiotherapy department."

Mrs. C. attended my surgery regularly every week, had still the same complaints as before, and began, to my puzzlement, to be rather aggressively flirtatious with me. I then told her one day, rather abruptly, that there was little more I could do for her and that it would be best if she went back to her job as a sales assistant and would not come back to see me for some time, and I did not see her again until 1950. She came then with her old complaints of pains again, and in the attitude of a penitent child ("Didn't you miss me?" and "I hope you won't be cross with me any more"). She still came every week, again became flirtatious and tried to put her foot on mine, and one day put her hand on mine. I rebuked her then, and she cried; went, only to come back the following week, and in subsequent weeks. She received five to ten minutes' chat and a bottle of medicine on each occasion.

Since then, due to a greater awareness of personality disorders on my part, she has been given a one-hour interview in which, *inter alia*, she told of her childhood, of a father who was in the Navy and away from home most of the time, of a much loved younger brother who died at the time of the onset of her symptoms, of her dyspareunia since the beginning of her marriage, and of her complete inability to have sexual intercourse since her brother's death. Further investigations are in progress. Her attitude to me since that interview has much changed, there are no more efforts to flirt and there is an improvement in her symptoms. But it took four years to get to that hour, and an appendicectomy. *Mea culpa!*

CASE 2 (*reported by Dr. E.*)

Mrs. A. and her baby son, born July 1948. This woman's child has had frequent illnesses and ill health from birth; coughs, colds, tonsillitis, no appetite, screaming fits, prolapse of the rectum, and so on. Hospital investigations all nil. Mother always very worried about him and dissatisfied with his failure to improve. Home conditions bad. Family lived on top floor of an old cottage-type house, with no facilities whatever; water, coal, refuse and swill all had to be carried up and down stairs. Lower flat in house occupied by man of eighty-four with wife of forty-four. Up to the age of eighty very virile. At the age of about eighty he became ailing and made a great deal of fuss about losing his virility. About the time when Mrs. A.'s baby was born his health had just begun to fail and he was entering his final illness, which lasted about nine months. He was an unsatisfactory invalid, and was a nuisance to his wife, doctor and all the neighbours. Wife suffered a great deal of distress and emotional upset, which was reflected on the family upstairs. (The upstairs family looked up to the ground-floor family with respect and tried hard to accept their standards.) Complaints of noise of baby, etc., caused much disharmony, reflected in the anxiety of the mother upstairs and the illnesses of the baby. Since the old man died his widow has gone out to work. Her own mental health has improved considerably, and her relationship with the family upstairs has also improved. In consequence, the health of Mrs. A. has improved, and the child is also well. He is now an infrequent visitor to the surgery —enough to cause comment when he does attend—although he still has an occasional prolapse. January 1949 Mrs. A. changed her doctor, who did not see her at all until February 1950, when she returned to us.

Case 3 was reported by Dr. P. at one of our meetings in which we discussed patients who apparently cannot be helped.

CASE 3

A woman, aged sixty, not very intelligent. She has been to quite a number of hospitals to see various specialists. For some years she has had bronchiectasis. She now comes regularly with three complaints: headaches, pumping in stomach and giddiness. When I give her medicine for her headaches, she complains next time of her stomach, and when I give her something for her stomach she complains next time of giddiness. I tried talking to her, but it was no good. I brought her to tears one day when I pointed out that all these medicines did no good. I suggested that she change her doctor, but she would not. I have found that the only way to cope with her is to continue giving her medicine as she asks for it, and now she is quite happy. She is about to move from her flat, and for the last six months she has been saying to me, "You will be very happy to hear I am going away." I told her I was not, and that I really wished I could help her, and added that I would always be here whenever she wanted me.

CASE 4 (*reported by Dr. R.*)

A single woman of 47. She came to see the doctor for the first time in May 1953 complaining of watering of the right eye which had followed a cold in the nose. Apart from that she said that her general health was good. The only physical finding was a very slight angular conjunctivitis. She was very excitable, talked a good deal. The doctor suggested that there might be something else wrong, but she denied it. Drops for the eyes were prescribed and she was told to return in a week if she was not better. She did not return until September, when her doctor was on holiday—she saw his locum. She said she had a "disgusting complaint," which turned out to be bleeding from a small haemorrhoid. It was difficult to examine her, she kept talking about this "awful disgusting trouble." She was given suppositories and told to come back in a fortnight if not better. She returned a month later, complaining that she was unable to sleep at night and felt that her throat was "very swollen, as though someone is strangling me," and she was very worried. The doctor assured her that there was no evidence of any physical disease, but she insisted that the trouble must be anaemia, as she had always been anaemic. She was referred to hospital for blood tests. The pathologist reported that the haemoglobin was 110 per cent, and when the patient was told that she was normal she remarked, "Oh what a nuisance. . . . No, don't get me wrong. . . . I mean it would have been such a simple explanation for my not sleeping." The doctor replied that it seemed that she would really like to have anaemia, and her answer was, "No, I don't want to be ill, but what can be the cause of my symptoms?" When the question was repeated back to her, her comment was, "Well, it must be something mental I suppose." She followed this by saying that in that case she didn't need medical help, but that her "common sense would see her through." The doctor told her to come back to him again if she felt she would like to discuss any emotional problems or difficulties, as she declined to do so then. It was not until six months later that the patient returned to the doctor. She complained of recurrent sore throats for the previous one month. She had changed her job and was now an industrial nurse, but did not like it. There was a definite acute pharyngitis, associated with a raised temperature (100°F.). After simple medical treatment with lozenges and a gargle her condition had improved when seen four days later. She then volunteered the information that she had been very worried, and she felt that this "must have been the cause of my bad throats." Three weeks later she again attended the surgery, this time with a return of bleeding and pain on defaecation. Examination revealed a small fissure-in-ano. Simple local treatment was prescribed. While being examined she was much less difficult than previously. She remarked that her trouble "must be due to a psychological strain at work." She was asked to return in a week if not better, but at the time of writing (two months later, in July 1954) she has not been back.

Later, in Chapter V, we shall have to discuss some of the general implications for everyday medical practice of clinical observations of this kind. Here I wish to add that in the discussion that followed this last report it was once again recognized that the case history was typical. The patient seemed to offer various "illnesses" to her doctor, to which the doctor responded with the appropriate physical examinations, followed by rational therapy, thus exploding in turn each proposition either as unjustified or as unfounded. The doctor agreed wholeheartedly and produced the patient's medical card, which amply proved this idea. As the file of this patient tells a typical story, it is reprinted here as one representative of innumerable cases of this kind to be found in the practice of every doctor.

*Notes of previous doctor**

1948

December   Attended a teaching hospital c/o pain lower abdomen, diarrhoea. Chest X-rayed N.D.D. F.H. Negative. No chest trouble.

1949

26th Feb.   Sub-conjunctival haemorrhage. Spots in front of eyes.
4th Mar.   Improved. Pluravite.
16th Mar.   Nails brittle. Tonic prescribed.
8th Apr.   Improved. ? caruncle.
8th Sept.   Run down. Insomnia. B.O. regular. Appetite good. T.Ferr.Co. and K Br. N.V.
23rd Sept.   Fell on left hand last p.m. Bruises round mc-ph joint of left thumb.
10th Oct.   Improved. Sl. restricted flexion. M-C-ph-joint L. thumb
19th Nov.   Sl. increase in size L. thumb. Dressing.
6th Dec.   Worked up easily. Sleep only fair. Sedative.

1950

20th Feb.   Burn mucous membrane of palate. Painted and tonic given.
30th Mar.   Abdomen blown up? Nil on exam. Ex bread and potatoes.

*As this is an exact copy, all abbreviations are printed in the form used by the doctor.

17th May	Benadryl.N.B.G. Hy. (Illegible entry but apparently drugs which must have been for cold.)
15th July	Ointment for skin condition.
15th Sept.	Liquid paraffin for making bowels work.
21st Dec.	F.B. right eye. Given drops.

1951

13th Oct.	Cold 1 week. Cough; weak; no fever. Pulse regular. Blood trace on straining. Constipation. Takes Enos. Metatone. Cough mixture.
25th Oct.	T.N. Says Temp 99° in evening (6 p.m.) no cough, ulcer frenul. of tongue. Cauterised.
26th Oct.	Sub-mental glands enlarged. Temp. normal.
29th Oct.	Says T.100° last p.m. Fauces N.A.D. T.98.4. T.C.A. to-night. Ulcer of Frenul of tongue. Sloughed.
29th Oct.	T. 98.4.
2nd Nov.	T.98. Urine N.A.D. Neurophosphates.
5th Nov.	Per. commenced. — 3 weeks interval. T.98.
12th Nov.	Improved.

1952

5th Jan.	Improved.
31st Mar.	Cold. Glands L. neck. Rubella type rash on face and chest. ? German measles.
11th July	Ointment prescribed.
11th Nov.	Nasal catarrh and frontal ache.

1953

24th Jan.	Catarrhal cold. Dental extraction two days ago. Tired. Neurophosphates.
5th Feb.	D. and V. 3 days.

Notes of present doctor

1953

12th May	(Company secretary) c/o watering of r. eye—one month since a "cold" and "throat." General health is good.
	Wt. up a bit. Sleeps well.
	P.H. Rubella 1952.
	Ch. Pox.
	Opn. on R.Parotid Gland (? Calculus).
	Menses: Regular. 3/25. No pain.
	O.E. Mild angular conjunctivitis (R)
	(Anxieties for discussion?)

22nd Sept.   Has had this "disgusting complaint." Saw locum. He gave
            her suppositories. Hammam. et Zinc. Ox. B.O.R. O.E.
            Skin tags only.
            General discussion.

26th Oct.   c/o wakes up in night—only once—feels "my throat is
            swollen and going to choke." "Only highly strung." Very
            voluble. O.E. Hys. To Hospital for Hgb. and R.B.C's.

28th Oct.   Path report—110% Hgb. No anaemia. When told not
            anaemic she said "That's a nuisance. . . . No don't get me
            wrong. I mean it would have been such a simple explana-
            tion for my not sleeping. Well it must be something mental
            I suppose. My common sense will carry me through."
            Declined offer to discuss problems.

1954

30th Apr.   c/o recurrent sore throats—one month. Has changed job—
            industrial nurse—doesn't like it. O.E. Temp. 100° F.
            Pharyngitis. Tr. Troch. Potass. Chlorate 0.3.h. Gargle
            Glyc. thymol.

3rd May   Improving. Says has been very worried—thinks this
            might have caused her sore throats. (!) Tr. Metatone.

24th May   c/o Pain on defaecation associated with bleeding. B.O.R.
            (Bowels open regularly), but occasional strain. Volunteers
            that she thinks it is due to "a psychological trouble at
            work." O.E. Small fissure-in-ano (No fuss while being
            examined this time.) Tr. Ung. Nupercainal. Emuln. Liq.
            Paraffin o.n.

Before going further I wish to call attention to the remarkable
difference between the notes of the two doctors. Both are correct
and complete—but only as far as they go. The first consists of a
shorthand version of the complaints, the physical findings, and
the rational therapy prescribed—the whole modelled on the usual
case records of a busy hospital outpatients' department, with
everything not absolutely necessary left out. The second doctor
goes further. In addition to the factual data, he records some
details of the patient's characteristic utterances and emotional
behaviour—but nothing about himself, as if his own contributions
were either unimportant or so stereotyped that every trained
doctor would have behaved in exactly the same way. It is only
in his report to the seminar that we get some glimpses into the
developing relationship between patient and doctor and in consequence can form some idea of what was really happening. We

termed these important differences, "differences in depth or level," and we speak then of the depth or level of observation, of recording, depth or level of diagnosis, of therapy, etc. In several of the later chapters we shall return to this topic.

These four case histories convincingly illustrate our first thesis, which, I am afraid, will sound rather startling to some of my colleagues. But we can quote innumerable case histories in support of it. The four selected here are only a small sample. We think that some of the people who, for some reason or other, find it difficult to cope with the problems of their lives resort to becoming ill. If the doctor has the opportunity of seeing them in the first phases of their becoming ill, i.e. before they settle down to a definite "organized" illness, he may observe that these patients, so to speak, *offer or propose various illnesses*, and that they have to go on offering new illnesses until between doctor and patient an agreement can be reached, resulting in the acceptance by both of them of one of the illnesses as justified. In some people this "unorganized" state is of short duration and they quickly settle down to "organize" their illness; others seem to persevere in it, and although they have partly organized their illness they go on offering new ones to their doctor. The variety of illnesses available to any one individual is limited by his constitution, upbringing, social position, his conscious or unconscious fears and fantasies about illnesses, etc. Still, as in these four cases, despite these limitations, there are always several offers or propositions. *One of the most important side effects—if not the main effect—of the drug "doctor" is his response to the patient's offers.*

In this book I shall try to follow up the devious paths along which an agreed compromise between doctor and patient is reached, the various stages along this route, the many propositions, counter-propositions, offers, acceptances and rejections that take place. I shall pay special attention to the contributions by the doctor towards settling a patient who cannot get completely cured in an acceptable illness, and, last but not least, to the price that has to be paid by both doctor and patient for this compromise. Finally I shall discuss some of the alternatives available to the doctor to help his patients to become aware of their problems and to find a solution less costly than settling down to acceptable long-term ill health.

Now taking the four cases reported above, the contribution of each of the four doctors was different, although each acted and behaved as objectively as possible and certainly in accordance with the rules of medical science and practice. In Case 1 the practitioner, so to speak, accepted all the various illnesses that the patient offered him and sent her to specialists eminent in the respective fields to which the proposed "illness" belonged. The specialists too did their job as it ought to be done; they reported correctly that nothing could be found, or proposed a rational therapy when there was some justification for it. Still, all this was of no avail, because the patient needed something entirely different, and only when the doctor became aware of what was being demanded of him, and allowed and helped the patient to realize and express her real problems, did the whole situation—both the past failures and the present suffering—become intelligible.*

As we shall come back to Case 2 in Chapter IV, here I wish to point out only that during the whole period of observation this practitioner accepted every illness offered by the patient as well founded, prescribed the correct short-term therapy for each in turn, with the result that he scored short-term successes but could not contribute anything to the real cure. The final cure was brought about by external events.

Case 3 shows a well-known unhappy situation between a well-meaning, tolerant and understanding doctor, and his co-operative but apparently incurable patient. Although both tried hard, the one to help and the other to be helped, no real improvement could be achieved. One reason was that the patient had settled down to her organized illness, and another that, at that stage, the doctor found it impossible to get to the root of the trouble.

Case 4 illustrates, in almost classical purity—especially if we take the previous history into account—this haggling between doctor and patient for a possible compromise. In this case the doctor's response was somewhat different from that of the previous three. He not only accepted every minor illness offered to him and either prescribed proper treatment for it or exploded it by appropriate physical examinations, but also tried to impress on his patient that there must be a common cause for all these minor ailments. As more and more offers were exploded, the patient was eventually driven into a corner and had to ask, very reluctantly, whether this common cause was not perhaps "mental."

* See, however, the follow-up report in Appendix III.

Although this would have been a major therapeutic achievement if it had occurred earlier, at this late stage, when the relationship between doctor and patient had become somewhat tense and uneasy, the patient had to reject the help offered by saying that her "common sense would see her through."

When the draft of this chapter was discussed by our seminar it came under sharp criticism. The doctors agreed with my description and discussion of the dynamic processes but maintained that the basic problem was not brought out clearly enough. Finally one of them challenged me, if we asked each participant in turn, what in his opinion the real problem was, no two of them would give the same answer. I accepted, and the result apparently fully vindicated the challenge. According to one doctor the problem was, "What does the patient need from his doctor and what does he actually get?" Another asked, "What is it that the patient cannot get from his doctor so that he must keep coming back for it?" A third, "What is it that the doctor gives the patient that the patient does not want or need?"

I think all these formulations can be considered as variations of the same theme; my formulation being not more true nor more important than any of the others. How should the doctor "respond" to the patient's "offers" so as to avoid an undesirable outcome as described in the four preceding case histories? This question implies that the doctor's responses may and often do contribute considerably to the ultimate form of the illness to which the patient will settle down. Before going any further, I propose to illustrate the usefulness of this idea with a few more case histories.

CHAPTER III

The Patient's Offers and the Doctor's Responses

LET us take a rather simple case, one well known to every practitioner. Dr. E. in charge of Case 5 reported in June 1954:

CASE 5

Mr. U., aged 36. A highly skilled workman, earning about £15 per week, married, two children. Very happy, apart from the fact that the younger boy, four years ago, had acute nephritis and has been rather ill ever since. Mr. U. had polio when a child and his left leg is about four inches shorter, requiring a boot. He deals with his infirmity extremely well, however. The boy's illness is rather tragic, but he copes with it quite well, although the illness gets his wife down. He runs a car, and takes his family out for week-ends.

In February while he was at work someone tampered with an electric connection and he got a very severe shock. He was thrown clear, but was out for about fifteen minutes. He came round and recovered completely. I think he then saw the doctor at the works or perhaps they sent him to the casualty department of the local hospital. Two or three weeks ago he came to see me, complaining of pains all over the front of his chest, the lower part of his back, right leg and right hand, and saying that the pains were getting worse and worse. I examined him thoroughly and came to the conclusion that no organic damage had been done, although he thought that something had happened to him through the electric shock. As he seemed rather worried about it, I suggested that I get a specialist's opinion, which he accepted. He came to see me last night. He had had all the examinations. The letter to me from the hospital said that they could not find anything, and that "we would like the patient to be seen by our psychiatrist." I told him that nothing wrong had been found, and he said that was funny because his pains were much worse. He said, "They seem to think I am imagining things—I know what I have got." After talking a few minutes in a very pleasant manner, he said he thought the hospital might have made a mistake. He is definitely ill, and would like to know what condition he could have causing all these pains.

21

"What does the book say about it?" I did not answer, except to say that it was not a matter of looking up the books, that, for example, if he had a broken leg he would not ask me the cause of it, but would ask me to get it better. Finally I said that as he could not accept the view of the hospital, would he like to go to an entirely different hospital to be examined again? He was not keen, saying that they would do the same thing and would not find anything wrong. I was not sure how to get on, what was the next step, so I suggested that he should come back for further discussion in a week's time.

Of course, this is a trivial case, of the kind occurring time and again in nearly every practice. Simple as it appears at first sight, it raises a number of difficult problems, both theoretical and practical, which must be discussed at some length.

Let us start with the problem already mentioned: the patient "proposing an illness" to the doctor—a very important first step in the history of any patient. In this case, in different periods, we can study an accepted compromise, an offer by the patient, then one by the doctor, the rejection of both of them in turn, and finally some of the ensuing consequences.

First, the accepted compromise. A severely handicapped man achieves, with the help of his understanding doctor, a highly satisfactory mental and physical equilibrium—very likely somewhat over-pressing himself and over-compensating his physical shortcomings by high efficiency. Then, out of the blue, he is subjected to a severe electric shock, causing unconsciousness and possibly—in the psychological aspect—more than that. His reaction is a gradual development of pains in the whole front part of the body—the part which was facing in the direction from which the shock came—with the conspicuous exception of his damaged leg. The whole picture, i.e. the illness "proposed," strongly suggests a psychological reaction—a queer mixture of fear, admission and denial—as if he were saying, "Something terrible has happened—I am afraid I have been badly damaged on my whole front, possibly my already disabled leg also; but no, that cannot be; I have pains practically everywhere except in my left leg."

It is at this point that the doctor gets to work. Faithful to his training, he first sets out to exclude all possible physical complications, although there is no evidence to suggest any. After all, the accident happened in February and the patient did not come until the end of May. Still, the first move is to ask for a surgeon's opinion. As expected, this turns out to be negative, and the doctor's conscience about his responsibility is put at rest. He now tries to switch the patient to a second set of examinations, this time by a psychiatrist.

But what happened to the patient—and, still more important, in the patient—in the meantime? He came to his old trusted friend, the family doctor, prompted by pains, anxieties, fears, but otherwise in a trusting and friendly mood, hoping for help, understanding and sympathy. It is true that he received a fair amount of all of them, but was then put through the mill of a routine hospital examination, almost certainly with a number of white-coated strangers firing searching questions at him. Perhaps he did, perhaps he did not, realize that everybody was getting more and more concerned about a possible claim for compensation, or to use a more fashionable term, about a possible compensation neurosis, and trying their best to prevent him from sliding into it. What he certainly did realize, however, was that all the doctors were at pains to convince him that *there was nothing wrong with him*, i.e. *they were rejecting his proposition*. When he came back to his doctor with the hospital report, the previous trusting, friendly attitude had been badly shaken, the model patient had turned into a disappointed, suspicious, mistrustful man.

Could anything have been done to avoid this undesirable turn? In the discussion after this report it was suggested that perhaps the order of the examinations should have been reversed. After all, if a patient comes with symptoms strongly suggesting kidney trouble, one would not start by sending him for a chest X-ray or a barium meal. Perhaps in the same way patients probably suffering from psychological complaints should be examined in the first instance by a psychiatrist, and only if further examination should prove necessary, by a surgeon or other specialists. The best answer to this suggestion was given by one of the doctors, who pointed out that if a general practitioner referred such a patient to a psychiatrist in the first instance, he would certainly receive an indignant letter rebuking him for his negligence in not having had his patient examined physically first.

We shall return to the problem raised here, the proper order of the specialist examinations. Medical thinking is at present crucially influenced by the fear of missing some physical illness while concentrating attention on possible psychological causes. There are several reasons for this fear, and in the next chapter we shall discuss them and their effects on the development of the patient's and the doctor's attitude to the illness. Here I only want to point out that to neglect a possibly psychological illness for the sake of getting reassured that no physical processes are present may be just as deleterious to the patient's future as the usually quoted opposite, that is to say, concentrating unduly on psychological implications and consequently neglecting possible physical causes.

Perhaps a way of avoiding this undesirable turn might have been for the doctor to have said to the patient, "I think that your complaints are due to some psychological after-effects of the shock you suffered, and so our first concern should be a proper psychological examination; on the other hand, to be on the safe side and just as a safeguard, at the same time I shall ask a surgeon to have a look at your body." The psychological examination—in exactly the same way as a physical examination—could then be carried out either by the doctor himself or, if he does not feel competent enough, by a specialist.

In Mr. U.'s case everything went satisfactorily until he was sent for a hospital examination. Previously the relationship between the patient and the doctor, in fact between the doctor and the whole family, had been excellent, although a good deal of strain had to be borne on both sides because of the grave illness of the younger boy. Not even the "illness" provoked by the accident could upset the spirit of friendly co-operation. Only when the patient suspected that the doctors would somehow reject his "propositions," i.e. either did not understand his illness or, still worse, did not care to understand it, did the relationship suffer. The patient started feeling—dimly at first—that perhaps the doctors were no longer on his side, that possibly they were actually against him. The hitherto model patient was thus forced first into an argument with his doctor, an argument which might later develop into a major battle. Yet we should not forget that despite this strain and suspicion the patient is still frightened and lost, desperately in need of help. His chief problem, which he cannot solve without help, is: what is his illness, the thing that has caused his pains and frightens him? In his own words, "What does the book say?"

I wish to emphasize here that nearly always this is the chief and most immediate problem; *the request for a name for the illness, for a diagnosis*. It is only in the second instance that the patient asks for therapy, i.e. what can be done to alleviate his sufferings on the one hand, and the restrictions and deprivations caused by the illness, on the other.

Not paying attention to this order of importance is the cause of a very frequent form of irritation and of bitter disappointment in the doctor–patient relationship—another undesirable side-effect of the drug "doctor." When a patient, after a series of careful and conscientious examinations, is told that nothing is wrong with him, doctors expect that he will feel relieved and even improve. Admittedly this happens fairly often, but in quite a number of cases just the opposite occurs and the doctor's usual reaction to this—in spite of its frequency, always unexpected—event is pained surprise and indignation. This perhaps could be avoided if doctors would bear in mind that finding "nothing wrong" is no answer to the patient's most burning demand for a name for his illness. Apart from the almost universal fear that what we have found is so frightening that we will not tell him, he feels that "nothing wrong" means only that we have not found out and therefore cannot tell him what it is that frightens or worries him and causes him pain. Thus he feels let down, unable to explain and accept his pains, fears and deprivations. It would certainly be no help to him to know that occasionally his suspicions are justified; that the statement "nothing wrong" sometimes really means that medicine does not know what is wrong in his particular case.

My chief reason for the lengthy discussion of this trivial case is that here the conflict between doctor and patient is in the open. It is true that this is not fully recognized by either of them, but both know and feel that their relations are under strain. The patient asks, "What does the book say?" and instead of answering the question honestly the doctor replies, "Never mind your illness, be concerned only about your pains and worries which I can relieve." Leaving aside the doubt whether this promise can be honoured as completely as is implied in the doctor's answer, the misunderstanding between patient and doctor is clear. The patient's burning problems remain unanswered, his demand for a name for his nameless, frightening illness is left frustrated, that is, his "offer" is rejected. Moreover, he is not given the opportunity or freedom to express his fears and disappointments frankly. Instead he is given a questionable reassurance that nothing is wrong with him, capped with the "offer" of a second set of unpleasant examinations and with a vague, not altogether realistic, promise of help. Thus there is a dangerous confusion of tongues, each party talking in a language not understood and apparently not understandable by the other. This situation is bound to lead to arguments, disappointments, and often even to open controversy and battles. As mentioned, I quote this case because in it the controversy is in the open.

There are many cases in which—though the signs of a confusion of tongues between the patient and his doctor are painfully present—there is apparently no open controversy. Some of these cases demonstrate the working of two other, often interlinked, factors. One is the patient's increasing anxiety and despair, resulting in more and more fervently clamouring demands for help. Often the doctor's response is guilt feelings and despair that his most conscientious, most carefully devised examinations do not seem to throw real light on the patient's "illness," that his most erudite, most modern, most circumspect therapy does not bring real relief.

The next case will illustrate this point. I wish to preface it by saying that it was reported by a very thorough and conscientious doctor, a good diagnostician, sincerely interested in helping his patients. Apart from his practice, he was a part-time clinical assistant in the medical department of a large hospital. This case history is based on the doctor's report to the seminar and on the ensuing discussions, but the compilation is by myself.

CASE 6

The patient was a man of thirty-five, a company director, in the care of his present physician only for the past three months. He had been ill for several years, complaining of pains in his abdomen. He had consulted several eminent and expensive specialists, and had had innumerable X-ray examinations, test meals, etc. His appendix had been removed during these years. In addition he had had periodic diarrhoea, belching, and even vomiting; one of the many diagnoses was "spastic colon." The patient's family came to England as refugees a few years before the war and lived in very restricted conditions. At the outbreak of the war the patient joined the Pioneer Corps and was very happy there. After some time, however, he began to lose weight.

was sent to hospital, and eventually, against his wish, was invalided out of the Army and has been ill on and off ever since.

After his discharge he joined his present firm. As he had no capital he had to accept rather hard terms, such as payment chiefly on commission with a small salary and no security. Although he was hardworking and very successful, and had improved the business greatly, somehow he could not bring himself to face his employer and ask for better pay and more secure conditions. This was partly because of his own diffidence, but partly because of the personality of his employer, a hard, forceful man, himself very ill and under the same doctor's care. The employer used to give the doctor instructions how to treat the patient, and complained that the business was suffering. The doctor maintained, however, that he was not concerned with the business, but only with the patient. The employer's wife, a partner in the business, was an even harder slave-driver.

The doctor, thinking that the various symptoms were likely to be somatic expressions of the patient's anxiety about his insecure financial situation, strongly advised him to ask for a proper contract, but the patient was unable to follow this advice. Psychiatric treatment was then suggested, to which the patient agreed, but after one session with the psychiatrist he suddenly departed to the Continent to take the waters. He felt much better there, but relapsed after his return and was given sedatives to tide him over. He was then called on to fly overseas for an important business deal. Although previously he had enjoyed flying, this time he felt unable to face it, and was in such a state that the doctor declared him unfit to fly.

As it was rather an important affair, the employer moved heaven and earth to make him fly. The doctor was severely rebuked and heavy pressure was put on the patient. The doctor, although he was the medical attendant of the employer as well, remained steadfast and arranged for another of the innumerable "thorough" examinations, this time at his own hospital. The patient, however, could not bear the strain, agreed to fly, cancelled the hospital appointment, and booked his seat.

Two days later he came to his doctor in despair; he simply could not face the trip, the plane would give him claustrophobia. This time the doctor encouraged him to stick to his decision, gave him some more sedatives, and apparently succeeded in reassuring him, as the patient departed in a calm mood.

The doctor next heard that the patient boarded the plane, which, however, had to be stopped at the end of the runway because the patient had an acute attack of claustrophobia. An ambulance was called and he was taken to a nursing-home, where his former psychiatrist took charge of him. The general practitioner first decided to keep away, especially as the psychiatrist was quite confident that with pentothal abreaction he would be able to help the patient over his immediate difficulties; the patient, however, bombarded the doctor with telephone calls, until he agreed to take part in the treatment, although he remained doubtful whether the patient would be able to co-operate with the psychiatrist. The main reason for his doubts was the patient's character. Hitherto the patient had always agreed to whatever the doctor advised, but added that he would be unable to carry out the advice because his nerves would not stand the strain.

This was the situation when the doctor reported the case at one of our discussions. The problems were eagerly taken up by the group. Some time was spent on the possible reasons why this patient cannot solve his problems though he is fully aware of them and why increased strain leads to a deterioration in his physical condition. The main interest, however, was centred on the "right" therapeutic approach. The doctor then added to his description that the patient is an intelligent and very well-read man, rather argumentative, who can easily "fix" his doctor. Most of the group suggested a firmer handling of the case; the doctor should not "tolerate any nonsense," the patient should be given an ultimatum. The doctor declined to accept this; he thought his job was to help the patient and not to quarrel with any of his symptoms.

The doctor found it odd, however, that the patient was able to take difficult decisions in his business but not take them in his private life; and a further puzzling problem was that his patient was able to understand and accept intellectual explanations but that his intellectual insight had no effect on his neurotic behaviour.

Further details were reported and it soon became clear that the patient experienced difficulty only when dealing with strong people, especially men. His pattern was to accept sensibly any advice given to him and then to defeat the strong men by a deterioration in his condition, i.e. by an attitude of helpless weakness. In the discussion this pattern was compared, as it were, with an allergic state towards certain kinds of stimuli, and some doctors returned to their former view and recommended de-sensitizing the patient with a heroic dose, for instance by declaring that no more nonsense would be tolerated, banging the table, giving an ultimatum, and so on. Further discussion then revealed grave doubts about the wisdom of such a course; such a heroic dose would very likely mean falling in with the patient's pattern and he would no doubt respond with still more weakness and pliability. The doctor was very pleased with this turn in the discussion, and reported that on several occasions it had been easy to cure the patient's diarrhoea with some sensible drug, for a fortnight or so, but then it returned. Moreover, the patient was clever, and developed pains in places where there were no organs, i.e. he had "organs" where the doctor did not expect them.

Another suggestion was to tell the patient that he was suffering from chronic anxiety and that his body reacted to fear in a pathological way. Characteristically, the doctor agreed again but said that this too had been tried and proved futile. Moreover, when the doctor had admitted to his patient that he himself had had similar problems, i.e. somatic symptoms in an anxiety state, even this had not eased the patient's fears. Here a few more important facts were reported: the patient was happy among men (the short healthy period when serving in the Pioneer Corps), married the daughter of one of his comrades, but broke down soon after marriage. We then discussed the possibility of some latent homosexual trend in the patient which would explain the above facts, and also why he was afraid of being "treated" by a strong man, why he first gave in and then defied the strong man by an exacerbation of his illness, etc.

Next week the doctor reported that on the day of our previous discussion the patient had discharged himself from the nursing home as he could not face the thought of being given injections. The psychiatrist had been very annoyed and refused to do any more for the patient, so our predictions about the uselessness of an ultimatum were proved correct.

The doctor quickly arranged for another X-ray examination, which, however, turned out to be entirely negative. When told of this the patient was very annoyed and disappointed, and the doctor, in his embarrassment and in order to save the man from despairing of himself as a worthless malingerer, pointed to a very slight scoliosis in the X-ray report, blamed that for the pains, and prescribed a surgical belt.

In the discussion which followed, the doctor was severely taken to task for being insincere with the patient. He was told that it would have been better to be blunt. In addition, if the patient agreed, at the best he would have to look forward to years of spurious orthopaedic treatment, involving a great deal of inconvenience and expense. The doctor accepted this criticism, but said that he had had to do something because, to his mind, the patient was very near to a serious depression, even to suicide. The other question discussed was why we expect patients to be relieved when told that nothing organic is wrong with them. We have met this complicated problem already when discussing Case 5; I do not wish to go into all its ramifications here; it will be discussed later, in Chapter VI.

Towards the end of this meeting, the question of referring a patient to a psychiatric department for proper psychiatric investigation was raised, but we received the impression that the general practitioner was not very agreeable to this suggestion.

A week later, towards the end of the meeting, the general practitioner himself returned to the discussion of the previous week. It was obvious that the severe criticism meted out to him about his insincerity still rankled with him. He reported that he had given his patient another thorough examination, and that the scoliosis had turned out not to be so completely irrelevant; it now appeared that it was connected with regional ileitis. The doctor was obviously very proud of his diagnosis, but his satisfaction was clouded. He told us that his patient had often said that if any proper organic cause could be found for his symptoms he would immediately be freed from all anxiety; but now that the ileitis had been found the patient did not seem to be pleased at all.

All the general practitioners in the seminar congratulated the doctor on his success in having found the "real" cause of this elusive illness.* Only the psychiatrists were rather reserved and had to point out that, despite the discovery of some organic process, the psychiatric problem was still unsolved. The doctor agreed but—perhaps encouraged by his success—admitted his ambivalent attitude to all kinds of psychotherapy, and especially to psychoanalysis. He did not like to surrender his patient to any kind of therapy which was unknown to himself. We all agreed

---

* This case was reported in the very early period of our research. When discussing the draft of this book practically all the practitioners were unable to accept my description as correct. It is, in fact, based on a record of the discussions taken down at the time.

that this would be a high price to demand of a doctor. Nevertheless, it had to be asked whether this attitude was profitable to the patient. Even if the patient did not run away this time, but submitted to the operation and made a good recovery, it was extremely unlikely that his character and attitude towards life would be changed by the surgeon's knife. The doctor was more hopeful than the psychiatrists. He argued that in this case the pains had become a special aspect of the personality. Now that the diseased organ had been found and was to be removed, the pains would very likely disappear, proving to the patient that he had been genuinely ill and not neurotic. Such an experience might help him to recover completely.

I have to end my report here, as the doctor never turned up again at our seminars, in spite of several letters inviting him to do so. One interpretation is facile: events may have proved that the doctor was wrong and that we, the sceptical psychiatrists, were right. This may be so, but at the same time the case history also shows that we psychiatrists were entirely wrong in our treatment of the doctor. Our interpretations, explanations—that is to say, our treatment—were ineffective and unhelpful; the doctor could neither accept our advice nor see that he was heading in the wrong direction. Moreover, this case is a useful reminder not to expect too much from intellectual explanations, even when they are backed by undeniable facts. Everyone in the discussion group, psychiatrists and general practitioners alike, was aware of the possibility that things might go wrong with this patient, except the doctor himself. He remained convinced all the time that the proper course was to go on examining the patient until a proper organic cause could be found, and then treat the organic cause; the neurotic symptoms would then disappear without further ado. This is quite a general belief, leading to a number of not quite necessary, or even quite unnecessary, examinations, operations and treatments. Although this is a highly important problem of medicine, for our present topic it is only of secondary interest.

Here we found again a patient "offering illnesses to his doctor." Unfortunately, in this case, despite desperate need on the one side and conscientious, unsparing and circumspect work on the other, doctor and patient could not understand each other. As mentioned, the same was true of the doctor and the psychiatrists. In Case 5 this lack of understanding led to the beginning of a controversy,

here it led to a confusion of tongues causing a great deal of unnecessary suffering to everybody concerned.

There are a number of points in this case history which we
shall have to discuss later in greater detail. But before doing so
I wish to demonstrate by one more case history a special form of
this "offering illnesses" to the doctor. This is the form which we
called "the child as the presenting symptom." All the practitioners in our course agreed that in a large number of cases when
children, especially babies, are brought frequently to the surgery,
the person really ill is the mother (less often the father, very
frequently both parents). Usually the baby's particular illness can
be dealt with easily, but only to make way for another.

This is a most important problem for medicine in general. We
often speak of the hereditary nature of neurosis, or of neurotic
constitution, etc. I do not wish to deny that all this exists. But in
addition to the inherited constitution there is the direct condi-
tioning of the younger generation to neurosis by the older, a
handing over of neurosis from generation to generation, a phenomenon which could be described as *neurotic tradition*. The child,
as the presenting symptom of the illness of one, or both, parents,
is a readily accessible field for the study of this tradition.

Case 2 is a good illustration of our views. Because of its importance, however, I wish to report one more case out of a very great
number studied.

CASE 7 (*in charge of Dr. G.*)

Mrs. D., aged 32. (Irish). About two years ago I was called to see
her son, then aged five, who was having his first asthma attack; since
then he has had bad attacks about every three months and had to be
sent to hospital three times, when adrenalin could not relieve the
attacks. Mrs. D. came last week with another child and I asked how
Michael, the asthmatic, was. She said he had recently come out of
hospital and was fine. Then I said, "And how are you?" and tears
came into her eyes. It was the first time I thought there was any
psychological aspect to her case. I asked whether she would like to
come back and talk to me, after surgery hours, to which she readily
agreed.

She is a very presentable, nice, quiet young woman, looking twenty-
five although she is thirty-two. Has four children, boy eight, boy
(Michael) seven, girl four, and boy three. Michael had his first attack
of asthma in July 1952, and Mrs. D. had a baby in September 1951.

Michael is a very quiet, well-behaved child, in fact the best she has. He stays in rather than go out to play, and if he has any odd money he does not buy sweets for himself, but something for her, e.g. eggs. With regard to herself, she has been very depressed for some time, has had insomnia, headaches. She has always been very anxious about Michael, e.g. she sends to Ireland for eggs for him because she thinks they are better than English eggs.

Her father died in Ireland when she was six months old. She has six brothers and sisters. Mother remarried when she was three. Stepfather was very good, but she could never like him. There were four more stepbrothers and sisters. Mother died eleven years ago, which was an awful blow to her. Two days before mother died of cerebral haemorrhage Mrs. D. dreamt that she had arranged her funeral. She also had two consecutive dreams in which she was looking at photographs of her own father. When mother had stepchildren she said she felt second-hand. She does not communicate with stepfather. Her whole childhood was a struggle against poverty, and after leaving home she worked in domestic service. She knew nothing about sex before she married and it came as a great shock to her. She used to go to church regularly, always wanted to be a nun.

Her husband never takes her out; when she goes to the pictures she goes alone. The husband has no active interest in the children; he comes home, reads the paper and goes to bed. The children quite like him, but if he never came home for a week she does not think they would ask about him.

Certain things were fairly obvious. Just in the first short talk I pointed out that perhaps the disadvantage she had had in her own childhood made her anxious about her children. I also pointed out what asthma might mean; that the boy craves for affection; this business of buying things for her and not wanting to leave her is an attempt at buying her affection, trying to prove he loves her, and so on, on those lines. Certainly I could have mentioned other things, e.g. dream of mother's death, and photographs of her own father, but I thought I had better wait. She then mentioned that before one of his attacks Michael cut his hand. One wonders whether this was deliberate or an unconscious thing. I wish to add that only Michael had been the patient until then. He had been investigated really fully at two different children's hospitals. No-one has mentioned any psychological aspect of the case.

Obviously here we cannot go fully into the psychodynamics of this whole family, and in particular I do not wish to raise the vexed problem of the psychogenesis of asthma in children, although the case contains quite a number of interesting factors which might lead to important conclusions if properly investigated; for instance, in Michael's relations with his distant and withdrawn father (who, although on the doctor's list, has never been seen by him) and the finer details of his relations with his overanxious and efficient mother. Then there is the problem of why Michael should have tolerated without illness the birth of his younger sister and why the asthma started only after the birth of the next child, who was a boy.

In the same way some aspects of the mother's neurosis are fairly clear after this first interview, although by no means all of them. Perhaps the most important for our topic is her high degree of inhibition, especially with regard to self-assertion, to aggressive healthy egoism and, above all, to making demands. This, coupled with a fairly efficient ego, enabled her to carry on "quietly, without any fuss." This deceived the doctor for several years into focusing his attention exclusively on the child and thinking that the mother was in no need of help. In fact, almost certainly her efficient, sensible handling of the boy's serious illness was in some way a plea for help. This is best shown by her breaking down and crying at the doctor's very first, and in fact very slight, sign of interest. Here in fact we have the child as the presenting symptom.

When this problem was discussed, opinions among the practitioners attending the course were somewhat divided. Some of them maintained that if they had the opportunity and the time to investigate, it would turn out that practically all mothers who, with their babies, frequently visited the surgeries were psychological cases. Others were more cautious; but even the most cautious estimated that in the case of at least one-third, if not more, of the mothers who came because of their children's illnesses, the child could really be considered the presenting symptom of the mother's illness. How far one should suspect any involvement of the father it is rather difficult to say, since, as a rule, the father, as in the case reported, does not come to the surgery at all; the assessment must be made on second-hand information, which is less reliable. Still, there are a number of cases where the child is obviously the presenting symptom of the father's illness.

In the discussion a doctor mentioned a family consisting of a young couple, scarcely over twenty, and two children who had been almost brought up in his surgery. Their visits were so habitual that when father came alone the elder child, aged three, cried because she was not being taken. This is a good illustration of the cases we have in mind. In the discussion it was agreed that in about one-third of the cases in which children are brought to the surgery by their parents it is the parents who need treatment, that in another third both parents and child need treatment, and that it is only in the remaining third that it is the child alone who is in need of treatment.

Those who are acquainted with psychiatric literature will be suspicious when seeing this "one-third, one-third, one-third" proportion cropping up again. Admittedly our figures are based solely on subjective assessment, but they are an attempt to describe very important empirical facts. How to explain them is another matter. Possibly they describe only the proportion of people in the population at large with overt personality problems. Whatever the reason behind these figures may be, the fact remains that in many cases a child's illness is also the presenting symptom of the parents' illness.

But let us return to our main topic. Mrs. D. offered the illness of her son to the doctor, which he accepted. Mother, child and doctor then settled down to deal with the boy's asthma. Was this a good enough situation for an efficient therapy? The fact that in more than two years not much could be achieved—despite conscientious medical care and consistent co-operation by mother and child—makes us feel somewhat doubtful. Then the doctor's sympathetic question brought to light the highly neurotic background behind Mrs. D.'s efficient façade. The situation has definitely changed, but we have to ask whether it is for better or for worse. Some people will point out—quite correctly—that asthma in a young boy is usually a wearisome, very chronic illness, demanding a great deal of patience from the whole family; instead of breaking down the mother's defences, the doctor ought to have strengthened them; now, in addition to the asthmatic boy, he also had a neurotic mother to look after, and in any case a general practitioner cannot do much in such difficult cases and the prospects of getting specialist treatment for Mrs. D. are not very high.

On the other hand, it must be admitted that his diagnosis of the case before the event, although correct, was rather superficial and incomplete. On the whole, one would expect a deeper, more comprehensive diagnosis to enable the doctor to make a better, more exact assessment of the case, and perhaps also to give more efficient treatment.* We shall come back to this problem later.

For our present topic the important point is the doctor's responses to the presenting symptoms. His first response centred the attention on the boy's asthma and excluded the mother's illness. His second response brought the mother's illness also into focus. This was a considerable change in the situation, and it was brought about by the doctor.

These three cases, then, clearly show that the doctor's response to the patient's offers, or to the presenting symptom, is a highly important contributory factor in the vicissitudes of the developing illness. In the following chapters we shall examine some of the more important aspects of the doctor's responses, or some further side-effects of the drug "doctor."

* See follow-up in Appendix III.

CHAPTER IV

Elimination by Appropriate Physical Examinations

IN the previous chapters we have seen that when becoming ill some people offer their doctor various potential illnesses (including illnesses of their children), out of which he may or must choose an acceptable one. In this chapter we shall discuss one aspect of the doctor's responses to the patient's propositions, the aspect which in medicine is traditionally called diagnosis.

Let me recall the case of the baby boy (Case 2) who was brought to the doctor by his mother once or twice a week practically for a whole year. The doctor very properly diagnosed the various minor illnesses present, such as tonsillitis, cold, influenza, coughs, bronchitis, screaming fits, etc. Quite conscientiously he entered all these diagnostic tags into his notes, prescribed the appropriate treatment for the particular ailment, and on paper the case was finished for him. He knew that the real cause of the illness lay not in the boy but in the mother–child relationship, which could not develop freely because, in her anxious insecurity, the mother overburdened it by restricting her boy's freedom more than was tolerable for a healthy child. But this diagnosis, the real one, was only in the doctor's mind and, although he was aware of its importance and himself brought the problem up for discussion, it took some time and effort to convince both him and the group of doctors attending the seminar that all the other diagnoses were in a way superficial and incomplete, perhaps merely a kind of short-term convenience.

As I have no doubt that some of my readers will also feel reluctant to accept this view, I propose to discuss at some length the arguments for and against it. Let us take a simple instance. The child had a temperature, was run down, complained of sore throat, and the doctor saw an inflamed pharynx and enlarged red tonsils with white follicles. His diagnosis, follicular tonsillitis, was then confirmed by events, i.e. the boy got better in a week or so. I propose to leave out of consideration the possible refinements of this diagnosis, such as the identification of the strain or strains of cocci present in the throat and causing the pathological changes; or, on the other hand, the changes causing a diminished resistance in the boy, such as an increased allergic state, disappearance of the antibodies from the blood, impaired local resistance in the tonsils and pharyngeal mucosa, and so on. Even if any or all of these changes had been ascertained and embodied in the diagnosis, it would not influence my main argument.

First, the point of agreement; the diagnosis "follicular tonsillitis" was correct so far as it went, and so were all the others. Each described adequately the present state of the patient, led the doctor to prescribe an effective therapy, and allowed him to predict with considerable accuracy the course of the particular illness under his treatment. This is one possible level of diagnosis. What all these diagnoses did *not* do was to enable the doctor to form a general view of the whole situation, to predict that this boy would not develop well, would get all sorts of minor ailments, and—most important of all—they did not enable the doctor to prescribe a comprehensive treatment that would not only cure the present illness but would prevent the development of any further illnesses. This kind of diagnosis obviously belongs to a different, deeper, or more comprehensive level.

The major cure corresponding to this deeper level of diagnosis was in this case achieved by external events which removed some of the mother's fears and eased her anxious and restricting way of handling her son. We all know of such sudden changes, for the better or for the worse, in our patients; usually not understood. What raises this case above such experiences is that here the doctor was able and had the courage to make a complete, or deeper diagnosis *ex juvantibus*.

Nevertheless, in spite of his courage and insight, even after arriving at this more complete, deeper diagnosis, he did not care to change or correct on his cards his former, admittedly superficial and incomplete, diagnoses. Moreover, even when in the discussion we asked him whether he would change or correct them now, he flatly refused and, which was equally interesting, he was wholeheartedly backed in his refusal by the whole group of doctors.

Undoubtedly here we are faced with a major issue. A doctor usually feels embarrassed, even somewhat ashamed, if his diagnosis is found to be faulty, not quite correct, or even only incomplete, and certainly would not hesitate to enter the correct diagnosis on his cards, either as a correction or an addition. Here by common consent all this was refused. One reason put forward was professional considerations; suppose the doctor has to give a certificate, or to refer the boy to a specialist, or—in the event of the patient moving to another district—to surrender his card to another practitioner, etc.; in any of these events it would be easy for him, and would be understood by his colleagues, if he speaks or writes of tonsillitis, bronchitis, etc., but it would be considered rather peculiar, not quite proper, if he used long-winded psychological descriptions. The wish to be understood and accepted by our colleagues is one of the reasons for sticking to these incomplete physical diagnoses.

This respectful attitude towards diagnostic tags is, of course, also a legacy of our training. General practitioners have been trained in hospitals by specialists. Specialists know how to cure illnesses belonging to their special field if they are curable, and know also the limitations of their skills; but they are less concerned with, and one may even suspect they do not know enough about, the total personality of the patient.* We must realize that in general practice the real problem is often the illness of the whole person—as every medical student has had preached to him on innumerable occasions. The inevitable consequence of this teaching, however, is but very rarely mentioned, i.e. that the illnesses described by the hospital tags are only superficial symptoms, and the tags themselves, as learnt in the teaching hospitals, are of limited help for the understanding of the real problems facing the doctor.

This means that *there is a cleavage between medical science as practised in the hospitals and general practice in the doctor's surgery.*

---

* When discussing the draft of this chapter one doctor mentioned a case as follows—"I had to send a patient to an orthopaedic surgeon. He did not find anything, but he began to talk psychiatry, with the most disastrous results. Being really excellent in his own job, he thought psychiatry was just common sense, so he trespassed on to a subject he did not know anything about but did not realize it. That is quite a common attitude of specialists." One ought to add that this is true mainly with regard to psychiatry and general practice. These are the two free-for-all fields, whereas all the other specialities are usually carefully respected.

There are quite a number of cases where the two—medical science and general practice—think and act in the same way, to the great benefit of the patient; but there is a wide field—we are just beginning to realize how wide—where the two ways of approach diverge. Our knowledge of the problems met with in this other, not well-charted, field is less certain, and our skill in dealing with them is unfortunately based chiefly on empiricism and hardly at all on science. Perhaps the most important reason for this unfortunate state of affairs is that consultants have, so to speak, only second-hand acquaintance with the problems described in the previous chapters. On the other hand, general practitioners, who were trained by the specialists, are overawed by the successes of their teachers in their respective specialities, and in consequence tend to think almost exclusively along the lines of their highly respected consultant-trainers in their own field of general practice, in which the latter have but little experience.

Another important reason for this unhappy cleavage is the lopsidedness of our scientific language. We have a most useful set of technical terms for describing the experiences that specialists meet in their practice. This is an exact, unequivocal language, understood equally well by the consultant and the general practitioner and used by both with ease and safety. One speciality, admittedly one of the youngest in medicine, has not yet been able to develop such a language, and this is psychiatry. It shares this shortcoming with the oldest speciality, general practice.

This want of a proper language is one reason for the unsatisfactory and often irritating lack of understanding between the general practitioner and the psychiatric consultant. We psychiatrists cannot yet give the general practitioners the badly needed set of technical terms which they could use confidently and which would help them to understand the deeper personality problems of their patients. For the time being our descriptions of pathological states are vague, complicated, long-winded, easily misunderstood when not backed by lengthy explanations, and, what is worse, any general practitioner who uses them feels some uneasiness for being highbrow, *recherché* and self-important. To develop a set of terms for the description of the pathological involvements of a whole person, a set of terms as good as that of the hospital specialists for describing specific illnesses, will be a hard task and will take a long time to achieve. It will need close

collaboration between the two specialities primarily concerned—
general practice and psychiatry. One of the aims of this book is
to point out this need and perhaps to contribute a little towards
meeting it.

What, then, is the function of this level of diagnosis, for the
doctor on the one hand and for the patient on the other? For the
patient illness is always an uncanny experience. He feels something
has gone wrong with him, something that might, or certainly
will, do him harm unless dealt with properly and swiftly. What
"it" is, is difficult to know. Often "it" becomes identical with
its name, and for the patient the function of the diagnosis is to
supply the name by which this uncanny, malevolent and frightening something can be called, thought of, and perhaps dealt with.
The importance of recognizing this need is well illustrated by
Case 5. In other words, being ill is still often thought of, and is
certainly felt, as meaning being possessed by some evil, and the
belief is rampant, not only amongst patients, that the devil can
be driven out only if his name is known. We all know that this
is far from being always true.

Diagnosis has as reassuring an effect on the doctor as on his
patient. The present attitude in medicine is that treatment should
not be started before having arrived at a diagnosis. This attitude
is justified and fruitful if the diagnosis really describes the pathological processes, that is to say, if it gives much more than just
a name into the hands of the doctor.

The diagnosis "neurosis" or "neurotic" we all know can be
made by anyone and it provides the doctor with hardly any
indication of what his next step should be. It is a kind of magic
name only, and not a diagnosis in the proper sense. If we are
sincere, we must add that "neurosis" is even less of a diagnosis
than pains, vertigo, constipation, headaches, etc., etc., which are
so justifiably abhorred by every teacher of medicine. Perhaps we
may also add, rather humbly, that in general practice we have
not so seldom to content ourselves with such inferior diagnoses.

Moreover, doctors, conditioned by their training, generally
think first of "physical" diagnosis. The reasons generally put forward are that a physical illness is more serious and more dangerous
than a functional illness, that is, more harm can be done by overlooking a physical illness than a functional one. This is a dangerous
half-truth; in some cases a physical illness represents in fact a more

serious threat to the patient's well-being, but in others the functional illness is definitely the greater danger, as, for example, in
Case 5 and Case 6, etc. As a consequence of this half-truth doctors
generally feel very ashamed when they have missed even a minor
or utterly irrelevant physical diagnosis. (A good illustration is
Case 11.) Another reason for this preference for physical diagnosis
is that such illnesses have something more definite and manifest
about them. Partly because of the state of our knowledge, but
partly also because of the bias in our training, doctors know more
about physical illnesses, and their better knowledge makes them
feel safer and on firmer ground than when they have to deal with
functional or neurotic diseases. Furthermore, and perhaps this is
the most important factor, if the doctor arrives at a correct
physical diagnosis, even if his therapeutic effort is unsuccessful or
no proper therapy exists at all for that particular illness, he feels
reassured because the patient's suffering can be accounted for,
can be explained, which in turn means that it can be accepted by
the doctor without guilt feelings. He will feel, and quite rightly,
that he has done a good job; he has found the true cause of the
suffering. For the rest, he is not responsible even if there is not
much he can do. Any lack of therapeutic success can be ascribed
to the "present state of our knowledge."

This kind of thinking compels the doctor, when diagnosing an
illness, to follow a curious, almost obligatory, sequence of steps,
a sequence which is obeyed mechanically without even examining
its drawbacks or its advantages. (See Case 1 and Case 5.) We call
this sequence of events, with slight exaggeration, "elimination by
appropriate physical examinations." Conversely this means that
the diseases are arranged in a kind of ranking order roughly
corresponding to the seriousness of the anatomical changes which
can be demonstrated or assumed in them. Unfortunately, not only
the diseases are given this kind of rank, but also the patients, so
to speak, attached to them. Patients whose complaints may be
traced back to demonstrable or assumable anatomical or physiological changes rank higher, and neurotics are in a way the dregs
left over after everything else has been drawn off. Thus it is
understandable that every doctor, when confronted with a new
patient, tries to give him a good rank and will relegate the patient
to the class of neurotics only if he cannot find any justification
for giving him a respectable status. A corollary of this state of

affairs is the fact that every physician is proud of a spot diagnosis of an organic disease but confesses only with some uneasiness to a spot diagnosis of neurosis. This, too, is understandable if we remind ourselves that the diagnosis "neurosis" can be made by anybody, whereas diagnosing a physical illness requires expert professional skill, enabling the doctor to feel a justifiable pride in his achievement.

Another corollary, which really belongs to Chapters XVI–XVII, on the doctor's *apostolic function*, is that as a result of this attitude all our patients are trained right from childhood to expect a more or less thorough physical examination. They are not trained to expect any psychological examination and very often may become frightened, put off, or even offended at any such suggestion or attempt. The attitude of some doctors in this respect is reminiscent of my student days, when we had to learn to auscult or percuss, especially women, through a vest or a towel because, without compelling reasons, no well brought up woman could be expected to expose her breasts, even to her medical adviser.

There is another fallacy in the approach of "elimination by appropriate scientific examinations." It is implied, although not stated, that the patient is not changed or influenced by the process of "elimination." Case 5 is only one of the innumerable cases which prove how utterly untrue this statement may be. The patient's attitude to his illness is usually considerably changed during and by the series of physical examinations.* These changes, which may profoundly influence the course of a chronic illness, are not taken seriously by the medical profession and, though occasionally mentioned, they have never been the subject of a proper scientific investigation. In any case, I do not know of any hospital where even as much routine attention would be paid to these psychological needs of a patient as is paid, for example, to

* May I use a simile to show what I mean? The analysis of the mineral contents of any living organism is highly important and, if carried out correctly, gives basic data which must be taken into full consideration in any theory of life or of a particular physiological process. But this analysis can be carried out only after the living organism has been completely incinerated. Though not quite so drastic, the "appropriate physical examination" of a patient is equally unable to apprehend and respect subtle, psychological processes, and may even play havoc with them. Anyone who cares to sit down for half an hour and listen to a patient during a so-called "week's stay in hospital for observation" may get some idea of the apprehensions, anxieties and uncontrollable fantasies to which he is prey during this time.

the regular opening of his bowels. The most that a patient can expect is reassurance—routine, well meant, usually wholesale, and as often as not ineffective.

To sum up, in general doctors prefer diagnosing physical illnesses, using the tags learnt from their consultant-teachers, rather than diagnosing problems of the whole personality. As we have seen, there are several reasons for this preference. First there is no really useful set of terms available to describe the personality problem of a non-psychotic patient; in practice those which are available amount to hardly more than a handful, such as hysteria, obsession, neurosis, anxiety, depression, and so on. Hardly any professional skill is needed to arrive at a diagnosis of this kind; or in other words, in this field the man in the street is nearly as good an expert as a trained doctor. Whereas a real diagnosis leads the doctor directly to a more or less rational therapy, the diagnosis of personality problems hardly ever does so. Then there is the belief, as often as not unfounded, that physical illnesses are more important than personality problems. The result of this way of thinking is what I have called "elimination by appropriate physical examinations" and the "ranking orders" of diseases and patients.

CHAPTER V

Incidence and Evaluation of Neurotic Symptoms

THE first object of this chapter is to show that the "elimination by physical examinations" and the "ranking order" as described in the previous chapter really do exist. One way to do so would be to observe the doctor at work in his surgery. Unfortunately, the presence of an inscrutable, non-participating, detached observer would considerably influence the atmosphere of the surgery, perhaps even change it basically. If we are to avoid this risk, the only course is to ask the doctor to be the observer himself. Accordingly the practitioners attending the Tavistock Clinic seminars were asked to note down on an agreed day all the patients seen during one surgery session, mentioning their complaints, the diagnoses, the psychological background, and the treatment prescribed.

Of the lists of patients seen I have chosen two, which will be reported in full. I wish to add that the two practitioners whose lists were chosen are both conscientious doctors, both are interested in the psychological aspect of their patients, and devote a considerable time to minor psychotherapy. Both work in busy partnerships, with large lists and some private practice, which means that they must get on with their jobs and cannot devote unlimited time to satisfy what their partners consider to be their psychological hobby.

LIST NO. 1 (*reported by Dr. M.*)

(1) Mr. Y., toolmaker, 19. Came two weeks ago with conjunctivitis. I do not know him very well. Said he wanted to go back to work and wanted N.H.S. certificate and two private certificates, one for insurance company. He had improved last week, but said he didn't want to go back to work then. Obviously wanted to get a little more money out of it.

(2) Mr. B., a cleaner, 63. My partner's patient. Suffers from psoriasis. He was very triumphant. My partner had told him his illness

was incurable, but had suggested a "desperate" remedy—liver extract injections. This has practically "cured" him. He said my partner would be very pleased when he sees him all clean and neat-looking.

(3) Mrs. F., 28. Married two years. Complained of dysmenorrhea. Obviously hysteric. Always cheerful and smiling, flirtatious type. Also suffers from frigidity and is sterile. Half wants, and half does not want a baby. Before last period I gave her tablets to take and she had no pain. She was doubtful whether tablets would always do the trick. Two years ago saw a lady doctor who gave her tablets which did not do any good. I gave her another prescription for her next period and she is going to come back afterwards.

(4) Mr. E., clerk, 25. Big, strong man, very unclerky looking. Had a septic toe and wanted to go on holiday; asked if it would be all right. I gave injection of penicillin and let him go on holiday.

(5) Mr. H., labourer, 41. Chronic sufferer from asthma. Very un-intelligent man. Wife suffered from acne rosacea. They had a mentally defective spastic child eight years ago which died four years ago to their great relief. When they had the child the wife was often ill. Since the child's death the wife has not been ill but he is often ill with asthma. He comes from time to time wanting bottle of medicine and a few days off. Then he is better for four or five months. This time he got his medicine and a few days off.

(6) Mrs. N., 28. Ante-natal examination. Baby due four weeks' time. First baby. Very well and cheerful. Took blood pressure and made urine examination. Went away very happy.

(7) Mr. B., 69, store-keeper. Father of five boys. Wife suffered from bad heart for many years. She was a patient of ours but never came to see us and never called us. Three or four months ago she suddenly died in a chair. The sons all suffer from headaches. They get certificates and stay off work and get better. In another year they come again. One son is particularly bad, but he gets great relief from pink tablets (aspirin) which I gave him some seven years ago. The daughter-in-law of Mr. B. is the woman I reported on in the seminar a little while ago—could not get out of mourning for her mother. Now Mr. B. cannot get out of mourning for his wife, though they did not live very happily together. I gave him tonic, and he will see me again.

(8) Mr. M., 23, labourer. A week before he had complained of pain in left wrist. I had it X-rayed and it was an old, ununited fracture of left carpal scaphoid. He could not remember having injured it. I asked what he wanted to do about it and he said he would leave it to me. I have sent him to orthopaedic surgeon. He says he does not want operation, mortally afraid of operations.

(9) Mrs. L., canteen worker, 44. Thin-looking, very poorly dressed. Septic finger for three–four weeks. My partner gave her penicillin injections. She told me every time she has periods she has terrible headaches, and could I give her tonic and tablets as my partner did. I did that. Then she was a bit doubtful whether it was really a good thing to see me, and did I think she would be all right now. She also wanted to go back to work for the money, I signed her off.

(10) Mr. M., gardener, 21. German boy who came here when thirteen—war-widowed German mother who went into domestic service here. He was put to foster parents. Has become complete Englishman, forgotten most of his German. Very happy at work; mother remarried, Englishman here. They all live happily together with his stepsisters. He is about six foot five inches, very broad. Said he had cold and headache and mother said he should come because he had some bronchitis before and did not want to get ill again. I told him that he was not likely to have bronchitis, and to tell his mother that, and go back to work. He went off relieved and still very infantile-looking.

(11) Mrs. C., with Susan, aged 7. She was moving from our district and came to say goodbye. She wanted to have some eardrops for the child and I gave her a prescription for that. She was moving from the district for the sake of the children. She thinks the constant colds they have are due to the damp in our district.

(12) Mr. W., 82. He had ulcers in the mouth for several weeks. Had tried mouth-washes and salt but they did not get better. In the end he had to give in and come and see the doctor. He went off happily.

(13) Mrs. W., 62, housewife. For several months has suffered from indigestion and bloated feeling in the abdomen. Very inarticulate. Difficult to get any history out of her. I examined her, found a very large abdominal tumour. I sent her to see surgeon. She was very anxious and worried about whether it was anything serious. What she implied was, was it cancer which would eat her up. I said I did not think it felt like that and she went away a little happier after I had reassured her.

Of the thirteen patients seen, three suffer from obvious neurosis (Nos. 3, 9 and 7, in the last of these the whole family, consisting of father, five sons and a daughter-in-law, all seem to be neurotics), three from some psychosomatic condition (Nos. 2, 5, 10). Of the remaining seven patients, at least two or three (Nos. 8, 11 and perhaps 13) show enough neurotic features to justify the assumption that a proper examination would very likely uncover a serious enough neurosis.

List No. 2

Dr. E. prefaced his report by mentioning that he happened to feel very sullen about his work that day; he resented having to be indoors on such a lovely afternoon.

(1) Boy 15, hemiplegic mother, neurotic father. Unsatisfactory family who usually attend my partner. He wanted a certificate for the Naval cadet authorities saying that he had not had enuresis for the last two years. I told him to get the Naval authorities to write and tell me what they wanted.

(2) Miss Q., an hysteric, 45-odd, who had operation five years ago. Living with ailing father of eighty. She said she came for his tablets but actually she was coming for some support and encouragement for herself. One of her complaints is weakness of the back since her operation. She got the tablets for father and also some reassurance for herself, but very scantily. Normally she gets much more.

(3) Mrs. Z., aged 28, English, married to a former Italian P.O.W. She has recurring dermatitis on the palm of her hand. It clears up and then comes back. I have never been quite able to understand her. She made one significant remark, "I don't put my hands in water. My mother has been washing up the last month or two. All this trouble is hardly worth it." I asked her what the trouble was and she said, "Not washing up. It's a great strain for me not to wash things up straight away." I put her off for another week.

(4) Mr. I., saturnine Welshman, aged 34. Brought boy to be immunized against diphtheria and whooping-cough—four years late. Complained himself of central abdominal pain which sounded very much like gall-bladder dyspepsia. Then in his son's presence he said, "By the way, after intercourse I have a strong burning feeling in the stomach and sometimes I do not want intercourse just to avoid this." I felt he had problems to discuss, but I put him off too. Sister a schizophrenic. (P.S. a fortnight later: Barium meal has now revealed an active duodenal ulcer.)

(5) Mrs. U., working-class woman of fifty. Complained that her vision had got worse and she wanted an "eye certificate." She said she could not read books after a day's work. As she was going out she said it was much worse whenever she had her periods and did I think that was anything to do with it. I fobbed her off too. Am leaving it to the eye test. She already has glasses and this was to change them.

(6) Mr. Z., aged 60, hypertension and Parkinsonism. Came for repeat of tablets. Has very real illnesses, but is also an extremely anxious man, and would like to stay and talk. He only refers to somatic symptoms, but he is very anxious.

(7) Mr. A., aged 32. Irish labourer. Muscular pain in the back. On examination it seemed just an honest muscular sprain. I left it at that.

(8) Miss Y., 48, looking after ailing mother of eighty. She came to tell me her stomach was better. She has a duodenal ulcer at times. She is not taking medicine since meat came off the ration. Came for mother's tablets. She makes little doll puppets out of aspirin bottles and corks, very attractive. A fortnight ago she produced half a dozen and asked me to choose one for myself. She wanted me to have one.

(9) Mrs. K., 72. Came in very cheerful and friendly. Much better than last year. I don't remember having seen her before but she knew me very well. She complained of eyes watering. The trouble was she and her new husband (been married for a year) are being persecuted by two spinster landladies who live in the same house. Her family approve of the remarriage, very much so.

(10) Driver B., soldier, Irish family, seven children. Peculiar family —extremely handsome mother—extremely coarse, rough, uneducated father. All the girls are very beautiful. Two sons are very uncouth and ugly and two are rather handsome, fine homosexual-looking young men. Patient was on leave from the Army, complained of toothache and wanted me to arrange for him to have it out, so that he could have as much leave as possible. He appeared to have some real problem that he was unable to bring out.

(11) Mr. Q., sweet wholesaler. Does not come very often. Complained of his throat, which gets worse every evening. Thinks it may be due to having been talking all day. His throat was infected and very red. There was something else; he was anxious about something but I did not get it, I was not in the mood. His wife is forty. Severe headaches this last year. Full investigation at K. hospital, negative.

(12) Mr. P., 28. Has seborrhoeic dermatitis. Came complaining of irritation of skin round ear. He is very fat. He has been coming during the last few weeks fairly regularly with this complaint. When I told him to go on diet and stop eating things he likes, he was satisfied. He seemed to need to be deprived of the things he likes by the strict doctor.

(13) Mr. Q., 32, poor working class, four children. Born in slum home in London. Saw one of my partners last week complaining of acute illness with temperature. Now wanted to go back to work the next day. He is a very anxious neurotic man, and he said that he thought his illness was due to nerves. He has changed his job since I last saw him and now he has to lift heavy weights, which he thinks is connected with his illness.

(14) Miss F., 12. Pain in foot, took off shoe to show me. She said it was much better when she wore proper shoes and not sandals.

I told her to wear shoes with heels. I asked her about her hay-fever. She said she had not got it. I reminded her that she had it last year but she said "No." Her voice was nasal and chest was catarrhal, but she persisted that she did not have it. I could not understand that.

(15) Mr. F., marital problem; both wife and mother severe hysterics, frequent visitors to the surgery. He complained of impotence last year and after he had been investigated his wife became pregnant. He insisted baby was not his. He is a man with a great deal of violence in him. When he sits down on his haunches and gets up again he is dizzy and sways back, but when he is high up—he works at something like a steeplejack—he has no symptoms. He had some sort of mental breakdown after being hit on the head in the Army and they did not want him back. I saw him for about twenty-five minutes. We have had discussions before. He told me how he wanted to leave his wife. He is afraid he might kill her if he allows himself to lose his temper with her. Normally I refer these problems to the probation officer or solicitors or F.D.B., but in this case I agreed they should consider separation.

(16) Mr. I., 20, police constable. His wife has just gone into the A. hospital and he wanted to know how long she would be there and what he would have to pay. I told him he would have to pay four guineas. Then, when he was going, he asked what I thought was wrong with his wife and how long she would be ill, and did I think it was due to his mother upsetting her. I did not accept that invitation, put him off, and told him to come back later.

(17) Mr. F., man of low intelligence. Varicose ulcer. Comes for viscopaste bandage every week. He has mentally deficient mother-in-law, is taking her on holiday with them. He expressed great concern about her.

(18) Mrs. Q., 32, poor intelligence, two adopted children. Chronic hysteric, cannot go out of house, controls her acute anxiety with sodium amytal. She came for tablets and complained she was too sleepy. She has been able to go back to her job recently—works in a laundry—and is getting along quite well. She has been referred to the psychiatrist at K. hospital and is waiting to go into a group there. She has been waiting two years. I sympathized with her, altered her tablets a little so that she would not be so sleepy.

(19) Mr. U., Irishman, 32. Upset and depressed. He had had chest X-ray a week or two ago and it was negative. He is still anxious about it, worried about what was wrong with him. I have arranged to see him again.

Of the nineteen patients seen, seven suffer from obvious neurosis (Nos. 2, 3, 4, 13, 15, 18, 19) and a further nine (Nos. 1,

5, 6, 8, 10, 11, 12, 14 and 16) show enough symptoms to suggest that neurosis is very likely present. Only three cases (Nos. 7, 9 and 17) are reported as showing no neurotic symptoms, but one is left with the impression that this is only because the doctor had not enough time or was not in the mood to probe further. The two lists show about the same general picture.

There is another respect in which the two lists agree. Both record with conscientious accuracy the physical signs and symptoms as well as the treatment prescribed for them. The lists also mention the presence of neurotic symptoms, but only as if they were of secondary importance, and in the notes hardly any therapy is mentioned for them. It is worth repeating that both doctors have a real interest in the psychiatric aspects of their patients and devote a considerable part of their time to psychotherapy. Conversely this means that they are likely to note more quickly and more readily than the average doctor signs of a psychological involvement and will attach more importance to them. Yet if we neglect the notes about the psychological backgrounds and the signs of uneasiness in the doctors at not having tried to do something about it, we cannot avoid feeling that, even by these two doctors, on the whole, patients with mainly physical complaints were given a better status or perhaps even a better treatment than those with only neurotic symptoms. Perhaps the only exception is No. 15 on the second list. If doctors who are genuinely interested in psychological problems discriminate between their patients in this way, we may assume with considerable certainty that the average doctor will do the same. I think this justifies my contention that the "ranking order" described in the previous chapter really exists. The same is true about the "elimination by physical examinations" which is, so to speak, the operative clause of the ranking order.

I expect that these lists will produce an uneasy feeling in a number of people. It is likely that some will try to deal with their uneasiness by reassuring themselves that all this is unnecessary, empty talk about psychological problems. Apparently it does not lead anywhere anyhow, so it would be much more sensible if general practitioners got on with their anyway overcrowded time-table instead of spending so much time on inessential frills. For instance, if a father brings a child to be immunized (No. 4 of the second list) the doctor should do so and then see the next patient, who has probably been waiting for quite a long time. Why bother about the parents' not entirely satisfactory sexual life or the unpleasant feelings reported by the father? In any case, that is not the general practitioner's job. Yet, if we bear in mind what we have found about the "child as the presenting symptom" we begin to wonder whether this attitude is really correct. Usually it is the mothers who bring their children; moreover, a four-year-old child is several years too late for immunization. Should the general practitioner notice these symptoms at all or not? If he should, is it then his duty to investigate them in order to evaluate their importance, or is it better to turn a blind eye? The answer is not easy. A test case quoted on innumerable occasions in our seminars was that of a young pregnant woman complaining of occasional sweating and a slight cough—there is no question but that every conscientious doctor would carefully examine her chest and arrange for an X-ray and even a sputum test. Should slight neurotic symptoms be considered as similarly significant or as negligible? Are they the first signs of a serious, slowly advancing process which may culminate eventually, say, in an involutional depression, or in prolonged absenteeism caused by an endless series of minor ailments, or only in a general lack of zest for life?

Or, must we assume that a large part of the whole population is exhibiting symptoms of personal problems, that is that a large part of the whole population is more or less neurotic? In this case the presence of slight neurotic symptoms would have no greater significance than a positive Mantoux in patients in their late twenties. Of course, if this is the case the two lists are devoid of importance for the general practitioner.

But the Mantoux reaction shows the presence of antibodies in the skin; that is to say, except when it is positive in very high dilutions it indicates that the infective process has been successfully overcome. Is the same true of the symptoms suggesting neurosis? Are they signs of past conflicts successfully dealt with or, on the contrary, do they suggest that the pathological process is still active or has been reactivated? This is a searching question which, in most cases, every physician and not only the general practitioner, will find difficult to answer. Any answer obviously means a different kind of diagnosis from that of an acute abdomen, of a 'flu, a septic finger, or varicose veins. This difference is what we have tried to describe as a different depth or level of diagnosis. There are some signs that not only doctors, but the general population also, are beginning to be aware of this new way of thinking. According to some of the doctors who attended our courses, patients who some time ago came for a tonic nowadays say, "I am depressed, can you help me, doctor?"

If the latter alternative is nearer the truth, that is to say, if the presence of neurotic symptoms means that the pathological process may be still active or may have been reactivated, then one must expect to find them more frequently in people who come to general practitioners than in the general population. Unfortunately we have no reliable data, based on statistical research, about the incidence of neurosis either in the general population or in the population frequenting the doctor's surgery, so we have to leave this question unanswered. But I think we may say with only slight exaggeration that the two lists could almost be a record of a psychiatric outpatient session. I wish to add that these lists were not selected, but were taken at random from many presented at our course.

There is, however, a third possibility. The doctor's personality and subjective interests may have a decisive influence on what he notices and records about his patients; he might, for instance, be super-sensitive, especially if he has had some psychological training. This might work in two ways. He would notice more, and by directing his patients' attention—let us say unnecessarily—to their neurotic problems, would hear more about neurosis than his average colleague. Moreover, the rumour of the doctor's odd interest would soon spread, and patients needing this kind of neurotic exhibitionism would come and pour out their hearts to his sympathetic ear. There may be a good deal of truth in all this, but even so, that does not detract anything from the importance of the real problem.

Obviously, if a doctor has learned how to use a stethoscope, he will use it more often and he will hear more than an untrained man, and by using it constantly he will train his patients to expect this kind of examination. The obvious result will be that he will have more data on which to base his diagnosis than a man without a stethoscope. Exactly the same is true of every new diagnostic method such as chest X-ray, electrocardiogram, intravenous or retrograde pyelography, and so on. All these methods produce a wealth of new data which would be inaccessible without them. Not all data thus provided have diagnostic significance, and the medical profession has had to learn how to evaluate them, and how to integrate their message into existing knowledge. Thus the problem is not personal bias or supersensitivity, but evaluation of the data arrived at by a new skill.

Conversely this means that the presence of neurotic symptoms —however slight—ought to be taken seriously. It does not mean, however, that their mere presence automatically clinches the diagnosis and with it the direction that a rational therapy must take. On the contrary, neurotic symptoms must be evaluated in the same way as physical signs or symptoms. A systolic murmur over the apex does not necessarily mean a mitral incompetence; as often as not its presence is not significant. On the other hand, a diastolic murmur is always pathological, that is, it has incomparably greater diagnostic importance. In general the same is true about neurotic symptoms. Some of them are pathognomonic, others are without much significance. Their proper evaluation, however, requires experience and professional skill, exactly as the reading of an X-ray picture needs them.

If it is true, as has so often been repeated in the literature, that at least one-third of the general practitioner's time is spent in dealing with neurotic people, then the evaluation of the various neurotic symptoms appears as a major problem. The problem involved is—which of the two attitudes is the more economical, to deal with the neurosis in the hope that the minor ailments will then disappear, or, as is generally done nowadays, to look after the minor ailments with conscientious care while turning a blind eye to the neurotic involvements about which we cannot do much in any case? Before we can give even a rough answer we must find out how to understand neurotic conditions and how much we can do to cure them. This latter question will be discussed in the second part of the book, after which we shall have to return to this major problem.

CHAPTER VI

Level of Diagnosis

IN the previous chapter we came to the conclusion that it is advisable for the doctor to aim at a more comprehensive, deeper diagnosis. By this I mean a diagnosis which is not content with comprehending all the physical signs and symptoms but tries to evaluate the pertinence of the so-called "neurotic" symptoms.

I shall now quote a few cases to show what is meant by this level of diagnosis, i.e. how we have tried to evaluate the various neurotic symptoms. Case 8 was reported by Dr. Z. in June 1954, as follows—

CASE 8

Professor E., aged 49. I have had the whole family as patients since the end of 1949. I have seen very little of him, mostly the two small children and the wife. She also is a lecturer. Exceptionally nice family. Professor E. had left nephrectomy for renal calculus a few years ago. I saw him once for sebaceous cyst and once for sore throat. August 1953 he came complaining of fortnightly headaches, since the previous November; he had a feeling as if the veins in his head were swelling. Blood pressure was 190/120. (A previous record showed it as 145/95.) I felt he had been doing too much and he agreed. He is doing a good deal of administrative work and still keeps on with research, which is his vital interest. He lives under high pressure but enjoys it. I thought he would settle if he went a little more slowly. I gave him amytal and kept him under observation for quite a while. As I went on seeing him he felt much better, then he got a little worse again. He had a good holiday, came back, hated the thought of work, and felt worse. I began to ask a few more questions, then last week I had him up for a long interview.

He thinks he has been overworking for about ten years and that he rather had to drive himself to work while his wife took everything in her stride. She is very competent, efficient, with a real sense of duty; he obviously admires her very much. His great interest in life was to be a literary critic, and everything else had to take second place. He has been interested in literature and painting since a child.

Although under very restricted conditions, he had a very happy boyhood. Has never been bored in his life. He used to paint and draw for hours. Always contrived to be popular; was not athletic. He said he was really a pervert. Some masturbation after marriage; he did not have any other women before or after. He thinks he has never been a good lover to his wife though she deserved something better. I got the feeling that both might have been better with someone else. He said his wife very much wanted children, although she has a horror of lust. He, however, feels it is the only thing he is good at. He thinks he has been too selfish and that he does not think he is deeply trustworthy. Stopped sexual intercourse years ago. Occasional masturbation.

I asked him about his present difficulties. He said he has recently had troubles in relation to his deputy, an immensely powerful woman, who is now retiring. He does not feel he is frightfully good on administration. At an earlier interview he said he might retire earlier in order to concentrate on research.

The patient was then sent to a cardiologist, who reported confirming the diagnosis of benign essential hypertension, blood pressure 190/120, heart normal, renal X-ray normal, blood urea 33. According to the specialist the condition did not call for any special treatment, but the patient should come up periodically for a check. Dr. Z. added to this report that in the meanwhile he had about two or three talks with the patient and the result of these seemed to be that the patient had been able to organize his life better and was steadily improving. For instance, although he had a lot to do at the end of term with students and all sorts of administrative affairs, he tolerated them without any further headaches.

I expect that after reading this case history a number of my colleagues will have a feeling of "much ado about nothing." The case is as simple as it can be. One kidney had had to be removed, and, perhaps conditioned by this, a benign essential hypertension developed, causing minor disturbances to the patient, such as headaches, but otherwise well compensated. Both the doctor and the specialist did the right thing—prescribed some sedatives and advised the patient to take things rather more easily. The results of this therapeutic regime were fairly good, and when there was a minor disturbance the doctor acted very wisely in asking for the specialist's opinion, which obviously reassured the patient. It might even be added that the only thing that might be objected to was the doctor's unnecessary probing into the patient's intimate affairs, above all into the delicacies of his sexual life. In the first place, it must have been most embarrassing to both doctor and patient, and secondly, the data brought to light did not contribute anything to the understanding of the case or to the treatment adopted.

Is this argument valid? One part of the objection, the unnecessary probing into the patient's sexual life, I shall have to deal with *in extenso* in Chapters XVI–XVIII on the apostolic function of the doctor. Here it suffices to say that every examination, physical or psychological, may or may not be embarrassing. The difference depends mainly on the doctor's approach. If he is convinced that the examination is necessary and approaches it in an understanding but objectively professional way, any embarrassment will be diminished to a tolerable amount.

In the present context the other argument, that of relevance, is the important one. My contention is that even the scanty data revealed by this "questionable" probing threw much light on the whole situation and enabled the practitioner to arrive at a much deeper understanding of the real problem.

First, the general impression of the happy marriage mentioned in the report gives way to a more precise picture of a mutual adaptation of the partners, perhaps at the price of hypertension in the man and, as the practitioner added during the discussion, of occasional attacks of migraine in the woman. It then appears that in his youth this man had the choice of at least two possible ways of life. One was represented by his desire for lust, prompting him to devise his various sexual pleasures, and the other by the reassuring security offered by his understanding, kind and highly efficient wife; the latter solution, however, also meant renouncing the satisfaction in his marriage of his need for lust. The material produced by the interview does not allow us to conjecture why he chose the second path, but it allows us to realize how he dealt with the necessary renunciation. Masterful, domineering activities in the outside world became more and more uninteresting and distasteful for him; he had difficulties with powerful people, especially powerful women; and instead of dealing with these external problems he withdrew from them. The withdrawal was greatly facilitated by his excellent powers of sublimation. He found ample gratification in painting and academic research. His illness fits well into this general trend; it will prompt the doctors to advise him to lead a quiet life, to do less administrative work, which corresponds exactly with one of his fantasies, namely, to retire early and concentrate on research.

The great question which the doctor has to decide at this level of diagnosis is whether the wish to withdraw, to lead a quiet, contemplative life, dedicated to painting and research and without sex, is a sensible solution which ought to be encouraged, or whether it is another symptom of a general neurosis of which the patient ought to be cured, or at least offered the opportunity of getting cured if he wanted to.

The objecting colleagues mentioned above may now add to their arsenal the further argument that probing deeper into the patient produced nothing but this problem, which was highly unpleasant, put the doctor into a most unenviable situation, and showered on him responsibilities which he had not asked for and which perhaps it was not even his duty to shoulder. We may sympathize and even agree with part of this argument, but we must ask what the alternative is. If the doctor does not try to get these data, his decision will be blind. Although he will not know what he is doing, his advice will be no less decisive for the patient's future. In other words, the only difference will be that he will have to take a responsible decision without knowing the nature of his responsibility.

An important factor in this kind of blind decision is the doctor's own conscious and unconscious attitude towards life. If he is one of the modern doctors, who believes in the overriding importance of a satisfactory sexual life, he will probably try to convert his patient to his beliefs, i.e. to prevent a complete withdrawal into the sphere of sublimation. Otherwise his advice will almost certainly be prompted exclusively by the physical illness.

When we discussed this case and the therapeutic approach to be adopted by the doctor, feelings ran rather high. Some wisely recommended great caution in view of the hypertension and the fact that Professor E. had only one kidney. Any attempt at re-adjusting this man's sexual life would stir up highly charged emotions, not only in him but also in his wife; possibilities certainly not without danger in hypertension. Others, more psychiatrically minded, emphasized the possibility of a slowly developing serious depression, which perhaps had already cast its shadow in the form of the gradual withdrawal from the external tasks of life into painting and research. Lastly, some recommended that all these problems should be discussed openly with the patient. After all, he was now near fifty, he had not much time to readjust himself if he wanted to do so. Failure at this point to offer him what might be his last chance might later bring serious reproaches against the doctor.

In the end it was Dr. Z. who decided to adopt the first mentioned attitude, namely, not only to allow, but to recommend, a quiet life. His reasons, in addition to those mentioned, were as follows—Professor E. had outstanding intelligence and took a high degree of pleasure in research and painting. In other words, his potentialities for sublimation were very good and could perhaps be trusted to provide a sufficient outlet for all his energies, including the sexual ones. Lastly, he told us that the possibility of psychotherapy had been mentioned casually to Professor E., who, however, did not seem very keen to accept the suggestion. I must add that very likely the doctor's way of approaching the problem of psychotherapy also had an important influence on the patient's decision. Dr. Z. is somewhat doubtful of the efficacy of psychotherapy and recommends it only in selected cases, rather reluctantly. Here we have another instance in which we can see the working of the apostolic function, which will be discussed in Chapters XVI–XVIII.

At the same time this case illustrates the great importance of the name given to the illness. The whole atmosphere, in fact Professor E.'s whole attitude to life, will be profoundly influenced by whether he is told that he is suffering from a benign hypertension or from a neurotic solution of his basic personality problem. The first "plays into his hands," is easily acceptable to his conscious personality, in fact is an external sanction relieving him from some of his responsibilities, especially towards himself. The other, it is true, opens up new possibilities but questions his solutions and, instead of sanctioning them, demands from him a decision based on a conscientious revision of his past life and attainments on the one hand, and of his future hopes and possibilities on the other. Perhaps this case may also help us to understand why patients have such a great need to be told what their illness is, what sort of fears may be rampant in them if no name is given, and, last but not least, what the inevitable implications of any diagnosis, however innocent-looking, may be.

Here, in contrast to Cases 5 and 6, on the surface there is no struggle, no confusion of tongues between the patient and his doctor. The illness proposed by the patient was accepted by the doctor, an agreement was easily and speedily reached. As just mentioned the situation would have been utterly different had the doctor decided to go beyond the diagnosis of hypertension. Whether the agreement will be durable or not is difficult to say as the scales—so far as we know the situation—are fairly evenly balanced. The next case, though similar in some ways, will show us what happens if no agreement, not even a compromise, can be reached.

Case 9 was reported by Dr. D., in February 1954, as follows—

CASE 9

I have a patient, Miss K., aged twenty-three, who is a problem; she goes from one to the other of us in our practice of three partners. Not very high intelligence. She is the elder of two children, the other is twelve or fourteen. Working-class family, mother and father living. I have known her for three years and the symptoms have always been the same. She says she has soreness at the back and side of the tongue. When I have examined it it has looked a bit red but that was all. No treatment or reassurance has any effect on her, as she is convinced it is going to turn to cancer. She gets mother to look at it every night to see if it is changing. She has given up a job as a secretary, says if she is going to die anyway it is no good going on with a difficult job. She has never really had any emotional affair with a man but she dresses herself up in an elaborate way. She never goes out in the evening.

She has been to an E.N.T. surgeon and he can find nothing wrong. She had previously been sent to a general physician with the same result. She is someone with a fixed hypochondriacal idea who might become psychotic or suicidal. It is difficult to get her to accept the idea that there is any sort of psychiatric problem at all. She always wants to know what is the matter with her tongue. As she is not very intelligent I have not been very anxious to get her back for a long session. I might have tried harder though.

This girl could have been one of the cases included in the two surgery lists discussed in the previous chapter. In her case history we can study the workings of all the forces mentioned previously. We see the patient offering an illness to the doctor, and the doctor first accepting it as a possibility. She is then sent to various specialists, who confirm the doctor's finding that there are some slight physical symptoms but the whole illness should be considered as hypochondriacal. Both doctor and patient agree, so to speak, that there is something wrong, but neither of them seems to be able to find out what the trouble really is.

In the discussion it was pointed out that several highly interesting psychological factors were not taken into consideration when arriving at a diagnosis, these are—

(*a*) The patient giving up a good job and withdrawing into solitude to the extent of not going out in the evening.

(*b*) Her giving up all attempts at having any emotional contact with men although still dressing up in rather an elaborate way.

(*c*) Her going from one doctor to the other, especially when one tries to get in touch with her in order to make her talk about her problem.

(*d*) And most important, her obsessional demand on her mother to look into her throat and reassure her that it is still the same, that it has not got worse.

To obtain a better understanding of the problem it was suggested that we should suppose that the patient had some similar trouble with her genitals and went from doctor to doctor asking to be examined in order to alleviate her fears. In that event we would all jump to the conclusion that she was an exhibitionist, afraid of normal sexual life, and that she was producing her symptom to get into the kind of situation, though in an unpleasant form, which she was frightened of and desired at the same time. If we assume that this case is a doubly displaced exhibitionism—she shows her throat instead of her genitals and she has to show it to her mother instead of to a man—there is a strong suggestion that we have to do with some hysterical elaboration of repressed sexual fantasies. This impression is reinforced if we take into consideration that she has to perform her obsession every night in order to be reassured that inside her throat everything is all right. Her dressing in an elaborate way may be another pointer in the same direction. This may explain why she cannot allow anybody to have a positive *rapport* with her, i.e. to get near her, as this might lead to her talking about her awful secret. On the other hand, by her persistence she obtains reassurance both from her mother and from the doctors that no irreparable damage has been done.

Under the weight of our criticism Dr. D. promised a new and more detailed examination, including a proper psychological examination. We heard nothing more about this girl for about six months, when in August the doctor reported as follows—

At times he had tried to get the patient to talk, but she was absolutely unwilling to accept any suggestion that physically there was nothing wrong with her. Then in April she was referred to a dermatologist, who also found nothing and on his own initiative referred the patient to a psychiatrist. The psychiatrist reported that the cancer phobia, which seemed to be the main complaint, was only one symptom in a very disturbed girl. In addition she had rheumatism all over her body, pain at the bottom of the spine, and so on. The prognosis was very guarded, as it was assumed that severe mental disturbances might follow such a severe hypochondria in a young girl. The psychiatrist finally suggested that the patient should be given as little treatment as possible for her various symptoms, otherwise her fear of cancer would only be confirmed. Since that time the patient has seen only the most junior of the partners, and Dr. D. did not know whether this was by chance or by design. All told, she has been fourteen times in the surgery between February and August, i.e. on an average rather more often than once a fortnight, complaining of all sorts of aches and pains. The doctor added that he had been definitely cured of his tendency to believe that there was something physically wrong with this patient, unfortunately neither his patient nor his junior partner had been.

This case illustrates well the drawbacks of what we have called "elimination by appropriate physical examinations." The slight sign on the patient's tongue was taken seriously and she was sent in turn to a general physician, then to an E.N.T. surgeon, and lastly to an eminent dermatologist, all of whom examined her tongue but not her personality. Eventually, more by chance than by design, she was seen by a psychiatrist, but his report was not very helpful either. The history shows that *there is a danger, not only in missing a physical sign, but also in finding one.* During these physical examinations about three to four years have been wasted, but that was only the less important part of the loss; the more important was that the physical examinations confirmed the patient in her belief that there was something to be looked at on her tongue. The psychiatric examination, thrown in too late and not by design but just as an extra, failed to shake the patient's confirmed belief.

In this case we can clearly see the struggle between doctor and patient. The patient tries to impress the doctor that she is physically ill, and the doctor, backed by all his consultants, tries hard to impress on her that she is not. We see also that she is not given a name for her illness, her need for it remains unrecognized, and in her despair she has no alternative but to cling to the only possibility that she can think of, that she has a developing cancer.

There is another interesting aspect of the case, an aspect which we shall discuss in detail later (Chapter XVIII). We refer to it as *the self-selection of patients according to their doctors*. Some patients go from doctor to doctor until they find one who is in a way congenial to them. If there is a partnership with several doctors of different views and opinions, all this may happen, as in this case, within the partnership. After some vicissitudes the patient seems to have settled down with the junior partner, who is probably the most organically minded of the three. One may wonder, however, for how long.

I do not wish to give the impression that this girl would be an easy case. On the contrary, it is certain that she is a very disturbed girl who is gradually withdrawing from life under the burden of her severe illness. I am also fully aware that in her case it would by no means be as easy as in Professor E.'s case to obtain information about her intimate life. But I wish to emphasize very strongly that the "elimination by appropriate physical examinations" caused the patient a good deal of unnecessary suffering and involved the doctors in a good deal of unnecessary work.

By chance at the same meeting another case was reported which shows the same problem from an entirely different angle. This patient also offered various organic illnesses to her doctor, Dr. R., who, however, did not pay too much attention to them but, using a kind of shock tactics, tried to bring into the open the psychological conflict which he thought was the real problem. He succeeded to a degree, but at a price. He reported as follows—

CASE 10

Miss M., aged 19, a girl who persistently said she had nothing to worry about. I first saw her in November 1953, when she registered as a new patient. She had had a sore throat for the last four days and when she got up that morning she collapsed, could not go to work, felt so ill. She looked very anxious misty-eyed, no make-up, hair very simply dressed in a pigtail with a bow at the back. I examined her thoroughly and found nothing except what could have been early pharyngitis. She had acne on her face which she said worried her. I asked if anything had upset her and she said "No." I gave her symptomatic treatment for throat, and certificate to stay off work. Four days later she came back, felt better, but had a cough. I looked at her throat and it was much the same as before. I asked her if she felt like going back to work and she said she still felt very run down and had a swelling in her leg. She had a minute prominent varicose vein. I remarked that she was very preoccupied with herself and she said she felt run down and would like a tonic. I gave her Metatone and told her to come back to see me when it was finished. She went to work. She did not come back to see me till yesterday, i.e. two months later, complaining of sore throat and loss of weight for some months. I looked at her throat and found nothing wrong. On questioning, she said her appetite was quite good, though not as good as it used to be, and she had not been sleeping well for a few weeks. She still said she was not worried about anything. Then she said she had been working very hard (shorthand-typist) going to evening classes three nights a week and perhaps that was why she was run down. On further questioning she said she had been living on her own since father died eighteen months ago, he was sixty-nine. Mother, still alive aged fifty-two, lives in the country. Mother was very upset at father's death but was all right now. Patient was not upset when father died although he meant a lot to her. I pointed out that she had not been upset at the time but for some weeks she had not been feeling all right and not sleeping well. She still insisted it did not worry her. Then she said that when she broke off her engagement it upset her. She was engaged to an Armenian, he was twenty-seven, she nineteen. He was Greek Orthodox, she Church of England. Her parents did not like him, and his parents had written to say they did not like him going with an English girl, so they broke it off. She still sees him nearly every day, still wants to marry him. I asked her how often she had intercourse. She said, "about . . ." and then burst into tears, ". . . once or twice a week." She said she did not want to tell anybody about it. I think it was the only way to get it. She broke down and cried and was very upset and angry, but she got over it. I said it was good to tell someone, as she had no father. Then she asked me what I thought about her marrying the Armenian, and I said, "What do you think?" She put forward the different standards of living; her fiancé had said she did not know how to cook in the oriental way, and she could not speak Armenian. It was getting late and I told her I had better see her again. Then she said she did not think it was right to talk about personal feelings in this way and I said it was for her to decide. Then she asked when she could come to see me again—she is coming next week.

Although Miss M. is obviously much less ill than Miss K., the two cases show a number of similarities. Both are of about the same age, of about the same social background, and have the same occupation. Both offered physical illnesses to their doctors. In Case 9 the physical illness was first accepted as a possibility and then, after the process of elimination by appropriate physical examinations, rejected. No other illness was offered, however. As a result of this procedure the patient had to go from doctor to doctor until she found one who accepted her as really physically ill and then she settled down to a real chronic illness. In Case 10 all the physical symptoms offered were treated as minor, unimportant incidents; the real emphasis was put right from the start on the psychological implications. The patient was not happy about this approach, she resisted the doctor's attempts and did not co-operate at all. Dr. R. then adopted shock tactics; the patient was taken unawares and had to disclose relevant information about her sexual problems, but afterwards highly resented it.

In the discussion the doctor pointed out—and I think rightly—that in his opinion he did the proper examination and even achieved some real therapy, that is, he broke down the patient's resistance. Some of his colleagues, including the psychiatrist, had grave doubts about what the price of these shock tactics might be, and they wondered in what way it would influence the future of the doctor–patient relationship. They felt that though Dr. R. was perhaps going in the right direction, his speed was excessive for the patient, and the patient was probably not allowed sufficient time to catch up with the doctor.

In spite of these warnings, the next week when he saw the patient the doctor continued to use the same sort of technique. Miss M. came saying that she did not see any point in discussing her personal affairs with him; a discussion would not make any difference to her illness. She complained again, as always, of sore throat and loss of weight. While examining her Dr. R. asked quite casually what contraceptives she used. Angrily, she repeated what she had said the week before, that she did not use them regularly. The doctor then said that it looked to him as if she wanted to become pregnant so that her fiancé would be forced to marry her. As the patient became rather angry and cross Dr. R. did not pursue the matter further. Moreover, as Miss M. did not want to come back for further interviews, the doctor arranged for a chest X-ray, hoping that this might bring the patient back so that he would have a further opportunity to get on with her case. As expected, the chest X-ray turned out to be negative, but the patient did not come back for the result. Several months later, in February 1954, she turned up again quite casually, complaining this time of a small cough. The doctor examined her chest and throat, but no signs of a physical illness were found. He then asked if she would like to talk about anything to him, but she emphatically said "No" and that everything was all right. She still saw her fiancé regularly.

I think both Case 9 and Case 10 must be considered as partial failures, although the level and the degree of failure—or lack of success—is different. In Case 9, although the discussion in the seminar gave the doctor some idea where to look for possible psychological implications, partly due to his own personality and partly to the severity of the case he was unable to gain a proper contact with his patient and to clinch the diagnosis. By "clinching" I mean obtaining indications which of the ideas put forward in the seminar were correct and which incorrect, and by this "clinching" to get some hints for a rational therapy. The patient rejected the doctor's half-hearted overtures towards discussing her worrying problems, and "self-selected" herself to the other doctor in the partnership, to the one who did not bother her with psychological examinations.

In Case 10, the doctor assumed, probably correctly, that the patient's real problem was her unhappy love affair and the worries and fears raised by it. Unable to solve her problems, she escaped in the direction offered her by her constitution, namely, into the psychosomatic field of minor respiratory ailments. The doctor, assessing correctly, in my opinion, the danger that the patient might develop some chronic psychosomatic illness of her respiratory system such as chronic bronchitis or pharnygitis, asthma, or even a flaring up of a tuberculous infection latent at present, did his best to get to grips with the real problem. Unfortunately his pace was too fast for the patient and she refused collaboration.

With regard to what we termed "level" of diagnosis, it is obvious that, in Case 9, hypochondria is a correct but much too superficial description of the illness. It does not in the least help the doctor to choose a rational therapy, and does not give the patient a helpful name which would be of some assistance in her struggle with her fears and worries. Hypochondria is, in fact, so superficial that it is almost useless. May I add that almost the same criticism must be made of the psychiatrist's report. The description of the case does not contain any new information and the advice offered is entirely negative; it tells the doctor what *not* to do, which is of only very limited help.

In Case 10, the doctor went deeper with his diagnosis than accepting the physical symptoms offered by the patient and attaching a label to them, but he could not give a name acceptable to the patient to the real illness which was troubling her.

One more, and rather important, point. All medical teachers emphasize: no therapy before diagnosis. These two cases demonstrate the limitations of that doctrine. *In a number of cases of this kind no diagnosis is possible without some therapy.* The reasons why the two doctors had only limited success with their patients was their inadequate therapeutic approach. In Case 9, because of the doctor's half-hearted approach, hardly any help was offered to Miss K. What was offered was only a *negativum*; there was "nothing physically wrong" with her, which meant a rejection by the doctor of the illness proposed. Beyond that she was given no positive indication of what was expected from her, or of where she could look for further symptoms, fears, sentiments, ideas that would shed some light on her problems and would enable her and her doctor to co-operate in order to find relief and even some kind of solution. As the result of this failure, the only course left to her was to cling to her idea of physical illness, to reinforce and overcharge it.

In Case 10, the doctor's somewhat impetuous therapeutic approach broke down the patient's resistances at one point and led to a confirmation of the supposed diagnosis. This, however, resulted in raising other resistances, such as indignation, resentment and suspicion. Henceforth—at any rate for some considerable time—this patient will very likely mistrust her doctor, and be on her guard against offering him any opening. Certainly an undesirable development, the more to be deplored as the doctor did his best to offer acceptable help to his patient in her distress.

And lastly, these three cases (Professor E., Miss K. and Miss M.) demonstrate the importance of the doctor's response to the patient's offer. With Professor E., the doctor after due deliberation accepted the illness offered, gave it a name and came to an agreement with the patient. It is true that the patient had to pay a price for this agreement, but the price, at any rate in the considered judgment of the doctor, was reasonable. In Miss K.'s case no agreement could be arrived at, and the patient had to change her doctor. The new doctor and the patient agreed, at any rate for the time being, but only at the price of a chronic incapacitating illness, from which it is uncertain whether the patient will ever be able to emerge. Miss M. rejected her doctor's counter-proposition, that her symptoms were due to some mental strain, and thus no agreement was reached. She did not change her doctor, but persisted in her two main symptoms, loss of weight and catarrhs of the respiratory tract. In Chapter XIII, we shall study the further development of this case.

In all these cases the "deeper" diagnosis enabled the doctor to arrive at a better understanding of the case, although admittedly not at a better, more effective therapy. In Professor E.'s case the therapy remained the same, in Miss K.'s case, after an unsuccessful attempt at achieving something, the patient was allowed to continue with her "organic" illness, and lastly, in Miss M.'s case the offer of psychotherapy turned out to be unacceptable to the patient, at least in the form offered. These results would obviously warrant the criticism, "much ado about very little." Fortunately we can point to quite commendable therapeutic successes founded on what we call "deeper" level of diagnosis. Some of these will be described in Part II—Psychotherapy.

Apart from an undeniably better understanding of the patient the "deeper" diagnosis has another function. This is the reduction of the number of cases in which the doctor has to take a blind decision based only on a physical diagnosis. Such blind decisions, hardly influenced by the patient's emotional situation and by a proper control of the doctor–patient relationship, allow free play to the doctor's personal bias, unconscious sentiments, firm convictions and prejudices, i.e. what we have called his "apostolic function." One of my aims is to throw some light on this aspect of our everyday work, and to enable the doctor to obtain conscious control over at least part of it.

CHAPTER VII

The Collusion of Anonymity

IN difficult cases, the general practitioner does not, as a rule, carry the burden of responsibility alone. Usually he asks and receives help from his specialists. The difficulties which prompt him to ask for help may be also described (viewed from a psychological angle) as crises of confidence. Either the doctor feels that he may not know enough to be able to help his patient, or the patient has doubts about the sufficiency of his doctor's knowledge and skill. In the first case the doctor's confidence in himself has to be increased, in the second the patient's confidence in his doctor. Or, in other words, in the first case, the need is mainly for a more accurate diagnosis; in the second, for reinforcement of the doctor's therapeutic potential. In both cases the appearance of consultants introduces a number of new factors in the doctor-patient relationship; the complications caused by them will be discussed in this and the following chapters.

In order to have concrete material for discussion, let us again start with a case, as reported by Dr. Y. at one of our seminars.

CASE 11

Mr. K., aged 54, was introduced to me in 1950 by his wife, who complained of being run down through constant worry about her husband. (Here we have the wife as the presenting symptom of the husband's illness.) He was never well, very excitable, and demanding a lot of attention to his food. His trouble started in 1934 with appendicectomy followed by peritonitis, necessitating a two-stage operation and a subsequent third one for the repair of the hernia.

Mr. K. is a tall, heavy man, with a certain elegance of appearance. He lives with his wife and daughter in a lower middle-class house. The atmosphere of respectability is relieved by a number of books and several musical instruments. He is a minor civil servant, started work at fourteen as a messenger-boy, and now is in a clerical administrative position. He never liked his job, though he is not certain what he would have liked to do instead. He reads and writes poetry and short stories. He also plays the flute and the cornet, and belonged for some years to an amateur orchestra. When he was thirty-five years old he took a correspondence course at Ruskin College in English and Literature, followed by General Psychology. His father was a farm labourer who later became a clerk. He was a born musician, and played the fiddle without being able to read music. One brother, a fire-brigade man, writes novels; one sister started to play the cello at forty-five.

His home life seems happy and affectionate apart from the fact that both wife and daughter are tyrannized by his ill health. His wife shows an undercurrent of rebellion by exhibiting increased menopausal symptoms; his daughter shows signs of frustration, but struggles to overcome them.

When I saw him he complained mainly of abdominal pains on and off; the pain often doubled him up and was followed by diarrhoea. He usually suffered severe pain before defaecation, sometimes the motion causing a burning sensation. In 1940 his former doctor sent him to see a surgeon, who suggested after due investigations that his trouble might be due to adhesions. He was given luminal and atropine.

In addition to all the symptoms mentioned above he complained of giddiness and added that he was afraid of crowds, going to the cinema, going to the barber to have his hair cut. His clinical history was complicated through a fall, with a fracture of the spine, in 1939. Since then he also complained of twitching in his right leg, with prickly-heat sensations. This happens only at night.

Mr. K. visited me once or twice a week regularly over a long period. On clinical examination I could not find anything organically wrong that would justify his ill health. The search for psychological causes always led back to his dislike of his work. He always improved very quickly on sick leave.

In February 1951 I sent him back to the surgeon, who again could not find anything abnormal in his alimentary system. In June I sent him to Dr. S., hoping for enlightenment from a psychiatric specialist. Mr. K.'s symptoms persisted, and he sometimes felt near collapse even without pains. Once or twice he was taken to the casualty department of a nearby hospital. In October 1951 he attended the teaching hospital, where Dr. S. is head of the Department of Psychological Medicine, for a narco-analytic session. I could never extract a report on this. He was, however, referred to the Medical Outpatients' Department, where the possibility of gallstone was considered. I was rather shocked that this should have been overlooked all the time and might have been the cause of his symptoms. After further investigations he was operated on in January 1952. After his operation he was fit and entirely free of complaints until the middle of April. Then he returned to me with recurrence of spasm, diarrhoea, pain under left costal margin, giddiness. I tried to convince him that we had left no stone unturned, that now after the removal of his gallstones there could be no organic cause, that his symptoms were entirely due to psychological factors, that he had to overcome his anxieties and dislikes in order to cope with his problem. I did not give him any more medicine.

I saw him again two days ago. He was in a happily resigned mood. I went once more with him over his whole life, and this time tried to discuss also his sexual life. There seemed to be no clue at all, or probably I was not successful in overcoming his resistance.

Here, unlike the case of Mr. U. (Case 5), on the surface there is no controversy, no battle. The patient came meekly and appreciatively since 1950, just as he had come to see Dr. Y.'s predecessor in the practice since before the war. Dr. Y. too remained patient and was always willing to start thinking anew. In this superficially undisturbed good relationship, the patient offered his doctor a great variety of symptoms which remained about the same, only the intensity of the one or the other changed. The doctor did his best to find the right answer to the patient's complaints, even to the extent of sending him to a psychiatrist, but somehow something did not click—the whole picture strongly reminiscent of Case 6, though less tense and less dramatic.

During these superficially untroubled years, an interesting episode occurred which throws sharp light on present medical thinking and practice. When, in the autumn of 1951, the chief assistant of the psychiatrist could not find anything, he referred the patient to the medical outpatients' department of his own hospital. They suspected cholecystitis and gallstones. Dr. Y., according to his report, felt terribly ashamed at not having thought of this possibility and, prompted by his guilty feelings, sent his patient in a great hurry for an X-ray, and, when this showed the presence of gallstones, in an equally great hurry an operation was arranged in the hope that at long last the real solution of the case had been found. The operation was followed by an uneventful recovery and three months' freedom from complaint, whereupon the patient relapsed into the state he was in before. This is a not infrequent outcome of abdominal operations decided upon on some slight, or even not so slight, positive physical evidence, without taking into full account the whole personality of the patient, especially the part his illness has played in his life. In this sense, too, it is a counterpart of the case of the company director. (Case 6) which, because of our unskilful handling cost us a doctor.

But it is not for this reason that I have reported the case. My main aim is to contrast on the one hand the doctor's feeling of shame at having failed to notice the presence of gallstones, and his lack of shame at not understanding his patient's problem; and on the other hand, the speed and confidence with which the operation was arranged, and the rather defeatist and complacent attitude towards the real, psychological problem.

This case, and that of the company director just referred to, show well some of the drawbacks of responding to the patient's propositions by diagnosing a physical illness whenever possible. Although to some the operations might appear as possibly the most spectacular drawbacks, I do not think they are of great importance, especially in our present case. On the one hand Mr. K. made an uneventful recovery and was actually free of complaints for three months; on the other, the symptoms and signs were highly suggestive: abdominal pains in the right side, at times doubling the patient up, more often than not at night, could be provoked by jerky bus rides, occasional diarrhoea, presence of gallstones proved by X-ray, etc. Even if we assume that the gallstones had nothing to do with the real illness (as is well known, they may be found at post-mortem in people who had no abdominal complaints whatever throughout their lives), both the diagnosis and the operation were justified and they did not cause much harm. The real drawback is the way of thinking, the "elimination by physical examinations" which cost this patient about twenty years of his life. Those twenty years were spent in chasing an elusive, and perhaps never existing, "proper" physical illness, while paying no proper attention to possible psychological causes. During these twenty years this case—I wish to add—might have been one of the patients mentioned in the two surgery lists (Chapter V), the possible entry being: "well-known patient, frequent visitor to the surgery; abdominal pains, giddiness, diarrhoea; prescribed his usual medicines: atropine and phenobarb."

There is another important point in this case, however. The doctor in charge was not alone. Being a careful man, time and again—as we learnt from his report—he referred his puzzling patient to various specialists. There were many of them, and in consequence there were many reports. As their spirit, their way of thinking, is most important for my argument, I propose to quote some of them. To give a coherent picture I have chosen all the reports of the dramatic period leading up to the operation, i.e. from February 1951 to March 1952.

Surgeon, writing from H. Hospital.   23.2.1951.

Dear Dr. Y.,

<u>Mr. K.</u>

Thank you for sending this patient to see me again.

Gastroscopy shows a normal stomach apart from a small fine scar.

Barium enema shows a normal colon.

I have reassured him that there is no evidence of any growth. He is still over-weight. I think he would be more comfortable on a light diet.

Psychiatrist, from his consulting rooms.   5.6.1951.

Dear Dr. Y.,

Yesterday I saw your patient Mr. K. on your kind recommendation, for which many thanks.

I originally saw Mr. K. on October 2nd, 1944, when he was complaining of cramps and tremors, and other symptoms which might have had a spinal origin. He had fallen on the ice and injured his back in 1939. X-ray revealed a fracture of the 11th dorsal vertebra and he was four months in a plaster jacket in hospital. His cramps started in the right foot about seven months after the accident.

I formed the impression that he was an hysteric, but, in order to be on the safe side, especially as both ankle jerks were absent (they still are), I sent him to Dr. Z. (a leading neurologist at J. Hospital). I never had a report from Dr. Z., who I understand referred the patient to Dr. I. at Y. Hospital.

Mr. K. still complains of cramps, especially before going off to sleep, and more particularly in hot weather. He does not pay much attention to this symptom nowadays. His chief complaint of late is of pain in the right half of the abdomen. This symptom follows or precedes an action of the bowels or is apt to be associated with any situation likely to cause anxiety or tension.

He also complains of panic-states characterized by tense attitudes of the body, when eating in company or sitting in a barber's chair. He has always been highly strung and subject to nervous dyspepsia since 1934. He is strangely complacent about his symptoms, almost to the point of belle indifference.

In so far as his symptoms are consciously motivated, I think that they provide a "cover" for his various failures in life; and I do not think that he is likely to be very responsive to psychotherapy of any kind.

However, I will have him registered at the Z. Hospital and add his name to our psychotherapy waiting list, which, by the way, is fantastically long, as you might expect.

Physician in charge of M.O.P., Z. Hospital.   30.11.1951.

Dear Dr. Y.,

Re Mr. K.

This patient was referred to me by Dr. E. of the Department of Psychological Medicine on behalf of Dr. S.

He gives a history of abdominal pain coming in attacks, four of which have occurred in the last year, and are associated with pain in the right side of the stomach. He has no vomiting. The attacks last four to five hours and generally mean admission to a hospital. He volunteered the statement that the jolting of a bus worried him also.

On examination he looks fit, but has a dirty tongue. There was resistance of the upper abdomen, and two scars from an acute appendicitis associated with peritonitis, for which he was operated on in 1935. There was no obvious enlargement of the liver or gall bladder, no renal discomfort and he had not lost weight.

I feel that he does require further investigation, but, as you know, X-rays are difficult at the present time. He states that he was X-rayed this year at the H. Hospital, a barium meal, and I would very much like you to send us a copy of the report they sent you. I feel that the possibility of gallstones must be excluded, but again there is the X-ray difficulty, and I would like to wait a period of three months. In the interval will you put him on Pil. Cholelith (Parke Davis & Co.), the number controlled by his bowel motions, and I will review him again at the end of this time.

(Copy to Dr. S.)

Physician, E. Hospital.   16.12.1951.

Dear Dr. Y.,

Re Mr. K.

Many thanks for letting me see this patient. I think the reports from the various doctors are almost more interesting than the patient. I disagree with my illustrious colleagues at Z. as regards the absence of the knee-jerks. There is no doubt that they are present, but I could not elicit the ankle jerks beyond doubt.* The Plantars are flexor. Babinski's sign is not present. This, together with normal abdominal reflexes and pupil reactions, can be taken as almost conclusive evidence against central or peripheral neurological pathology.

He was vaguely tender in his abdomen, more on the right side, but certainly

---

* (Cf. Psychiatrist's letter of 5.6.1951.)

nothing decisive and localized. I could not convince myself of a tenderness over the gall-bladder. P.R. I noticed a tender internal pile on the right side and an ampulla filled with spastic scybala.

The beginning of his trouble dates back to the time not long after his abdominal operations, and with this in mind I have asked for a barium meal and follow-through to clarify the picture as much as possible.

If any medication is required it should be spasmolytics as it is already done. He might benefit from Vichy water tablets two to four times a day for ten days at a time.

Surgeon, E. Hospital. 12.3.1952.
Dear Dr. Y.,

<u>*Re Mr. K.*</u>

I saw the above-named patient of yours again in the O.P.D. on 10.3.52. He was an inpatient from 22.1.52 to 18.2.52. I removed his gall-bladder and found chronic cholecystitis with gallstones. Convalescence was uneventful and he is now free of complaints. I have discharged him.

This case is a very good example of what we call the "collusion of anonymity." No-one was really responsible for the decision to perform the operation. The first surgeon examined the patient conscientiously, but did not find anything, and fobbed him off with some "reassurance" and a light diet. The patient then saw a psychiatrist privately who did another lot of physical examinations and, though not very confident about psychotherapy, put him on the waiting list. Next, the patient was, in due course, seen by the two chief assistants to the psychiatrist (these two did not write reports) was whisked off to a physician, and the suspicion of gallstones emerged. The doctor was ashamed of having missed the "right" diagnosis, a second opinion was asked, the physician disagreeing with the psychiatrist but agreeing to the gallstones, and in consequence the patient's gall-bladder was removed. The second surgeon is the last—proudly discharging the patient after operation, free of complaints. Nobody mentioned, and perhaps nobody was even interested in, what happened inside the patient while he was being whisked from doctor to doctor, eventually landing on the operating table. Who was now responsible for the patient—the general practitioner, the surgeon, the two physicians, the psychiatrist, or his two chief assistants? I wonder how many of the specialists involved in this treatment took the trouble to follow up the results of their recommendations. The one who

cannot help knowing the results is, of course, the general practitioner, but he is exonerated as he was acting strictly on the advice
of his eminent consultants.

In any situation of this kind, that is to say, when the patient
offers a puzzling problem to his medical attendant, who, in turn,
is backed by a galaxy of specialists, certain events are almost
unavoidable. Foremost among them is the "collusion of anonymity." *Vital decisions are taken without anybody feeling fully responsible for them.* The serious operation in Case 11, just reported, is
only a rather dramatic example of this kind of decision, but there
are others at least as important.

Although Mr. K.'s case is quite a common one, demonstrating
impressively the existence of the collusion of anonymity, I wish
to quote a few more cases to show its manifold consequences.

CASE NO. 12

Miss F., aged 24, was referred in March 1954 for a psychiatric
examination by Dr. C., who had treated her for more than a year—
following the instruction of an eminent physician on the staff of a
London teaching hospital. The doctor was highly dissatisfied with this
complicated three-cornered situation, especially as the results were not
very good; moreover, the patient developed further symptoms. When
she let slip that she thought the cause might be "nerves," he seized on
the opportunity and arranged for a psychiatric examination.

Miss F. came from an upper-middle class country family. Her
present illness started at a boarding school with food poisoning which
affected several girls. All except Miss F. returned after a few days to
normal school life. She recorded the subsequent history of her illness
in her application form for the psychiatric examination. As this shows
poignantly her share in the collusion, I shall quote her application
verbatim.

"When I was fifteen at boarding school I had food poisoning, but
only fairly slightly. I became very thin indeed and worried myself a
good deal because I feared I should get behind my form in work, in
fact I had a nervous breakdown and my hair fell out badly. I stayed
at home for a year and gradually put on weight, returning to a smaller
boarding school when I was much fitter. It was at this school that I
began to notice my legs swelling and they became gradually worse
over a period of time until my doctor prescribed Mersalyl injections,
but these only slimmed my legs temporarily. Since that time I have
had numerous injections also to get my monthly periods going again
(*which completely disappeared after the food-poisoning illness when I was*

fifteen). The hormone injections did a little good as I had a slight sign of a period now and again, sometimes at six-month intervals. I worried a good deal about the lack of periods and even more the fact that my legs swelled up so badly caused me great worry and lack of confidence. About a year or eighteen months ago I started a very nasty irritable rash. The skin specialist diagnosed this as due to nervous tension. This will not go altogether and seems to come in spasms especially if I am going to a party and want to be clear. I also worry about finances. I broke off an engagement nine months ago as I felt my fiancé was losing interest in me. This upset me a very great deal and my rash increased, and also the swelling of my legs. I felt it was due to my legs and the unsightly rash that I lost my boy friend. Mummy was ill in the spring of this year and had a serious operation. I went home to nurse her. She has now completely recovered. I did not earn for four months and I worried a good deal about finances. I find it very difficult to relax and I work myself up very much when going out anywhere to a party or anything. I find I lack confidence."

She mentions one doctor and a skin specialist in the whole of this lengthy report and completely omits that she consulted doctor after doctor, preventing anyone from taking full charge of her. In fact, ever since her food poisoning she has been continuously under medical treatment. Among the numerous doctors who saw her were the family doctor in the country and a friend of the family's, an eminent physician at a London teaching hospital. As she was living in London, the latter referred her to a London practitioner, asking him to take her on his list and to prescribe her the drugs, give her the injections and sign the National Health certificates. The recommended treatment consisted mainly of long courses of hormone injections to regulate her periods and mersalyl injections for her swollen legs. As time passed, Dr. C. became more and more discontented with his rôle, especially as Miss F. kept on complaining to him, being highly critical of Dr. Z., the eminent physician. Eventually, at a time when Dr. Z. was on a long holiday, her complaints became so insistent that the general practitioner referred her for psychiatric examination. I quote his letter of referral—

This girl came to me a year or two ago when she had for some time been under the care of a consultant physician. She only wanted me to prescribe on the N.H.S. various drugs which he had recommended. He was treating her for amenorrhoea with complicated glandular combinations. I was not asked to do anything else. Her home is in the country and she works during the week as a secretary. She also has a family doctor in the country.

Then she developed other symptoms of obviously nervous origin, cramps in the fingers so she could not type, rashes which came on during emotional upsets, etc., and she volunteered the information that she thought the whole of her troubles were nervous. She responded eagerly to a suggestion for treatment, as physical treatment had done no good.

She is an only child. Father retired, aged 68. Mother 55. The patient's menstrual periods started at 13½ and were quite regular till she was 15 when she started to worry, about a scholarship she says. The periods vanished for many months and even with gland treatment have appeared at rare intervals since. She is pleased when she sees one.

She is a pleasant, friendly, rather plain girl, who gives the impression of childishness and immaturity. She won a scholarship to a good public school, so she is above average intelligence. She is superficially cheerful, but numerous physical troubles seem to point to a lot of concealed misery. Her swollen legs coming on at adolescence without cause seems to be Milroy's oedema, supposed always (as far as I can find out) to be caused by severe psychological damage.

I have taken no psychological history. I don't want to treat her myself as I feel her case may be difficult and prolonged. I am sending her for assessment with the idea of group, or more likely, individual, treatment.*

This is a fairly typical situation which develops all too often when a number of doctors are involved and no-one is really responsible for any decision. The family doctor was consulted only when Miss F. visited her parents and had little share in the treatment. Dr. Z. saw her only occasionally and rather cursorily; moreover, he was concerned only with her physical symptoms; while the general practitioner who really carried out the treatment, although highly critical of his eminent colleague for neglecting the psychological side of the illness, found it awkward and perhaps thought it useless to tell him firmly that he thought the exclusively physical treatment was of very little use.

The psychiatric examination revealed that this difficult situation was as much the making of the doctors as of the patient. Prompted by her psychological make-up—I do not propose to discuss this in detail here—Miss F. had to behave as an obedient, dependent child accepting any advice or instructions without resistance, but afterwards playing off everyone against everyone else so that in the end no advice was of any help. Everybody was induced by her dependence to try his best to help her but was manœuvred

---

* It was an agreed arrangement at our research seminars that, when referring a patient for psychiatric interview, the doctor had to state explicitly whether he wanted to continue the treatment of the patient and was asking only for advice or whether he wanted the Clinic to take the patient over. This arrangement worked to the satisfaction of all concerned.

into a position in which with the best will in the world he was made unable to help.

After the psychiatrist's report the seminar discussed at length how the doctor could extricate himself from his uneasy position. His problem was that on the one hand he genuinely wanted to help the patient; on the other hand, although critical of Dr. Z., he did not wish to do anything which would disturb their amicable professional relations. In the discussion it became gradually clear that the only hope of solving this situation was to get in touch with Dr. Z. and convince him of the necessity of presenting a common front to the patient, so that she would not be able to play off one against the others. In addition, although the psychiatrist was more than doubtful, we arranged that the psychiatrist should offer help to the patient provided she wanted it. Everybody agreed, and most, though not all, of us thought that things were moving in the right direction.

It is very instructive to follow what actually happened. Dr. C. reported at our next meeting—

I wrote a full letter to the physician telling him exactly what had happened, that she had been referred for a psychiatric examination and what the report was. I added that I would send the report if he wished it—was he agreeable to her being treated psychotherapeutically or did he still wish to carry on his physical treatment? He replied very briefly and politely that she had told him an appointment had been arranged at the Tavistock Clinic, but she did not say she had already been there. He wrote, "She has spoken to my secretary several times, but never disclosed the fact. I think there is no doubt that she has organic lesion with periodic water retention and urinary disturbance." She came to me then, and I told her that she could have psychiatric treatment, and she said, "I think I ought to go to Dr. Z. again, he has been so kind," and she insisted on this. I pointed out that there were four or five doctors concerned already and she was playing off one against the other. In the same way, although she spoke to Dr. Z.'s secretary on several occasions, she did not mention that she had been seen by a psychiatrist and is now considering accepting the proposed treatment.

Some weeks later we learned that Miss F. accepted the treatment in principle but asked to be allowed to postpone starting it as she wanted to go for several weeks' holiday. During that time she consulted a gynaecologist, who prescribed further medication. On her return to London she started psychiatric treatment and whenever anything was pointed out to her responded, "My doctor (meaning the general practitioner) said this, or said that." After four attendances she broke off treatment saying that she was feeling remarkably well. The doctor reported that on seeing him she said that she dropped the treatment not because she was so well but because she could not go regularly and she did not think it was fair. Several months after these events, in June 1954, Dr. C. reported—

She comes regularly for injections always at inconvenient times. Still goes to gynaecologists for tablets.

After about a year, in May 1955—

No change, I am still the dispenser and do not know how to get out of it.

And last, in October 1955—

I asked her in August about her periods, and she said they had been pretty regular for a year. But she had never mentioned it, and if I had not asked her presumably would not have thought of telling me, though she had seen me about every week. She is now more spasmodic in her attendances, her legs still swell, she still has the same ugly skin rashes and her personality is completely unchanged. I am doing my best to keep up the hopeful attitude recommended at the last meeting when her case was discussed, and bide the time when she will ask for something more than hormones. In the meantime she has collected at least two more doctors, one from a London teaching hospital.

This case appears to be more complicated than Mr. K.'s, but this is only because the report includes the patient's rôle. The "collusion of anonymity" rules the situation not only as far as the doctors are concerned, but the patient has her full share in it, too. Everybody is trying hard, is expanding his energies in a futile way, but nobody can be held responsible for the management—or mismanagement—of the case.

CHAPTER VIII

The General Practitioner and his Consultants

I WISH to remind the reader that, as stated at the start of our journey, we set out to study why it happens so often that despite earnest efforts on both sides the relationship between the patient and his doctor is unsatisfactory or even unhappy, what the causes of this undesirable development are and how it could be avoided. That means that the greater part of the book will be mainly critical. In studying a pathological process one has to concentrate on the diseased part of the body, but this is not tantamount to saying that the whole body is equally affected.

To return to the complications caused by the entry of a consultant into the patient–doctor relationship. In the previous chapter we studied the working and the drawbacks of the "collusion of anonymity." This may lead, and unfortunately much too often does lead, to a dissipation of responsibility. Important, often vital decisions are taken without anyone openly accepting full responsibility. Often, in fact much more often than one would expect, the patient is a willing party in this tacit collusion. Our previous case, No. 12, shows this situation well.

In every case of collusion of anonymity, if the two doctors involved are a specialist and a general practitioner, certain other factors also operate, making the situation still more difficult to deal with. They can be summed up as the *perpetuation of the teacher–pupil relationship*. The general practitioner looks up with ambivalent respect to the consultants, who by their standing ought to, and often even do, know more about certain illnesses than he. If this is not confirmed by events, the general practitioner feels highly critical and dissatisfied but is prevented from taking appropriate steps because of the respect which the consultants inherited from their predecessors in the teaching hospital.

It is true that some consultants are more than willing to preserve this teacher status. At our seminars doctors often read out consultants' reports, especially those they found unsatisfactory. The commonest reason for dissatisfaction was that the consultants gave opinions and futile pseudo-psychiatric advice on a sorely inadequate basis instead of stating squarely and sincerely that they found no illness belonging to their special field which would account for the patient's complaints, or in other words: that in this instance their specialist services were not needed and could be of no use. Many consultants, being the successors of the doctors' teachers, obviously feel obliged to pretend to know more than they actually do.

The next case, No. 13, well illustrates all these undercurrents: the shedding of some of the burden of responsibility, the consultant giving perfunctory advice, and the discontented, grumbling practitioner paralysed by his ambivalent respect. The case was first mentioned casually by Dr. Y. when the seminar was discussing patients who demanded an X-ray as a reassurance.

CASE 13

She came on my list three years ago. Had been married happily to farmer, lived in country, had two children now grown up. Husband met with an accident, had ear abscess which was operated on, but as a consequence of which he became psychotic. Shortly after patient also had mastoid which was operated on; was terrified the same thing would happen to her but she recovered all right. At this time (about 1940) they lived near R.A.F. aerodrome and she fell in love with a man stationed there and decided to marry him. She got divorce from husband on mental grounds (though he was not as bad as she made out) and came to live with this man in London. The man had wife and two children but his wife refused to divorce him. They lived in his parents' house and there was constant strife between patient and man's mother. When I first saw patient, about 1950, she came with severe backache which I thought might be due to slipped disc, but on investigation this was disproved. Her symptoms were considered hysterical. In April of 1953 she suggested she might have X-ray and I reported on this case then. When I was on holiday in the summer my locum saw her; she had been on holiday to Isle of Man, was standing in a bus which gave a terrific jolt, she hit her head on the ceiling, felt giddy and sick, but said nothing about it as she did not want to spoil the holidays of her companions. From then on suffered from bad headache and insomnia. I sent her to Z. Hospital and got a letter from them dated 10th July—"She certainly has post-concussion syndrome. X-rays show some shadow in part of brain yet to be determined. She also has mitral stenosis. I have arranged to see her later. . . ." On the 17th July they wrote—"This lady's post-concussion syndrome persists. What she needs is really a long holiday. It would also help if she could sleep better, so perhaps you would give her phenobarbitone gr. 3 per day until she gets better." I had returned from my holiday by then. She came frequently to the surgery looking ill, could not sleep, headaches terrible; was worried whether it might have anything to do with previous mastoid operation. I suggested it was queer she had mastoid after her husband had had his accident and did she not think that that had affected her mind. . . . She replied that she was perfectly happy and never thought of her husband. In August I wrote back to the physician at Z. Hospital, gave her present history and asked for his opinion. He replied, "She is still suffering from severe insomnia with depression and loss of appetite. This is all very odd because her head injury was not severe. Moreover, she had not developed diplopia. No doubt her symptoms have hysterical origin. I don't think we need worry a psychiatrist yet and I suggest she goes back to work to see if it does not improve her. May I suggest you give her a mixture of chloral and bromide in place of barbiturates?"

Here again we see the futility of referring patients for specialist examination as a routine without proper "screening." This routine is just as futile as if every case of a broken leg or measles were referred for thorough examination by a psychiatrist. We see also how misleading consultants' reports can be. And lastly, we see the general practitioner looking up to the specialist as to a superior being and allowing him to treat the doctor as a kind of dispenser of drugs—almost as in the previous case of Miss F. Moreover, it is interesting to note in passing the attitude of the general practitioner. He noticed the inconsistency in the letters. The shadow "in some part of the brain" mentioned on July 10th was apparently completely forgotten by the consultant and his assistants at Z. Hospital, and the general practitioner in tacit collusion with them omitted to enquire further about it. This is surprising enough, especially to those who know how con- scientious Dr. Y. usually is. It is still more surprising that his ambivalent respect for the consultant so inhibited him that he was unable to use his knowledge to refute the consultant's super- ficiality. The consultant advised "I do not think we need worry a psychiatrist yet." The doctor grumbled, but he needed a fair amount of pressure by the seminar to divulge that he knew the following facts—First, a considerable amount of conscious guilt feelings in the patient about her husband; in a way she accused herself and denied at the same time that she had left him much too unconcerned about his illness, perhaps he was not so psychotic after all. Then the doctor knew of the patient's chronic conflict with her own daughter. The daughter, though devoted to her mother, doubted whether mother had really been justified in divorcing her husband; she was convinced that father was not really a mental case and went on visiting him. Moreover, the daughter, like her mother, lived with a married man who could not obtain a divorce. The mother felt rather sore about it, perhaps the more so as, being at fault herself, she could not show her disapproval. And lastly, there were the constant rows with the man's family, especially with his mother. All these suggest that the patient has not been able to solve her problems satisfactorily either in relation to men or, obviously, still less, in relation to women. Taking all these things into consideration, it was highly unlikely that either sedatives or tonics would help. The consultant's advice, given in complete ignorance of all these significant facts, could not be anything but futile and useless. And still, so great was the doctor's ambivalent dependence on his respected consultant that he needed quite some help before he could free himself sufficiently to be able to criticize the consultant's—and his own —rôle in this collusion.

Although it appears on the surface to be just the opposite of tacit collusion, my next topic is only another symptom of it. It happens not infrequently that the general practitioner and his consultant differ about the way of life desirable for the patient. A frequent instance of this kind of disagreement is the management of a patient with hypertension, especially if there have been some small premonitory signs. For instance, the general practitioner, knowing the whole background, the patient's personality, his ways of reacting to any restriction of his freedom, his proneness to hypochondriacal fears, and so on, might think that the best way to help him would be to preserve his zest for life and his capacity for work, even if it meant taking considered risks. The specialist, having only a cursory acquaintance with the patient's personality and judging mainly on the basis of his physical findings and his subjective impressions, might conclude that a cautious and quiet life was indicated. Devising ways and means by which the two partners—consultant and practitioner—can inform each other of their motives and aims presents a most thorny problem.

The general practitioner, however apprehensive of the consultant's possible bias, is compelled by the circumstances to ask for a specialist examination in order to find out, for instance, how far the heart muscle is involved, how much reserve power it still has, whether the kidney function is affected or not, and so on. He simply has not the facilities for obtaining these data himself. Another source of apprehension is that the doctor is always uncertain what his patient will be told during or after the examinations. Verbal instructions, particularly in a busy outpatients' department, are often given not by the consultant himself but by one of his registrars, or perhaps even by his houseman. The general practitioner has no control over them at all and at any rate, according to our experiences, consultants do not go out of their way to supervise this extremely important field of their services. Usually the written letters containing the physical findings are checked carefully to ensure that the results of the examinations are accurately described. Perhaps somewhat less care is given to the therapeutic recommendations to the doctor; more often than not they appear somewhat schematic. But what the junior staff say to the patient after all the examinations have been done is—with rare exceptions—left to their "common sense" or power of imitating the "great white chief's" *ipse dicta*.

Most general practitioners do not dare state their *desiderata*; still less do they dare instruct the specialist how to talk to the patients referred to him, what to tell them, or what not to tell them. And even if they did, I wonder how many consultants would follow such instructions and how many would go into an indignant huff at such lack of respect. The correspondence between Dr. C. and Dr. Z. about Miss F. (Case 12) is a good, though mild, illustration of this point.

The result of this mutual evasion is a reinforcement of the tacit collusion of anonymity. The consultant grumbles about indolent general practitioners who write perfunctory or nonsensical requests for examinations and are of no help to him and his hard-pressed staff; or, on the other hand, write long-winded verbose epistles as if the consultant had time to read all these outpourings and *desiderata*. Especially in London it is very seldom indeed that general practitioner and consultant meet face to face and find time and opportunity to learn each other's views, concerns, therapeutic aims and the ways chosen to achieve them. On the rare occasions when the general practitioner plucks up courage and rings up the hospital, or even goes there to discuss his patient, it happens almost invariably that he finds himself confronted with a registrar and not with the consultant. As often as not the registrar, though possessing higher postgraduate qualifications, is junior in years— and perhaps also in experience—to the general practitioner, which does not make the situation easier. Usually the registrar, to hide his diffidence, tries to be politely superior and non-committal, while the general practitioner is apologetic and irritated. On the rare occasions when the general practitioner is admitted to the presence of the consultant, the time is so short and their relation so tense that a thorough discussion of the case is seldom possible and the two part without either having explicitly undertaken full responsibility for the management of the case, thus conserving the rule of the collusion of anonymity. Case 27 in Chapter XVIII is a good example of this situation.

Another example of disagreement masking the collusion of anonymity occurs when the general practitioner and his consultant differ fundamentally about the therapeutic method to be applied in a particular case. Case 14 is a striking illustration of this unpleasant situation. At the same time it shows again how the patient's unconscious mental patterns first help to create, and then make use of, this collusion, causing the two doctors to become much more personally involved than they desire and certainly more than is expedient for the treatment. Dr. B. reported in October 1954 as follows—

CASE 14

Mr. I., aged 33, is under the care of a psychiatrist and has been having methedrine. For three hours after the methedrine injection he sits and writes down experiences and recovers all sorts of memories. Then he takes this material to the psychiatrist to read. I have known him for some time. On several occasions he has had acute breakdowns. This time I was seeing him because he developed bronchitis and sore throat. In the course of dealing with the physical illness we started discussing his mental problems. He has now reached a point where he collapsed, he has completely given in, gone to bed.

He is one of four children. Father was a business tycoon, kept very strict control; the patient had a very close attachment to one of his brothers who was killed in the war; after that he had his first break-down. Then he got married for the first time, to the sister of his favourite brother's wife; but quarrelled with his wife constantly. He came to see me one and a half years ago when in a highly tense nervous state. I saw him a number of times and he got over the acute phase. The next thing I learnt was he got married three months ago (summer, 1954) for the second time.

What is happening now is related to his second marriage. The present episode started because his wife wore a necklace which she had got from a previous boy-friend. He gets into a state of very acute aggressiveness which he is unable to control and today he said he felt he might hurt his wife. He got into a state of depersonalization. He was due to go for treatment last week but he did not go. An appointment has been made for this Saturday. I feel that the treatment he has been having has mobilized a lot of unconscious anxiety material which has not been dealt with at all. He is being made much worse by methedrine. I phoned the psychiatrist and asked him whether it would not be better for him to have analytic treatment. He said he did not think that was of any use in depressive cases and that the patient would have these attacks from time to time and that methedrine treatment would relieve the acute anxiety. I am not sure what to do with this man now.

On questioning we learnt from Dr. B. that it was the psychiatrist who boarded the patient out of the R.A.F. Dr. B. had advised analytic treatment already eighteen months ago, but the patient—when a breakdown threatened—had gone to the psychiatrist for help without first consulting his doctor. Some doctors in the seminar held rather strong views about this and declared that they would refuse further contact with a patient who behaved in this way. Dr. B., however, maintained that the man was his patient, suffering from an illness with physical as well as mental symptoms; the fact that the man had gone to the psychiatrist against his advice and behind his back, was merely a piece of emotional acting out, just another symptom. He then reported in detail what had actually happened recently.

I discussed the situation with the patient. I said that as his G.P. I must make decisions about his whole treatment and that I would get in touch with the other doctor, and the patient agreed to this. But when I spoke to the psychiatrist he was completely unco-operative. He was very antagonistic to my suggestion that there was any alternative treatment. He more or less implied that I as a G.P. did not know about psychiatry.

It was then pointed out that the patient must have some part in the plot, possibly by playing off the two doctors against each other. Dr. B. agreed, "And now he is playing up to the fullest possible extent. He has got control of the situation. He has got his wife terrified, his two doctors quarrelling politely, and I have to do something about it." He then added, "When he first came to me, before he got married for the second time, we discussed a great deal his relationship to the brother who died. It was quite obviously a nearly homosexual relationship. The brother was also substitute father and the Oedipus anxiety was bound up with it too. After his discussions with me he took flight from his anxieties into marriage instead of analysis."

After his marriage, to which by the way the doctor was invited, the patient did not consult his doctor for quite a period. Then he came complaining of sore throat and bronchitis and the present situation developed.

In a long and involved discussion the seminar arrived at the following picture of the dynamics of this case—the patient had a fairly strong feminine-submissive attachment to his brother, and he was probably the passive, expectant partner in this relationship. After his brother's death he looked for another strong man who would take the brother's place. Dr. B. might have raised expectations in the patient that he would be the strong man who would look after him, but instead of satisfying these expectations Dr. B. fobbed him off by advising analytic treatment. The disappointed patient first carried on for some time but then looked around for another strong man. He found a strong psychiatrist who—quoting Dr. B.'s report—"pushed all sorts of injections into him and made him work for three hours." In this relationship he was again the little brother. Then something went wrong. He broke down and came back to Dr. B. with a physical disease, again as a little brother, pleading for help. To his plea Dr. B. responded by assuming again the rôle of the big brother—"Now I will take everything in hand."

All this, however, was complicated by compulsive patterns set up on the model of the two brothers' relations with their father; the little brother, the patient, oscillating in his loyalty between father and big brother. The most important feature, which made the situation so difficult to handle, was that the two doctors accepted their allotted rôles and competed in reality for the patient's confidence and loyalty.

A further complicating factor was the wife's provocative flaunting of her past, to which an uncertain man like Mr. I. could not help but react with excessive emotional outbursts. Dr. B. was fully aware of this complication and took care to avoid becoming in any way involved with the wife and thereby provoking the man's suspicion.

I hope that enough convincing details have been reported to explain why the two doctors were at loggerheads. Apparently the disagreement was about the right method of psychiatric therapy. As his final argument the specialist produced the difference in professional status between him and Dr. B., which left the latter with nothing to reply, except his indignant anger. As we have gained some insight into the dynamics of the case, we can see the hopelessness of this kind of dispute. What usually happens in such a situation (as is shown by the two previous cases, 12 and 13) is that both specialist and doctor go on grumbling and pushing the responsibility on to the other. In this exceptional case the general practitioner was sufficiently versed in psychological medicine to become aware of most of the dynamic picture himself. He was thus in the unusual position of feeling confident that he was better informed than the particular consultant and had the courage and the perseverance necessary to solve the knotty problem. Moreover, when the discussion at our seminar reassured him that quite a number of his colleagues did not consider his going against the psychiatrist as a breach of etiquette, he took over full responsibility for the case. It is perhaps interesting to quote verbatim his retrospective description, dated March 1955, of this period—

From the beginning my way of dealing with my relationship to him (Mr. I.) was interpretative. That this was successful was clear from the fact that after the first interview he was a little less acutely anxious. The dynamics of the situation as it developed, so far as I can remember, was that I exposed his anxiety about continuing the injections and discredited the method of inducing massive recollections of past situations without the possibility of integrating them into his whole experience as should happen in analysis. I gradually openly expressed my own feelings about the value of physical psychiatric methods of this type and attempted to demonstrate to him the kind of help that could deal with his anxieties specifically, and illustrated it from the immediate situation to myself, to his wife, and to the psychiatrist. What I believe clinched the matter of his going on with the psychiatrist or with me was that he discovered for himself the relation of his present illness to rage at seeing his wife wearing a necklace given her by a former boyfriend. I was able not only to show him that this was a repetition situation in which he was developing intense guilt feelings over his threatening rage against his wife but that in fact the exploring of this material brought about a real relief of his symptoms. I was also aware that to some extent I was intervening. The opinion of the seminar was, I think, that I as his general practitioner had to take charge of all aspects of his case and it was as a result of this that he decided to put himself entirely in my hands, cancelled his appointment with the psychiatrist and, after considerable parley with various relatives, we arrived at the solution that I should try to find him an analyst. He is now making good progress in his analysis.

Mr. I.'s case shows a rather unusual solution of this well-known unpleasant situation. A more common solution of the same situation will be described in Case 27 in Chapter XVIII.

CHAPTER IX

The Perpetuation of the Teacher–Pupil Relationship

AS every doctor will recognize, the few cases discussed in the two previous chapters are only a minute sample of innumerable others with similar structure. In all of them the most important factors causing complication between the general practitioner and his consultants are—

(1) The prevalent preference in present-day medical thinking for diagnosing physical illnesses if at all possible.

(2) What we have called the collusion of anonymity.

(3) The ambivalent and not entirely genuine teacher–pupil relationship between the general practitioner and his specialists.

As we have discussed the first in the previous chapters, let us now turn our attention to the other two.

It would be easy to decree that the collusion of anonymity should cease forthwith and that one doctor only should be in charge of any one patient. This one doctor must obviously be the general practitioner, certainly at least as long as the patient is in his charge, that is, is not in a hospital. Unfortunately, the situation is much too complicated to be dealt with by a simple decree. In our research we were able to expose in detail some of the causes of this complexity. We experimented with a system which not only permitted but demanded that the general practitioner should remain in full and unrestricted charge of his patient. Although this arrangement preserves, even enhances, the practitioner's dignity, it is only with great difficulty that he can accept it. One reason is the burden of responsibility, sometimes really severe, that it involves. It is so much easier to farm out responsibility, to say, "I have asked all the important specialists and none of them could say anything of importance; I really need not be better than the bigwigs." No such escape was permitted in our research set-up. Although the opinions of specialists were asked for and listened to, they were not accepted as final or binding; they were criticized for what they were worth, and then the doctor in charge was asked to decide what was to be done with the patient and to accept undivided and unmitigated responsibility for his decision. Often the decision influenced the patient's whole future. This fact, too, had to be accepted.

No wonder that the practitioners, as often as not, do not like shouldering this heavy burden. What is more surprising is the willingness of all the specialists, including the psychiatrists, to enter into a collusion with the general practitioner in order that this responsibility may be dissipated, if I may say so, into thin air. The patient with psychological complications is often seen by several "eminent" physicians, each of whom gives his opinion about one aspect or another of the problem, but the final responsible decision is seldom explicitly stated even if it has to be taken. If possible no decision is taken; things are left in suspense until fateful events intervene and make the decision anonymously, allowing everybody to feel that after all it was not his word that counted. On the other hand, if things turn out well every doctor concerned may feel that his contribution was highly important, if not the decisive one.

One feature of our scheme was to lay bare this anonymity by making the practitioner accept that he is and must remain in charge of his patient. If the doctor needed more help than the case seminars could give him he was free to refer his patient to the Tavistock Clinic for consultation only, that is to say, if he was willing to continue the treatment.* The patient was then tested by a psychologist and interviewed by a psychiatrist (usually the leader of the seminar). The results of the tests and of the psychiatric interview were then reported at our conferences and mercilessly scrutinized. The final test of their value, which kept psychologist and psychiatrist alike on their toes, was the standard question of how much help in his further treatment of the patient the doctor got from their reports.

This is a severe test indeed, as I can testify from first-hand experience. Neither I nor the psychologists who took part in this research found it easy to accept that some of our reports were

---

* Of course in severe cases, where treatment was beyond the possibilities of a general practitioner, the patient could be referred in the normal way to the Clinic and was eventually taken over; i.e. ceased to be the doctor's responsibility.

merely nice phrases, repeating in somewhat different form the facts known only too well to the doctor, and giving him hardly any help in his difficult task.

The "collusion of anonymity" discussed above provides an excellent way out of this often trying self-criticism. The specialist need not realize the futility of his reports, and may remain securely perched on his "eminent" pedestal; the doctor may grumble and feel that his contemptuous opinion of the useless and pretentious specialist is justified and no-one need do anything. Our scheme, by bringing face to face as equals specialists and practitioners, has made this escape impossible. Admittedly we, like everyone else, have had cases in which very little or nothing could be done; this fact, too, had to be accepted explicitly and in full and frank responsibility.

There are, however, further reasons why it is so difficult to make any change in this respect. The "collusion of anonymity" dominates the field in medicine as in education—very likely for similar reasons. The burden of responsibility is much too great in both spheres, and everyone, including the patient, naturally tries to lighten it by involving someone else, or, if possible, a number of others. *This may be described as a process of dilution of responsibility.* Both education and medicine had to create readily available institutions and mechanisms by which this dilution may take place easily and smoothly often to the extent of ultimate anonymity. As the burden of responsibility is thus lightened all round, everyone concerned is willing to enter into the collusion of anonymity.

For the patient this situation is similar to the all too common one in which a single child has to face a whole world of grown-ups endeavouring to educate him according to their lights, which, in our terminology, means according to their "apostolic function." (See Chapters XVI–XVII.) Vital decisions concerning the child are made anonymously by "the grown-ups." If all goes well, all the grown-ups concerned—parents, relatives, friends, the school, the child guidance clinic, etc.—feel justly proud and gratified. If anything goes wrong nobody is individually responsible. Anyone acquainted, either in a professional or a private capacity, with the environment of a problem child knows how painfully true these two complementary statements are.

It is no wonder, then, that in a "problem patient" the similarity of the situation mobilizes all the anxieties, animosities, fears and frustrations, blind confidence and dire suspicions of his early years. This fact explains why so many patients regress to employing surprisingly childish methods in their relations with their doctor or doctors; such as complete subordination, swearing blindly by the doctor's words; or, on the other hand, an unrealistic, almost crazy rebelliousness, ridiculing and belittling anything and everything that the doctor suggests; and, lastly, a particularly annoying method, very adroitly playing off one doctor against the other.

Miss F. and Mr. I., Cases 12 and 14, are striking examples of this uncanny power in certain patients capable of paralysing the best-willed doctor by involving him in sterile conflicts with his colleagues.

Returning to the medical profession, the collusion of anonymity is one method of lightening the burden of responsibility. Another, equally important, is *the perpetuation of the teacher–pupil relationship*. It is only natural that the doctor, when faced with a difficult problem in his practice, should ask for advice, and it is equally natural that he should turn for advice to those who trained him, or to their equals—the consultants. He looks up to them with respect and admiration, and expects them to know more than he. He is reinforced in his expectation by the fact that present-day practice in medicine is hardly more than the sum total of the various specialities.*

It was in the various specialities that the immense successes of the last few hundred years were achieved, and under the impression of this long succession of very real triumphs doctors tend to forget that a price has to be paid for it. Nowadays everybody preaches that when a patient is ill the whole person is ill, not only his skin, his stomach, his heart or his kidneys. This truth, while constant lip-service is paid to it, is unfortunately ignored in everyday medical practice. Let us suppose that the doctor has come to the conclusion that the whole personality of a patient is ill, can anybody tell him which specialist to consult if any problem or difficulty arises? But let us compare this embarrassing problem with the ease with which a patient can be referred for a

---

* A very experienced and somewhat disillusioned practitioner said to me, "Nowadays it is enough for a doctor to know about twenty prescriptions and the addresses of about thirty consultants."

chest examination to this consultant, and the other for advice·on his duodenal ulcer to that consultant, and this woman for her skin condition to a third, and so on. No doctor has any doubt in these cases who are the few consultants among whom to choose; but if really the whole person is ill he is faced with nothing but doubts about where to turn for advice.

No wonder that, particularly in these awkward cases, the general practitioner is reluctant to accept full responsibility for his patient. It is equally understandable that the specialist who has been asked for his opinion and from whom help is expected prefers giving some advice to confessing that he cannot give any, and that he does not even know who could be asked.

Returning to the embarrassing question whom to consult when the general practitioner comes to the conclusion that the whole person is ill—why not ask a psychiatrist? After all, though we speak of mind and body, it is only the body which has been parcelled out among the various major and minor specialities; the mind—both in theory and in practice—has remained more or less undivided. It should be fair to expect that psychiatry would be the right answer to our embarrassing quest.

Being a psychiatrist I regret to have to admit that psychiatry also falls short of this expectation, often in a much worse way than the other specialities. The reason for this failure is that there are a number of difficulties due to the present state of psychiatry, which are absent in other specialities.

General practitioners frequently report that they experience much greater difficulties when they suggest to one of their patients that he should see a psychiatrist than when any other kind of examination is proposed. This undeniable greater difficulty is due partly to a general feeling shared both by the doctor and by his patient. We shall have to discuss this general resistance against psychiatry later. So let us disregard for the time being, the patient's fears and the doctor's own involvement in this problem. Obviously the doctor who believes that a psychiatric examination is a kind of stigma will have more difficulty when referring his patient than his colleague for whom a psychiatric examination is a matter of course. Apart from this personal, i.e. individual, problem, there is a general difficulty here, and in this chapter I propose to discuss only that part of it which is caused by the doctor's relationship with his consultants.

Sending a patient for a psychiatric consultation (or in fact to any consultant) is a much more complicated matter than asking for, say, a bacteriological test or an X-ray. The two kinds of request are similar only in that the general practitioner asks for an examination which he is not able to carry out himself; but while for a bacteriological examination only a specimen is needed, for a psychiatric interview the whole patient is required. This means much more than it appears to mean on the surface. A proper psychiatric examination must extend to all important human relationships of the patient, including those with his doctor; that is to say, in a somewhat exaggerated form, not only the patient will come under examination by the psychiatrist but, to a considerable extent, his doctor also. By this I do not mean only his possible mistakes in diagnosis but also, perhaps even foremost, his individual ways of dealing with his patient's personality problems. This kind of threat is to some extent present whatever the consultant's special field may be, but nowhere is it so marked as in the psychiatric field. Looking at the situation from this angle it is understandable why some general practitioners think twice before referring their cases to psychiatrists.

In addition to this subjective involvement, there are also objective reasons why a general practitioner hesitates before sending a patient to a psychiatrist. He soon finds out that in the majority of cases the psychiatrist's recommendations do not amount to much; moreover, these recommendations seem more to safeguard the interests of the particular psychiatric department than to help the doctor. Some of these routine recommendations may even have a fairly bad effect on the general practitioner's relations with his patient. This, I am afraid, is a severe indictment against us psychiatrists, so let us begin by reviewing some of these routine recommendations.

Suppose that the psychiatrist may decide that, in this case or that, "proper" psychotherapy (or psychoanalysis) is indicated, but he can offer no vacancy in the foreseeable future. What is the general practitioner to do in such a case? The patient has accepted his advice probably reluctantly and with apprehensions and misgivings, and has, so to speak, left the stronghold of his well-proved defences to get from the psychiatrist specialist help and treatment. To the patient this may mean, and in fact often does, that the general practitioner does not consider his own skill sufficient to deal with the illness. This opinion is then confirmed by the consultant, but no help is offered, either now or in the near future. In what sort of mood will this poor patient, who has now fallen between two stools, accept the inferior help which his general practitioner can offer him, and what should the doctor do in such a case? It is obvious that from this angle the situation has been changed considerably for the worse by the consultation.

Equally bad are the effects of the not infrequently given opinion, "We cannot do much for this patient now; he is not ill enough (i.e. for us)." Something of this kind often occurs with borderline cases referred to the outpatients' department of a mental hospital. Shall the general practitioner tell his patient to hurry up and get worse quickly so that he may get some help, or shall he tell him to go on suffering to avoid treatment? Here, too, the situation has changed for the worse by the psychiatric interview.

Then, every general practitioner has a practically inexhaustible collection of psychiatric opinions which do not go beyond recommending him to "reassure his patient and give him some sedative or a tonic—or even both." Although psychiatric interviews resulting in this kind of recommendation are not of much help to doctors, they readily admit that they prefer this kind of disappointment, because at least it does not worsen the situation drastically. It only means one hope less for the patient, but at any rate his confidence in his doctor is not impaired as the consultant did not know more either.

Another equally inexhaustible source of complaint is the psychiatric reports themselves. First, they are always too late. True, many patients expect their doctor to receive the result of the interview the next day. The reason for their impatience is clear. All specialist examinations, but especially psychiatric interviews, more often than not stir up fears and anxiety, and the result is awaited with trepidation. Any delay is felt to be ominous. Unfortunately, apart from this subjective lateness, the reports not so uncommonly are really late. Secondly, a large number of psychiatric reports are too short and contain hardly more, or even less, than what the general practitioner has known anyhow about his patient. The inclusion in the report of one or two diagnostic labels does not help the general practitioner either. He knows well, as I have tried to show in Chapter IV, that these labels hardly ever describe the real pathological process or give advice about a rational therapy. At best they are diagnoses of symptoms, not of illnesses. Their limited usefulness remains unchanged even if these diagnostic labels change according to the prevalent fashion in psychiatry. During my lifetime I have witnessed the change in fashion from neurasthenia to psychasthenia, then to neurotic character, and recently to anxiety or depressive states; but the help given the general practitioner by describing his patient by any of these names has not changed very much.

Lastly, there are the rather infrequent novelistic reports. As some psychiatrists have a good style, these novelistic reports often make pleasant reading. Unfortunately, they too end usually in the futile recommendation of reassurance, phenobarbitone and tonic. This book contains samples of both the short and the novelistic reports, showing that my description is not unduly exaggerated.

So far we have criticized mainly the consultant, which is certainly unfair. There are, of course, general practitioners who for some reason or other do not resent being restricted to the rôle of dispensers of drugs. According to the stories circulating among consultants and their registrars, these doctors are indifferent, bordering on indolent, or possibly even totally uninterested. The famous, always recurring tag, about "? heart—please see and advise" sums them up admirably. According to specialists the proportion of this kind of referral is fairly high; according to general practitioners the specialists treat most doctors, even those who welcome real discussion of their cases, as if they belonged to the indifferent class. Here again we find the shedding of responsibility, the collusion of anonymity.

It is impossible to establish what the real situation is, to decide to what extent either party is in the right or in the wrong. It would be a most valuable piece of research to collect and scrutinize a large number of the letters with which general practitioners refer their patients, and the corresponding reports by the specialists. This would not be an impossible venture, as almost all hospitals file this correspondence meticulously and so it could be looked up for many years past. That this research has not been undertaken by some responsible body such as the Medical Research Council or the British Medical Association is another symptom of the collusion of anonymity.

Still, whatever the true situation may be, it must be admitted that some general practitioners do not deserve and perhaps would not even welcome a detailed and well-argued report by the specialist. In their case the letters criticized in the previous two chapters are perhaps an understandable institution.

We have now to return to the question of how to deal with this awkward and embarrassing situation. Any proposition must be able to answer two very knotty problems which in reality are two variants of the same basic problem. The first variant asks who is to be in charge of the case and accept full and undivided responsibility for the patient? The answer one would like to give, is that it ought to be the general practitioner. This proposition, however, means that the general practitioner must become more independent of his consultants, and must undertake the added responsibility of screening his patients more carefully in order to be able to state in his requests for examinations the specific questions that he wants the specialists to answer. He must also learn to criticize firmly but sympathetically the specialists' reports and recommendations and assess them at their real value. Last but not least, he must learn to recognize the limits of advice and help that he may in fairness expect from his specialists. On the previous pages we discussed a number of reasons why general practitioners are not, on the whole, so anxious to shoulder this additional responsibility.

The other variant asks what should be the rôle of the consultant in relation to the general practitioner; should he be an expert assistant or a mentor, a teacher? The implication of this formulation is clear enough, but I propose to illustrate it with an example. If a doctor sends a specimen of blood to a laboratory he gets a report from an expert, the pathologist, who carries out an examination or does a test which the doctor cannot do. The reason why he cannot do so is irrelevant; it may be lack of time, of equipment, or of skill, etc. But, though the pathologist in these respects is superior to the general practitioner, he does not assume the right to give him any instructions. On the contrary, he merely does what he has been requested to do, and reports his findings. He is, in fact, an expert assistant doing his limited job. The picture is entirely different when the test or examination has to be carried out by another type of expert, say, a general physician or a surgeon. His report gives the result of his examination, but invariably goes beyond it, and states what the diagnosis in his opinion ought to be and also gives instructions about the treatment that should be carried out.

It is only natural that the doctor's relationship to the two types of expert will be different too. It is this difference that I wish to emphasize by asking whether the consultant should be a mentor or an expert assistant to the general practitioner. Specialists, as we have seen, are just as keen to adopt the rôle of mentor as general practitioners are to accept the *status pupillaris*. This is what we termed "the perpetuation of the teacher–pupil relationship," a very powerful partner to "the collusion of anonymity." They work together in providing ready mechanisms and institutions for the dilution of too heavy responsibilities. All of us being human, it is to be expected that the specialists will be as reluctant to divest themselves voluntarily of any part of their authority as general practitioners will be to add more responsibility to the burden they already carry.

It can easily be shown that this unsatisfactory situation is maintained on both sides for the sake of the unconfessed, small, but desirable advantages that it provides. The "? chest, please see and advise" type of referral requires much less thought and care than assessing the extent of the pathological process and, on the basis of this assessment, asking detailed questions which inevitably disclose the doctor's limitations. In the same way one rarely sees reports by specialists which clearly state the exact limits of the specialist knowledge and experience on which their advice is based and make plain at which point they have to resort to guessing or to well-meant but not so well-founded counselling.

From which quarter can a change be expected? In my opinion the general practitioner is faced with the harder task. It is exceedingly difficult for anyone to accept that he has really and irrevocably grown up, and that, though there remain still a few people in the world with superior knowledge in this field or in that to whom he can turn for limited advice, more often than not it is impossible to escape the full weight of responsibility. This burden is made the more difficult to bear by the fact that the general practitioner knows too well how much his decision affects the patient's future life and happiness. Moreover, for the general practitioner the patient is not only a patient but someone well known, including his family background, all his relatives, his past, his disappointments, successes and hopes, and quite often also his whole neighbourhood. The consultant, however sympathetic, is hardly ever involved to such an extent. Moreover, by forgoing the not fully justified rôle of a mentor equipped with overall superior knowledge and wisdom, the burden carried by the specialist will be lightened, and the weight of his opinion in his special field enhanced. So perhaps it is not entirely unrealistic to hope that it will be the specialists who will first realize the advantages of openly accepting the rôle of expert assistants to the general practitioner.

One of the many changes that this will involve will be that the phrase, this or that complaint is "of hysterical or of psychological origin" will no longer be considered a satisfactory end-result of a careful examination, as well-earned laurels on which to rest—but as a challenge. No conscientious doctor would, for instance, give phenobarbitone or a tonic for a complaint or symptom thought to be of tuberculous origin, but would insist on thorough diagnostic examination and specific treatment; in the same way phenobarbitone or a tonic, and even "reassurance," are more often than not useless in cases "of psychological origin." These patients are just as much in need of proper investigation and a rational therapy.

True, but who is to conduct this examination and provide the well-founded rational therapy? Today, broadly speaking, medicine cannot provide either, because it has been split up into many, admittedly highly efficient, specialities. None of these seems to be interested in complaints of "psychological origin," and still less to have worked out the proper methods for dealing with them. In a way psychiatry suffers from the same general predicament. In its way of thinking and in its pathological theories its orientation is primarily physiological. The same is true—perhaps even truer—or psychiatric therapy. Used far more often than anything else are either chemicals like alkaloids, vitamins, sedatives, insulin, etc., or physical methods such as E.C.T. or leucotomy. Thinking in psychological terms is very much in its infancy, and accordingly the provision for psychotherapy is pathetically inadequate all over the world, in this country as elsewhere. The coming of the National Health Service brought no change for the better in this respect; on the contrary, the situation has taken a turn for the worse as the demand has greatly increased while the facilities for psychotherapy have remained about the same.

A real change in this respect can be achieved only on the basis of painstaking long-term research carried out in close co-operation between the general practitioner and the psychologically orientated psychiatrist. This proposition in several variations will recur again and again as a refrain in this book, and we shall have to discuss it at some length in a later chapter. Here I wish to consider it only as far as it affects the relations between the general practitioner and his consultants.

This research into the pathology and therapy of complaints "of psychological origin," i.e. of the whole person, cannot, in my opinion, be carried out by specialists but only by general practitioners. This, however, requires a fundamental change in outlook, as research as well as teaching has been almost exclusively in the hands of the specialists for the last few generations. It is true they have deserved this privilege by their undeniably great success in both fields as is demonstrated by our greatly enhanced therapeutic possibilities and our much sounder medical training. But the problems encountered in the field of whole-person pathology are—as I have tried to show in the previous chapters and will discuss further in those to come—largely unknown and even inaccessible to the specialist. On the other hand, they are *the* problem of general practice and, to a considerable extent, of psychological medicine. That is why I believe neither the general practitioner nor the psychologically orientated psychiatrist has any choice but to accept this heavy honour and that the research must be carried out by them jointly, although the lion's share is bound to fall on the general practitioner. I wish to add that he will not be alone in this task. He will certainly be able to call on the co-operation and help of his consultants, but they can only be his expert assistants. That will be no novelty in medicine. In exactly parallel fashion present-day specialist research needs and uses the help of chemistry, anatomy, physiology, pathology, radiology, bacteriology, and so on, but all the time the specialist, attending his patient, remains at the centre of the research. In the research into the pathology of the whole personality, the novelty will be that the centre will be occupied by the general practitioner and *his* patients. The demand for this research is there, and is very pressing. What is needed is for general practitioners to respond to the demand.

To sum up, some of the more important factors in the doctor-consultant–patient triangle, which make relations between them unnecessarily tense at times, are—

(1) Preference for diagnosing physical illnesses and if possible recommending physical treatment or operations, even in cases where these are not fully justified.

(2) The overwhelming burden of responsibility to which all three parties react by shedding some of it on to the other two, resulting in an almost institutional collusion of anonymity.

(3) The perpetuation of the teacher–pupil relationship between doctor and consultant well beyond what is realistic.

(4) Lack of sufficient understanding of the patient's regressive tendencies in this triangular relationship, especially his playing off one doctor against the other or others.

(5) The unhelpfulness of many specialists' reports, especially if they touch on psychological aspects—reports by psychiatrists being no exception to the general rule.

A real change for the better can be expected only as the result of long-term research into the pathology of the whole personality corresponding to what was described above as the deeper level of diagnosis. As the problems belonging to this field constitute *the* problem of general practice, no-one but the general practitioner can undertake this research.

PART II

Psychotherapy

CHAPTER X

Advice and Reassurance

IN the previous chapters our main concern was the psycho-
dynamic aspect of medical diagnosis. That is, while we took
for granted the techniques and skills which a general practitioner is expected to possess, we examined critically some of the
most important psychological processes involved in making a
diagnosis. Our main field of investigation was the part played by
the doctor; that played by the patient—though not completely
disregarded—was only of secondary importance for our survey.

In our survey we saw the patient in his still "unorganized"
state making various "offers" of illnesses to his doctor, and the
doctor responding to these offers by rejecting some of them and
finally accepting one. An important aspect of the doctor's
response is the process of "elimination by appropriate physical
examinations," resulting in the establishment of a ranking order
both of illnesses and of patients. Under the impact of the doctor's
response a kind of "agreement" is more often than not reached
between him and his patient, and the illness thus enters upon its
"organized" phase.

Our next step led us to examine the complications caused by
the great burden of responsibility that a doctor has to bear on his
patient's behalf. If the burden becomes too great, the help of
specialists is called in. An unforeseen, but perhaps not entirely
unwanted, consequence of this is the "dilution of responsibility"
by the "collusion of anonymity" and the "perpetuation of the
teacher–pupil relationship."

By now we have reached therapy. What is the general practitioner supposed to do, and what does he actually do for his
patients? It is generally agreed that at least one-quarter to one-
third of the work of the general practitioner consists of psychotherapy pure and simple. Some investigators put the figure at
one-half, or even more, but, whatever the figure may be, the

fact remains that present medical training does not properly equip the practitioner for at least a quarter of the work he has to do.

Although the need for a better understanding of psychological problems and for more therapeutic skill is keenly felt by many practitioners, they are reluctant to accept professional responsibility in this respect. The reason most frequently advanced is that they have too much to do as it is, and it is impossible for them to sit down and spend an hour with a single patient at a time, week after week. This argument, impressive as it sounds, is not, in fact, firmly based. It is true that establishing and maintaining a proper psychotherapeutic relationship takes much more time than prescribing a bottle of medicine. In the long run, however, it can lead in many cases to a considerable saving of time for the doctor and for his patient (and of money on the drug bill of the National Health Service). Our case histories 12, 16, 18, among many others, are ample proof for this statement.

As we have seen in the previous chapters, what happens in practice in most so-called psychological cases is an almost mechanical prescribing of sedatives and tranquillizers if the patient is not depressed, and of some "tonic" and antidepressants if he is. When this fails, various specialists are consulted, usually resulting in "reassuring" reports that nothing organically wrong has been found. Eventually a psychiatrist is consulted, often not so much as a deliberate policy but as *faute de mieux*. This mode of action, however, is created as much by the difficulties of the psychiatrist as by those confronting the general practitioner. It is common knowledge that the psychiatric services are pathetically unequal to the ever-increasing demand; they are flooded with patients, and consequently the psychiatrist must pick and choose. If a patient is picked, he is put on the waiting-list, eventually accepted for treatment, and, more often than not, completely lost to the practitioner. If the patient is not picked, the report sent to the doctor hardly ever helps him in his psychotherapeutic task; except by advising him to prescribe sedatives or a tonic.

Thrown back on his own resources, the doctor, often shame-facedly, prescribes some *placebo*, and gives advice or a "reassuring" pep talk. (It is a common joke to ask: "Reassuring—but to whom?") Then there are the advocates of "common-sense" psychology who advise the patient to take a holiday, to change his job, to pull himself together, not to take things too seriously, to leave home, to get married, to have a child, or not to have any more children but to use some contraceptive, etc. None of these recommendations is necessarily wrong, but the fallacy behind them is the belief that an experienced doctor has acquired enough well-proved "common-sense" psychology to enable him to deal with his patient's psychological or personality problems even without attempting a proper diagnosis. But minor surgery, for instance, does not mean that a doctor can pick up a well-proved carving-knife or a common-sense carpentry tool and perform minor operations. On the contrary, he has to observe carefully the rules of antisepsis and asepsis, he must know in considerable detail the techniques of local and general anaesthesia, and must have acquired skill in using scalpel, forceps, and needle, the tools of the professional surgeon. Exactly the same is true of psychotherapy in general practice. The uses of empirical methods acquired from everyday life are as limited in professional psychotherapy as are carving-knife and screwdriver in surgery.

To demonstrate the limited usefulness of "common-sense" advice and reassurance, I wish to quote a case in which this method, and nothing else, was used. Dr. S., in spite of the severe criticisms of the seminar, did not go beyond the traditional limits of medicine: taking a history, carrying out a physical examination when he thought it necessary, "reassuring" his patient, and giving her "common-sense" advice in an avuncular way as his nature is. In this way Mrs. B. never had any psychotherapy and was not even examined psychologically. The many well-observed details of her history, however, enabled the seminar to get good glimpses into the mechanisms and the problems of her case. Thus we were able to follow the ups and downs of the history of her illness, criticize her doctor for his technique, and appreciate with understanding the limited success he achieved.

In May 1953 Dr. S. mentioned our Case 15—

CASE 15

Mrs. B., aged 24, whom I had known since she was 17, when she had an appendicostomy for colitis. She is the only daughter of a very neurotic woman who had kept her under strict control. Some years ago I advised the patient to get out more, go to dances, etc. She took my advice, and met her husband at a dance. They live now with her mother, who does not get on too well with her son-in-law. The couple tried to emigrate, but it was discovered that the husband had a shadow on his lung. The T.B. clinic could find nothing wrong at first, but one of the many samples taken was positive, and he was sent to a sanatorium. After four months he came home, and husband and wife came to see me a fortnight ago, together. She has nervous symptoms, palpitations, insomnia, and sometimes diarrhoea. She asked me whether it would be advisable to have a child, and I said it would, but the husband said he did not want a child, as he was not in a secure enough position, not having a house and not knowing whether they would be going to emigrate, as is their intention as soon as his health permits. This morning the girl's mother rang up to say her daughter was very ill with nerves. The patient then came to see me in the surgery, and told me she was obsessed with the idea of being changed from a female into a male and has to pray all the time that such a thing will not happen. She had read of such a case in the papers. Sexual relations with her husband are very infrequent. I examined her, and assured her that her genitals were quite normal and there was nothing for her to worry about. She felt happy at being told this, and said she would think no more about it.

Her husband is rather a peculiar man, has no friends, is lazy. He wants to wait six months to make sure his chest is all right and they will then try to emigrate. They have been married two years and he insists on having no children; contraceptives are used.

As the readers of this book will expect, Dr. S. was criticized on two counts in the seminar. It was pointed out to him that "reassuring" the patient by telling her that there was "nothing wrong" with her would have only a short-lived effect. Admittedly his prompt examination eased the patient's anxieties, but this was not necessarily a desirable result. He intervened therapeutically before establishing the correct diagnosis. He allayed Mrs. B.'s anxieties, probably only temporarily, but certainly missed an opportunity for finding out more about her problems and the causes of her anxieties. Dr. S. produced the ever-ready excuse of not having enough time just now, but promised to be more thorough when he saw the patient again.

A week later he reported—

I was called to see the girl, who was in bed with colitis. She told me that after the examination she thought she was convinced that she was not changing her sex, but since then she had changed her mind again, and she was not sure now. The patient's mother told me that her daughter is always wanting to compare her genitals with her mother's to make sure she is normal, but the mother will not allow this. Apparently my examination had not been sufficient to reassure the girl as I had hoped.

The seminar, and its psychiatrist leader in particular, triumph-antly pointed out to Dr. S. how short-lived had been the effects of his reassurance, that exploding one "offer" by the patient by a physical examination had resulted only in her producing another "offer" in the form of colitis, and lastly that it would be advisable for him either to do a psychological examination himself or to refer Mrs. B. to a psychiatrist.

A further week later we heard from Dr. S.—

Mrs. B. came to see me last Thursday, when she said she was feeling very much better, but she still thinks sometimes there is a possibility of her changing into a man. She is very depressed, her husband never takes her out. It was arranged that she should call to see me the follow-ing Monday. She is now training to be a shorthand typist and goes to school. She came on Monday with her husband, said she was very depressed, but she was very changeable—sometimes she is deeply depressed and then she feels very exhilarated. She even threatens suicide, but neither mother nor husband takes her seriously. She blames her depression on lack of friends and lack of entertainment. As the patient felt better, and I was very busy, she was asked to come again in a fortnight.

The "offer" of colitis apparently not having been accepted, Mrs. B. produced a third "offer"; depression and some slight threats of suicide. This third offer did not make much impression either. Mother, husband, and doctor alike refused to take it seriously. Dr. S. then admitted to the seminar that he was trying to mark time. As the couple intended to emigrate, it would be inadvisable to start probing into Mrs. B.'s problems; this might create highly emotional reactions, which could not be dealt with in the time available. As there was some truth in this argument, it had to be accepted, but Dr. S. was again warned that unexpected things might happen.

The next report came at the beginning of July, about seven weeks after the first—

Although she believes me when I say she cannot change her sex, yet she cannot help feeling sometimes that it might happen, and she has to pray to God. If the change happens, she feels perhaps it will be a kind of punishment because she was not nice to her parents when she was young. She said that when she was five she played with another girl, and they touched each other's genitals. She felt later on that it was wrong, and told her mother. Before she tells me anything she always discusses it first with mother, who usually says things are not important and there is no need to tell me about them. Mother is still very strict with her. Patient said she would like to go overseas to get away from her, but it is a little too far and she would rather go somewhere where she could visit her mother if she wanted to. Her general depression has been much less lately but she has attacks of disbelief about the impossibility of changing her sex. She was told to come back in a week. She says she likes to come and see me as when she leaves me she feels cheered up, because I listen to her.

Dr. S. then added "Patient does not talk about father much. He once had a slipped disc and was in bed for two weeks, and in January he was suffering from melæna, from which he soon recovered. He is a traveller, and often away. His wife domineers him and tells him what to do."

At long last, Dr. S. found time "to listen"* to his patient. Apart from repeating her doubts about changing her sex, some important material was produced. We got an idea of the closeness and tenseness of a mother–daughter relationship which went so far that a married woman of twenty-four had to report to her mother all the details of her sexual life, and even had to ask her advice about what to discuss and what not to discuss with her doctor. That this relationship was not exclusively one-sided, i.e. caused only by the domineering mother, was shown by the daughter's wish to compare her genitals with her mother's for the sake of the reassurance which that might give her. This, taken in conjunction with the sexual play with another girl at the age of five, plainly indicated a strongly ambivalent homosexual attachment to the mother. The obsessional idea and fear of changing her sex thus became intelligible as a fantastic method of escaping from the conflict of ambivalence, and also explained why it was felt as a punishment. If this train of thought is roughly correct, we can understand why a "common-sense reassurance"—which failed even to touch on her real problems—could not have much effect on her.

A week later a dramatic *dénouement* started. Dr. S. told us—

A couple of days ago I received an urgent telephone call from the girl's mother that the girl had had a row with her husband and had taken poison. She had really only taken six aspirins and one sleeping tablet. When I called, mother, father and daughter were in a room

* The meaning of this expression will be discussed in Chapter XI.

together, and they all started talking about the row. A few minutes later the girl's husband came in and said the matter should not be discussed in public, so the mother and father went out. The daughter then blamed her husband for not giving her a child, and threatened divorce. I told the husband that it was the primitive right of a woman to have a child, and that if his wife divorced him it would be his own fault. This morning the patient came in much happier. She said they had had intercourse three nights running, which she had enjoyed because no preventive measures were taken. However, after intercourse the husband said that if they had a child as a consequence, he would not like it, as it would be in the way and an unwanted expense; now she is worried about that. In spite of this, she still has fleeting ideas about changing her sex, and asked what she should do when she has these ideas, which question I did not answer.

Nearly all the doctors turned against Dr. S. for again giving premature advice before finding out what the real situation was. Dr. S. retorted that in an emergency such as this a general practitioner was entitled to use his personality; he simply could not sit and wait for results, he had to do something, and whether it was to the advantage of his patient or not remained to be seen. The urgency was admitted, but it was pointed out that the urgency had been partly created by Dr. S.'s procrastinating policy, which always found good reasons for not probing deeper at any particular moment.

In mid-August, Dr. S. reported—

Since last reporting on the case I saw her twice. She and her husband are now getting on very well, they have regular, satisfactory intercourse, and are looking forward to having a child. Patient has taken a job as a secretary and has passed her typing examination. She is feeling very much better and very pleased with everything, though I had not been able to reassure her completely that she would not change her sex. She asked me several times whether it was not possible that she had changed since I examined her, but I refused to make further examinations as it would mean loss of prestige for me, and the girl would think I was uncertain about it too.

Reluctantly the seminar had to admit that the advice to the husband to accept his wife's right to have children had not been so bad after all. Dr. S. had certainly succeeded to a certain extent, but how and why nobody knew. Still less was known about what the price of his success would be and who would pay it. So Dr. S.

was advised not to rest too contentedly on his laurels, but to watch for further developments.

In October we learnt that the young couple had found a flat several miles away from mother's and that they had come to say goodbye to Dr. S. Sexual relations were satisfactory, but the girl "still had silly ideas occasionally about changing her sex, but she was able to reject them straight away."

In May, 1954. we heard again about Mrs. B.—

Her mother came yesterday, and she was very nervy and full of aches and pains. She said her daughter was not happy in her first flat and she had moved to another place, where she was quite happy. Moreover, she is working and she is pregnant, but does not want to see her mother at all. Mother is very sad about it, the more so as Mrs. B. threatens that she does not want her mother to see the child either. Perhaps there is no need now for the girl to feel she is not a proper woman.

Now I wonder whether all this was due to the overwhelming mother, who talked for the daughter all the time and who had to be told all about the sexual affairs between the daughter and her husband? Was it this that made the girl so inconclusive about her own state? Now, not only has she become pregnant, which proves she is a woman, but she has become independent of mother.

In November 1954, Dr. S. received a letter from Mr. B. announcing that a baby had arrived without any trouble, and that Mrs. B. had never looked better. They had given up the idea of emigrating, and in a few weeks were moving to a house which was being built for them in the country. Dr. S. then rang up the mother and

congratulated her, and she was very surprised that I knew about the baby. They did not let her know about it at all, she heard from someone else in a roundabout way that her daughter was having a baby. She went to see her the day before yesterday and spent an hour with her. The daughter and her husband say they will not have anything to do with her, and they will not allow her to touch the baby. The mother offered to have the daughter with her for a week when she comes out of the home, but they refused point-blank. They made a complete break with the mother.

The neurotic conflicts had not been resolved, but only adjusted. But the adjustment was definitely there, and it was undeniable that Dr. S. had played a great part in it. This case history shows that "common-sense" methods may have successes, but not because they are "common-sense." They represent shots in the dark in a possibly correct direction. It may even happen that they get near the target.

We asked who would pay the price for the doctor's success. Recent events seemed to suggest that it would be Mrs. B.'s mother, but more was to come. In January 1955, we heard from Dr. S.—

The mother of this girl sprained her ankle soon after her daughter left her, and now she has broken her wrist. I think that is very interesting. She broke the wrist of the right hand, which ought to have hit her daughter. She was full of hate; she is a nervous wreck now.

One partner of the intense and richly ambivalent homosexual relationship had escaped into femininity and motherhood; the other had broken her wrist and become an overt neurotic. What were the chances of the young woman's remaining as healthy as she now appeared to be, and of the older woman's recovering from the severe trauma that befell her? No-one knew, and now it might be impossible for any one doctor to assess these chances in their mutual relation, as the two women were separated and under two different doctors. Was the present situation more favourable for therapy than that in which Dr. S. did a physical examination and "reassured" Mrs. B., or otherwise? Was it the right decision in the spring of 1953 not "to go deeper?" So far as we can tell Dr. S. and his advice helped the young woman to free herself at her mother's expense. Was it a fair price, or could a better bargain have been struck if Dr. S., instead of carrying out a physical examination and "reassuring" his patient, had embarked there and then on "going deeper?"

A number of further questions could be asked. For the time being, asking them is fairly sterile, as there is no answer. Proper research conducted by general practitioners is the only way by which reliable information about these most important problems can be obtained. I wish to reiterate, though it is pretty obvious, that this research can be conducted only by general practitioners; no-one else, certainly no specialist, has access to the patient material. The answers to questions of this kind can be obtained only in a close and constant relationship with the patient, which is the essence of general practice. The best follow-up service conducted by specialists is incapable of achieving the intimacy which is an essential condition without which this sort of information will not come to light. As we shall see in the next chapter, asking the patient questions, even in the most sympathetic manner, is not enough.

In spite of our almost pathetic lack of knowledge about the dynamisms and possible consequences of "reassurance" and "advice," these two are perhaps the most often used forms of medical treatment. In other words, they are the most frequent forms in which the drug "doctor" is administered. It will be easy to accuse me of being a trouble-maker, who sees untold dangers in something perfectly simple and human. What, after all, can be more natural than to sympathize with a patient in distress, and to try to show him that much of his distress has no physical cause? Moreover, the patient is often relieved by our sincere "reassurance," and afterwards things develop in a favourable direction. As everyday practice shows, these two statements are true—in a way.

That is why I reported Mrs. B.'s case *in extenso*. If we take the beginning and the end of the story, we cannot but be deeply impressed by what happened. Here was a young woman, unhappy, under the thumb of a domineering mother, receiving hardly any help and support, or even normal sexual affection, from her husband, thinking of divorce and suicide in her despair, and eventually developing a fixed idea, not knowing whether she was really a man or a woman. At the end of the story we hear about her as a happy mother, who has had an easy confinement, has freed herself from her mother, and is looking forward to settling down as mistress of her own home and of her own life. Undoubtedly Dr. S.'s therapy of reassurance and advice contributed considerably to these impressive changes, i.e. was both helpful and effective. That is my opponents' argument, and I readily concede that it is valid as far as it goes.

But it is only a superficial picture, which does not tell us anything about what really happened or why it happened. When we take into consideration the other details which Dr. S.'s frank reports enable us to follow closely, the convincing argument based on this case history dissolves into a haze of what, for the time being, are unanswerable problems, and Dr. S.'s simple and straightforward therapy appears to have been a lucky shot in the dark. Indeed, unless a detached observer made himself disagreeable by drawing attention to it, it would be easy to forget that one shot—the physical examination and ensuing reassurance—was a complete failure. On the other hand, the other shot—the advice to the couple to have a child—was a resounding success.

That too is typical of this situation. Failures are suppressed and forgotten while successes are proudly paraded. I should like to remind the reader that both therapeutic measures—the reassurance about the woman's sex and the advice that she should have a child—were "common sense." One had no effect, while the effect of the other was excellent. *So the question is not how much common sense is required but how better to aim it.* The answer must come from more research by critical general practitioners.

I base my whole argument in this chapter on one case history. True, it is a well-observed and frankly reported case history. Is this a firm enough basis? From one point of view it would be easy to quote a number of other cases. From another, because of the way in which our research was conducted, it would be very difficult. Advice on insufficient grounds is given much too often in medical practice, and we were able to study several instances of this. But it is not easy to see one's unhappy mistakes reported in print. That was the reason why I chose the one case in which the advice was not utterly futile, in which it achieved partial success. Most of the other cases would have made the doctor concerned appear in a much more unfavourable light.

CHAPTER XI

" How to Start "

IN the previous chapter we saw the limitations of advice and
reassurance, the two forms of psychotherapy most used by the
general practitioner. It must in fairness be added that they are
used at least equally often by specialists, and even by psychiatrists,
with the same limited results.

I wish to reiterate that advice and reassurance are not necessarily
wrong in themselves; they may even be very powerful therapeutic weapons. What is wrong is that they are administered
wholesale, without proper assessment of what their effect will be
in the individual case. During the First World War, as a young
medical student, I served in a busy military hospital. The medical
officer in charge of the ward had a highly efficient system of
prescription. If a patient complained about his head or neck, he
was given aspirin; if about his chest, codeine; if about his tummy,
medicinal charcoal; if about his legs, aspirin again. If the patient
did not recover after four or five days, he was transferred to a
special ward according to his complaint. The results of these
wholesale methods were about as good as those of the present
wholesale administration of advice and reassurance.

The similarity goes somewhat further. Aspirin, codeine, and
medicinal charcoal are all valuable and well-proved medicaments.
Their administration as practised by my medical officer may even
be called—with some forbearance—a common-sense method.
What is wrong with this kind of treatment is that a therapeutic
intervention is embarked on without proper diagnosis. In this
respect the advocates of wholesale common-sense advice and
reassurances are in a much weaker position than my medical
officer, because their therapeutic agent is not so innocent as
aspirin or charcoal, or even codeine, which is a scheduled drug.
We have seen in several of our case histories that the drug
"doctor" is a potent one with many untoward side-effects.

So the first principle should be: *Never advise or reassure a patient before you have found out what the real problem is.* More often than not, after the real problem has been brought to light, the patient will be able to solve it without the doctor's advice and reassurance. Another, almost equally important, empirical principle is that the doctor's verdict of "nothing wrong" or "nothing physically wrong" hardly ever reassures a neurotic, though it may reassure a patient who is physically ill.

Some doctors may be inclined to pooh-pooh all this. They may say that they have always known it, for it was dinned into them every day during their training, and every decent doctor observes the rule of no treatment before diagnosis.

Let us revert, once more, to diagnosis. Making the diagnosis, in ordinary physical medicine as taught in medical schools and hospitals, is entirely the doctor's task. True, he invites the patient's collaboration, but this need not go very far. It is possible to arrive at a diagnosis if the patient is unconscious or under an anaesthetic. These admittedly are exceptional cases, but the fact remains, as we put it in our jargon, that the doctor examines the patient in order to find out what the diagnosis is. *The doctor always takes the active part: the patient may remain passive, though co-operatively passive.*

In psychological terms, arriving at a correct diagnosis is a one-man task, the one person being the doctor. It may be objected that it is impossible to make a proper physical diagnosis without taking a proper medical history, and that taking a medical history requires the full collaboration of the patient. This is true. Indeed, it is impossible to take a medical history with an unconscious or anaesthetized patient. But it is equally true that every medical student has to learn the right questions to ask and how to ask them in order to arrive at a relevant history.

In essence medical history-taking means collecting answers to our well-tried set of questions. More often than not practically everything else that the patient tries to tell his doctor is pushed aside as irrelevant. While we were discussing this a doctor recalled the first medical history he took, knowing little about the correct routine. Then he stood in front of the class and read it out. In no time the lecturer interrupted him, saying, "Sorry, we can't be here all the morning. Almost all of your history is irrelevant for the diagnosis. If you want to tell the patient's whole history, we shall be here as long as the patient has lived."

This is a highly important point. Taking a medical history is a kind of borderland between the one-person situation—the doctor examining the patient for physical signs in order to arrive at a physical diagnosis—and the two-person relationship which is necessary for a psychological, "deeper," diagnosis. Hospital medicine has developed a highly efficient and reliable technique for use in this borderland. It may be called—"Structurizing the two-person situation according to the pattern of the physical examination." In essence this consists of a sequence of questions, starting with general enquiries, and the doctor using the answers to narrow down the field of his next questions till he arrives at a few potential diagnoses which can then be verified or refuted by physical examination. For instance, if a patient starts complaining of vague abdominal discomfort a few well-directed questions will, as a rule, enable the doctor to decide whether he should think of acute indigestion, chronic constipation, incipient pulmonary tuberculosis, mild coronary attacks, nervous flatulence, spasms caused by intestinal obstruction, first signs of pregnancy, etc., etc. To arrive at a sound diagnosis the first requisite is, of course, well-founded knowledge, i.e. the doctor should be able to think of all sorts of illnesses, and in the second place he must possess sufficient alertness and elasticity of mind to notice any unusual or unexpected answer to his questions and to be able to change his original ideas accordingly.

But all the time he is the one who asks the right questions in order to get relevant answers; all that is required of the patient is to understand the doctor's questions and to answer them truthfully. The personal relationship between the individuals involved, although somewhat more important than, say, while the doctor is listening to the heart-sounds or palpating a tender abdomen, is far from being in the focus of attention.

The technique of medical history-taking has not been as rigidly standardized as, for example, have those for identifying flowers and trees; nevertheless, it amounts to a systematic questionnaire. Unfortunately, no such systematic questionnaire exists yet in the field of the pathology of the whole person, the true field of general medical practice. Moreover, it is still doubtful whether it is possible to develop such a system in this field, especially for the "unorganized" stages of an illness. For want of a better technique, and as a matter of "common sense," doctors, when faced with patients who present problems beyond the field of hospital medicine, resort to that of medical history-taking. Although the results are not very encouraging, doctors have no choice but to continue with this method, as they do not know of anything else.

Psychiatry is in the same unhappy predicament; here, too, no adequate systematic questionnaire exists. As a matter of interest, the method adopted by one of our leading psychiatric teaching hospitals for dealing with this uncomfortable situation might be mentioned. As there is as yet no *rationale* which would enable the doctor examining the patient to choose his next question on the basis of the answers obtained to his previous ones, the solution adopted is to list *all the questions* thought to be relevant to *any* psychiatric diagnosis. The result of this conscientious, painstaking, safety-first method is, apart from a number of other documents, an eleven-page record book, called the "item sheet," which contains more than five hundred questions. The senior houseman or registrar needs two days' hard work to obtain from the patient all the answers to this list. This is hardly a procedure which the general practitioner could be called on to imitate.

Our experience has invariably been that, *if the doctor asks questions in the manner of medical history-taking, he will always get answers—but hardly anything more*. Before he can arrive at what we called "deeper" diagnosis, he has to learn *to listen*. This listening is a much more difficult and subtle technique than that which must necessarily precede it—the technique of putting the patient at ease, enabling him to speak freely. *The ability to listen is a new skill, necessitating a considerable though limited change in the doctor's personality*. While discovering in himself an ability to listen to things in his patient that are barely spoken because the patient himself is only dimly aware of them, the doctor will start listening to the same kind of language in himself. During this process he will soon find out that there are no straightforward direct questions which could bring to light the kind of information for which he is looking. Structurizing the doctor–patient relationship on the pattern of a physical examination inactivates the processes he wants to observe as they can happen only in a two-person collaboration.

This sounds rather odd and mysterious, so it will be advisable to illustrate more clearly the difference between this approach and that in medical history-taking. All the practitioners who attended our seminar were well aware of it. Nearly every one of them would say in the middle of a report on one or the other of his cases, "At this juncture I felt that there was more to it than meets the eye; so I asked the patient to come for a long interview and went into his life history." Asking the patient for a "long interview" involves a different approach and means starting something entirely new in the doctor–patient relationship.

To emphasize the importance of this change we termed it, "How to start." To show what we mean by it let me quote a case which shows both the routine situation according to the pattern of medical history-taking, and the "long interview" and its consequences. Dr. G. reported Case 16 in March 1954 as follows—

CASE 16

Mrs. O., aged 41, was originally a private patient of mine, but since the Health Scheme has been on my list with her whole family. For the last six to eight years has seen me regularly once a week or a fortnight. She complains of sweats, headaches, migraine, depression, fibrositis, pins and needles, pleurodynia, eyes feel heavy, tires easily, sinusitis . . . without any physical signs. The only thing she has had really wrong was a caruncle of the urethra, and she had it removed. She is a very presentable woman. Now she has waves of depression, and cries, complains of noises in the flat above, and cannot get on with housework.

I have always realised her illnesses were psychoneurotic, but I was afraid to enquire into them. She probably thinks I am a pretty good doctor in spite of still having these symptoms. She is terribly anxious about her two children; one boy, just left the Army, fourteen stone and fit; the other son, thirteen, just as tough. She is always asking anxious questions when they have a cold and that sort of thing. Her husband is a decent, tough sort of chap, but gentle and nice to her. Prompted by the seminar, I decided to enquire into the psychological aspects, and last week I asked if she would like to come after surgery hours.

She came and told me father was a drunkard, used to beat his wife, sometimes involving police action. On one occasion patient had to go to hospital with mother to have stitches put in. Mother had nine children, patient was the third eldest. Mother very hard-working, always ill. She died when patient was thirteen and she had to leave school and look after the rest of the family until nineteen, when she married. She never went out. Father worked at a fruit market, had to get up at 3 a.m. and always expected her to get up first, to get breakfast ready for him, etc. She remembers awful scenes at home. She and the other children were once out in the street in the early hours, terrified to go in, had to go to a neighbour's house, because the parents were fighting. Mother was a wonderful woman, always saw the children had enough to eat, whether father brought the wages home regularly or not.

Soon after mother died, father brought another woman into the house and married her; patient hated her and left home six months before her own marriage to get out of the situation. Father died in 1939.

She had known her husband since she was sixteen; she went to live with her in-laws when she left home and stayed there for some time after they were married. Her husband is very good, very generous, would do anything for her. She herself is frigid, intercourse is revolting to her, but her husband has no idea that she feels like that about it. She occasionally gets pain and feeling of tightness which suggests vaginismus. She thinks her two boys are normal—indeed they are, except that they seem to be following her pattern of rushing to me when they get any little thing wrong with them.

She was happy at school, but did not have much time to play with the other children. She remembers one thing when she was nine— she had just recovered from an illness—woke up in the middle of the night, felt she wanted comforting; went into parents' bedroom without knocking and witnessed them having intercourse. It horrified and shocked her; and she has never been able to get it out of her mind. She mainly felt guilty about not knocking. She immediately had a relapse of her illness. She has never mentioned this to anyone, not even to her husband.

Mrs. O. thinks her mother-in-law is an awful woman, she is filthy. She used to stay with them, but patient persuaded her husband not to let his mother sleep there; now she comes to see them sometimes, but does not stay.

Those are the main things. She spoke quite freely. At the end I wondered whether I was not right all the time in not doing anything about it. I seemed to come to a dead end.

This is an instructive case history, as it clearly shows all the details we are just discussing. We see the doctor attending conscientiously to all the changing ailments of his patient, using his well-proved skills, accepting every one of her "offers" and responding to them in positive and sympathetic fashion. It is true that by his acceptance he had helped his patient to "organize" her illness—whatever

its true nature may have been—as physical ailments. The relationship between them had remained untroubled in spite of two
interrelated facts—

(*a*) That the doctor had been unable to cure her but had
succeeded only in making her symptoms tolerable.

(*b*) That on the whole she had been a nuisance to him all these
years.

Patient and doctor, without noticing when and how, had
slipped into a tacit collusion, each accepting the frustrations and
irritations caused by the other's limitations and letting sleeping
dogs lie.

Then, under the weight of his experience at the seminar, Dr. G.,
early in March 1954, decided "to start" and offered his patient
a "long interview" after surgery hours. The result may be
likened to an opening of the floodgates, and the patient became
able to talk about things which she had not been able to mention
to anybody throughout her life. A vast amount of important
information was obtained which threw light on the real problem
in her case, and made it possible to understand why no physical
therapy had really been able to help her. I wish to add that all
this information surged up without much questioning; all the
doctor had to do was to listen.

Lastly, an equally important aspect: the doctor felt highly uneasy after the interview. On the one hand, as he later admitted
in the discussion, he felt guilty "for not having done anything
about the possible psychological roots for all these years;" on the
other hand, he felt he "had come to a dead end, and wondered
whether he had not been right after all in not probing deeper into
his patient's personality problems." When questioned by the
other doctors, Dr. G. admitted that after the "long interview"
the patient had appeared to be relieved, but he could not see any
way open for a sensible continuation of the work started. As his
uneasiness is a typical reaction of this kind of situation, I propose
to quote his words—

The thing about this case is that it seems to be different from any
others. . . . With the others I did feel I could get somewhere, or that
somebody would be able to do something, or if I knew more about
it I could. . . . But I do not feel it in this case. I am wondering whether
it was right to stir things up here, in spite of her pressing symptoms.
There was no more reason that I should do this now than any time in

the last three or four years, only that I felt I ought to be pulling my weight here in the group in presenting a case.

I wish to warn any doctor who may decide, without previous experience, to offer a "long interview" to one or other of his patients that he must be prepared for something of this kind. The sincere opening up of a patient's intimate life, with all its miseries, petty and profound fears, frustrated hopes, few and often very precarious joys, is a deeply moving experience. Moreover, the help that can be thought of or offered is often hopelessly inadequate to the real need. The result in the physician, especially in the early stages of his experience, as in Dr. G.'s case, is a feeling of indignant impotence, of injustice, of futility, though Dr. G.'s feeling of defeat did not turn out to be well founded. I must add that this kind of experience sometimes leads to just the opposite, to a feeling of well-earned triumph and of over-confidence. It usually needs time and considerable mental effort to adjust either reaction to the level of reality.

In the discussion all sorts of theories were put forward to link the patient's past with her present symptomatology, and Dr. G. was encouraged tentatively to interpret this or that aspect of the case on the lines of the various theories. Dr. G., however, flatly declined. He argued that he was a general practitioner and had no intention of becoming an amateur psychiatrist—a stand often taken at our seminars. In the end we all agreed that what he did could, and even should, be done by a general practitioner as an integral part of his services. Going further is a more complicated matter. General practitioners who are interested and have acquired some professional skill in psychotherapy may go further and experiment in their practice with minor psychotherapy. Dr. G. was neither interested, nor felt skilful enough, for this task, so he was right in deciding not to go further on his own initiative. On the other hand, he wholeheartedly agreed that he should remain available for Mrs. O. if she wanted to have further talks with him, and even that he should mildly encourage her at her next visit by some such question as, "What do you feel now after talking over these things with me?"

Next week Dr. G. reported—

I had a call to see her son, who was ill, genuinely, and after I had seen him she said with smiles all over her face, "I feel a lot better—

I feel a lot of tension has gone out of my head," and she was very pleased, and is coming to see me next week. Obviously something has happened there.

Nearly four months later, at the end of June 1954 Dr. G. mentioned Mrs. O. again—

I have seen her once since (the discussion) for usual physical things. Now I see her only in the street, she is very friendly, but she does not come in. From the question of relieving my big surgery it is a good thing.

Lastly, a follow-up report in October 1955, a year and a half after the "long interview"—

I see Mrs. O. from time to time—certainly much less than in the past. The relationship is especially good. She gets occasional migraine, but the whole atmosphere is now that "we understand each other's silent language," and that there is much more to it than is actually said, but both doctor and patient have agreed (silently) that we don't need to go into it. Friendly, encouraging chats do the trick, and the doctor is a real friend who makes things right by his understanding the hidden problems.

I would call this a very successful case, perhaps more so than some of the spectacular ones, even if only to have produced the relationship which exists. (She even walked in one day with a new patient to whom she had obviously been cracking me up.)

This case is an excellent *prima facie* answer to those physicians who argue that they have not the time for this kind of quiet listening. If we take it that Mrs. O. came to the surgery about three times a month, needing from five to ten minutes' attention on each occasion, her disappearance from the surgery saved the doctor between one and two hours' work in four months. Even if the "long interview" is set against this, the saving was considerable; moreover, the follow-up report showed that it continued. Another aspect is the cessation of the drudgery and irritation caused to Dr. G., and the relief to him when Mrs. O. changed from a complaining, depressed and dissatisfied patient into a friendly and cheerful acquaintance. Still more important, the "long interview" caused his understanding of his patient's problems to be better and safer. True, his responsibility also increased with his better understanding.

Because of the importance of this problem of "how to start,"

I propose to quote another, much more complicated case. This was brought up when we decided to discuss patients who come asking for an X-ray; the doctors were asked to report on all such patients who came during the week.

Dr. K. reported Case 17, in October 1955, as follows—

CASE 17

Mr. Y. has been on my list for some years; he is nearly fifty-five, and I know the family quite well. He is a very pleasant man, kind-hearted, and runs a shoe business. He has chronic T.B., which he was discovered to have in 1951. He has always looked a perfectly fit man. Had a long history for years of indigestion and winter bronchitis, and had been through hospital once or twice before he came on my list. They never found anything. His chest was not X-rayed, as nobody bothered much about the bronchitis. Anyhow, we did refer him to a hospital in 1950 or 1951, for a routine check-up; by the X-ray they found he had T.B. It was not considered serious and he took it philosophically. We thought he might be a little upset, but he managed to make arrangements and went to Switzerland for treatment lasting about a year. He is now back at work.

He is under the T.B. clinic and he had his routine check-ups now. He occasionally comes to see me for his indigestion tablets, which he has had for years. He has had barium meals before in the past, shown no ulcer, but he came in this morning at 10.30, just before I got out to do my rounds. He said, "I want an X-ray," so I just had to hear his story. He said he had had his usual not real pain, just a vague discomfort and a nausea feeling, and he said he would like to be X-rayed. I said, "Why have you come this morning?" He said, "I don't know, I would just like an X-ray now." I put on rather a fast question, I said, "What are you worried about, are you worried if you have got a growth or an ulcer?" And he said, no, no, he was not worried about that. I could not get out of him why he wanted the X-ray. I examined him, his tummy and back passage and so on, and reassured him. I said, "There is no sign of a growth here, or anything like that to worry about." He didn't seem particularly relieved. And then in the chat that followed he did a lot of the talking, most of the time. We discussed whether perhaps "it is really my nerves; when I am a bit worried it always goes to my stomach. If I had an accident in the car, I would feel upset; even if it is quite a trivial thing, my stomach gets upset." When he goes on holiday, without the stress and strain of business, he is all right. He went on with this line of talk, emphasizing really to me that he thought a lot of it was really nervous trouble. Then I said, "Well, look here, after all, what are you worried about, are you afraid of a growth?" He said, "No, no." Anyhow, I went on talking a bit, and then I said, "Well, I don't really know, there is not a lot of indication at the moment," which he seemed to take fairly well. I said I had been into it very fully, there was no sign of anything serious. He said he had run out of his prescription for tablets, and that he liked to have them by him (he only took one every day when he wanted it). Then, just as I was finishing writing the prescription—this vital thing always comes just as they are going to leave the surgery, at the moment when you are least responsive—he suddenly said something that did not quite reach me—I think he said, "A lot of my relatives seem to be getting a bit old now, and have arthritis and things, and then there is my daughter kidding me last week to come and see the doctor." (This is his daughter, just about nineteen.) Then he said, "She said, 'Now you must remain young, daddy, you go and see the doctor.'" And it seemed to me that he had come at that particular moment because his daughter was wanting him to remain young, and not like some of these ageing relatives. But he does look a youthful man, under fifty instead of fifty-five. So that seems to be the reason.

There are many characteristic details in this frank, totally un-prepared report. First among them is the faithful description of the confusion of tongues between doctor and patient. The doctor thinks that the patient is worried about the possibility of a cancer, and does his best to "reassure him that there is nothing wrong." In this case he can do so sincerely and truthfully, as he has found not the slightest suspicious sign after a careful examination. The patient, however, is not affected at all, he does not appear to be worried about cancer, neither can he be reassured. Still, prompted by his training and preconceived ideas, the doctor cannot "listen," and must go on with his reassurance. Thus a good half-hour is wasted in talking at cross-purposes. I may add that this was an exceptional case in that—as mentioned—we had decided at the previous seminar to look out for people who ask for an X-ray; during the week no-one had turned up with this request; Mr. Y. had dropped in at the end of the morning surgery of the day of the seminar. So Dr. K. may have been more careful than usual, knowing that he would be expected to report about this patient.

After the "reassurance," to round off the visit the doctor started to write out the patient's usual prescription. Then, when all medical history-taking and reassurance had stopped and there was a moment of silence, the patient started saying something to his trusted doctor. The latter, however, was still so busy with his work that he did not listen properly. Still, he was sensitive enough to prick up his ears, and some relevant information was given and received. By then time was so pressing—a busy morning round to be started a good forty minutes late—that the interview had to be terminated with the prescription.

Now, it is almost certain that the real motive which prompted this man to seek his doctor's aid was his fear that he was ageing. (Later we shall get some confirmatory evidence for this.) It is highly probable that in a normal routine, undisturbed by the influence of the seminar, the doctor would not have "listened" to the few half-hearted sentences spoken by the patient while writing his prescription. It is possible that the patient would have got his "reassurance," and in addition a chit for an X-ray. After all, Mr. Y. was fifty-five, complained of vague abdominal discomfort, and the doctor had the impression that he was worried—possibly about a cancer; a barium meal or enema would certainly have been justified, particularly if the doctor was on the cautious side. In any case, a negative finding should certainly have a healthy reassuring effect. But, as we have seen in the previous chapters, the doctor's verdict of "nothing wrong" as often as not has no effect. Here we have a case which shows one of the reasons why it cannot have any effect. The X-ray examination—whether positive or negative—had no connection with Mr. Y.'s problem, and was no answer to his "offer." However, innumerable X-rays are asked for and carried out, and innumerable prescriptions are written, on the basis of this kind of reasoning—with the same futile results.

However, we must be prepared for more to come. Dr. K. had "started" something which was bound to develop. One aspect of what was to come was the influence on Mr. Y.'s illness of the daughter-father relationship. He was fifty-five, his sexual powers may have been waning; he might, consciously or unconsciously, be jealous of his daughter, who was perhaps beginning to claim a sexual life of her own. On questioning Dr. K., we learnt that Mr. Y.'s nineteen-year-old daughter was an only child, and that her parents worked hard to assure her a degree of financial security. All sorts of other details about the family were revealed by Dr. K., who rounded his report off—

I think if I had been a stranger this man would not have told me of such a trivial thing as his daughter sending him round; it was only because I knew him pretty well that he let it out. He might have thought it was too stupid to tell a doctor. And he could not mention it at the beginning, he left this detail until the very end.

Dr. K.'s former assistant, now a principal, happened to be taking part in the same seminar. He continued the story—

I can add to this father–daughter relationship because I saw the daughter (when he was assistant to Dr. K.). She went abroad when she was quite young, she must have been only about seventeen, I think, and I rather gathered against the parents' wishes. Whilst abroad she contracted Bell's palsy. She had some treatment there for about a couple of months, and I think the parents rather agitated for her to come home, and reluctantly she came home. They were very worried about it, she was not. I fixed her up with some physiotherapy and electrical treatment. Again, she was quite satisfied, but the parents were not, and actually they both (i.e. father and daughter) came round, and they wanted to see somebody to have a private consultation. The father wanted somebody who really knew the subject. In the end I sent them to Dr. X. (a most distinguished neurologist), who said just the same thing, and reassured them. After that I did not see them again so the consultation seemed to satisfy them. She was a plain girl, but not unattractive. The palsy was quite noticeable but it was improving. Still, it was, I should say, a perfectly normal anxiety about his daughter.

It was pointed out here that perhaps the anxiety had other sources as well, although on the surface it appeared to be just normal. After all, we knew that the daughter left home against her parents' wishes, went abroad, and returned at the parents' urging much against her will. All this pointed to some latent conflict within the family. If one took the father's concern about his daughter's palsy in conjunction with the daughter's concern about her father's ageing, one could not escape the impression that there was a pretty strong attachment between the two. Our next question was about the mother's rôle and personality.

Dr. K. reported—

The mother is a very interesting woman, she looks rather priceless, has conspicuously dyed hair. They are all a very nice pleasant family, extraordinarily kind. She has nerves. I have not seen her for some time now, but she came perhaps two years ago for a nerve tonic. I never really went into it, though I would now. But I do remember giving her a bottle one week, and in the interval I hung up in my waiting-room a new, really modern picture. I was staggered that this woman, whom one would not imagine had any feeling for art at all, came the next week into my room really gasping, "I came here for another bottle of your tonic, doctor, but really that new picture has done me more good!" She was so moved by this picture. I would not have believed it possible that she had a capacity to receive what this picture had, which was an obviously very powerful emotion. She told me then of a previous exhibition in X. One particular picture there had given her the same tremendous kick which suddenly made her feel better.

We went on with the discussion, somewhat impressed that we had started with a man suffering from vague indigestion and asking, apparently not unreasonably, for an X-ray, while now we had a whole family on our hands. There was general agreement in the seminar about the diagnosis, but great uncertainty about the best therapy. As one doctor put it, "There are three people in this family, and they all have some neurotic trouble. Now, should all of them be treated separately, or which of them, or none at all?" Before we began discussing this question, Dr. K. drew attention to an important detail:

One point I would make is quite interesting. It is the fact that I missed the T.B. in the early stages. I ought to have thought of it before, of course, but Mr. Y. never really complained. He would come in with a stuffy nose or something, and the problem of his chest never really arose in a serious sense. Then I had the letter from the hospital, saying that he had T.B. If I remember now, I felt quite a bit guilty about it, because the person who was insisting on the X-ray was the patient. When the report came back positive, I felt absolutely shattered. I felt this man would now be cross with me, as he had every right to be. I felt terrible about it. But he is a man who likes a good relationship with people. He likes to do his work well, have satisfied customers, and to do his best for people. I thought leaving his little business would completely upset everything and might lead to utter chaos, but I was surprised how well he took it.

Here is another example which shows how painfully surprised doctors invariably are when a patient does not feel relieved on learning that there is "nothing wrong" with him, and conversely, when he does not break down on learning that he has a serious illness. Some, like Mr. Y., can take bad news in their stride; it is even possible that in some way it satisfies something in them.

We spent some time at that meeting discussing people's need to be taken seriously. A negative finding, capped by the unavoidable "reassurance," sometimes amounts to frustrating such a need, whereas finding a serious illness might satisfy it. It was even suggested that if Dr. K. had given Mr. Y. ample opportunity to talk, i.e. had taken him very seriously, say in 1947 or 1948, he might perhaps have prevented the flaring up of the T.B. process in 1950 or 1951. But, however that might be, it was felt that Mr. Y. must be taken seriously now, for he needed it badly. Reassurance and palliatives might force him to develop new, and perhaps more serious symptoms and illnesses in order to get the attention that he needed; in short, he should be considered as being on the danger-list. As one doctor summed it up, "Possibly this man must be taken seriously on one level or another. If one does not take him seriously, as it were, on a psychological level, sooner or later he will make demands to be taken seriously on a physical level."

We next asked Dr. K. how he had parted from his patient. He said that Mr. Y. had been given enough of his pills to last for about a month, and it was certain that, as usual, he would come back for more. The group, and particularly the psychiatrist, felt somewhat uneasy about this. Being left alone for a month might be felt by the patient as not being taken seriously and, furthermore, a month's interval would certainly make it rather difficult to reopen the important subject mentioned in the last minute of the interview. Dr. K. tried to reassure himself that his patient had been happy and unworried when he left. He was reminded, somewhat mercilessly, "that in 1948 or 1949 the patient would have been just as happy with a renewed prescription for an expectorant; if Dr. K. had been in our seminar then, he might have used exactly the same sentence as he was using now."

There followed a long discussion about the best thing to do. I shall sum up the conclusion only. Mr. Y. might be in a precarious situation. Nothing need be done in a hurry, but when he next came he should be given enough time to speak his mind, with hardly any questioning. Dr. K. should examine him again very carefully. After all this, the doctor should try to direct the talk to Mr. Y.'s family, especially the daughter, who was considered to be the next in need of attention. Mrs. Y., although obviously highly strung, was felt not to be in need of immediate help. Whether this assessment was correct or not we cannot yet say, as the case was reported only in October 1955. One of the reasons why it was included here is that it gives some idea how discussions developed in the seminar and in particular how a case becomes richer as the discussion goes on.

Returning to the problems mentioned earlier in the chapter, these two case histories well illustrate the difference between the results of medical history-taking and "listening." I think it fair to say that it would have been practically impossible to ask questions which would have yielded information such as that Mr. Y.'s daughter wanted her father to remain young; that Mrs. Y. had her hair dyed and could be deeply moved by modern pictures; that Mr. Y. was not at all concerned at his doctor's failure to discover his T.B. in time, but was deeply worried about his daughter's appearance, etc., etc. In the same way no questions could have elicited from Mrs. O. that she had witnessed both her parents' violent quarrels and their sexual intercourse (Case 16).

That is why we say that *if you ask questions you get answers— and hardly anything else.* What we try to foster is the growth in the doctors of an ability to listen to the events as they develop in the doctor–patient relationship during the interview. Later, in Chapters XIII and XVIII, we shall revert to the doctor–patient relationship, and in particular to its special form as it occurs in general practice and in no other field of medicine. This special form of doctor–patient relationship in general practice is conditioned by the often long and intimate connection between the two. We described it as a "mutual investment company"; it was this that enabled Mrs. O. to talk to her doctor on the first occasion offered her, and likewise enabled Mr. Y., though only at the very end of the interview, to mention what really had brought him to the surgery.

Then there is the vexed problem of "giving a name to the illness" (see Chapter IV). Part of Dr. G.'s uneasiness was certainly due to his inability to "name" his patient's illness after he had at last discovered it. Incidentally, before the "long interview" revealed it to him, he had no difficulty in giving names to all the minor ailments that Mrs. O. "offered" him. Moreover, his uneasiness was certainly aggravated by his inability to think of a rational therapy for it. The fact that in spite of his qualms the patient definitely improved made things no more palatable to

Dr. G., who is a sober doctor and likes to know where he stands.

Mr. Y.'s case—at least for the time being—was somewhat simpler. Though his illness cannot be given a name either, there was no pressing and immediate need for it. Mr. Y. was satisfied with calling it indigestion, and the doctor, knowing what he had to watch for, did not feel the need for a name.

Lastly, a word about the rôle of a consultant of any kind in cases such as these. Let us suppose any member of the Y. family had been referred for a specialist opinion. Miss Y. in fact saw a neurologist, who diagnosed a Bell's palsy, which was no news to the doctor or to the family. True, the neurologist successfully reassured the father—the daughter did not need reassurance—but was completely unaware of and uninterested in the real problem facing the doctor. The radiologist and general physician who carried out the barium tests on Mr. Y. were, if possible, still more remote from it. They were simply unaware of the facts, and it would have been difficult for any of them, using their skill in medical history-taking, to find them out. The family doctor was in possession of all the facts, not as the result of asking questions, but because he knew his patients. *He did not, however, listen to them*. What the seminar achieved was to bring the facts and the doctor (in Mr. Y.'s case two doctors, the principal and his former assistant) together.

This ever-recurring situation shows why it is so often futile for the specialist to adopt the rôle of a mentor and for the doctor to persevere in his old *status pupillaris*. In these cases the specialist has nothing to teach, because the general practitioner knows far more —if only he dared to use his knowledge. In fact, he could teach the specialist a great deal, but that is a far cry. First the doctor must learn to listen.

CHAPTER XII

"*When to Stop*"

IN the previous chapter we saw two doctors deciding to "start" and the unexpected developments that followed. The chief difference in the doctor's attitude before deciding to start and "when starting" is that he gives up asking questions and changes over to "listening." This, of course, is no more the whole of psychotherapy in general practice than diagnosis is the whole of therapeutics in clinical medicine. But I wish to stress that "listening" during a "long interview" represents a very large part of psychotherapy and is, moreover, an indispensable requisite, almost in the same way as diagnosis is indispensable for a rational therapy. Before going any further, however, I wish to examine the next problem: "when to stop."

This seems to be rather a far jump, a kind of *non sequitur*. In fact, just the opposite is true. The two problems, "how to start" and "when to stop," are closely linked and largely overlap. The reason is simple. When deciding "to start," the doctor automatically decides not to stop at that particular juncture, and when considering "when to stop" he is naturally influenced by the difficulties and risks of "starting" the next phase of the treatment.

Our first case is an illustration of a special aspect of this problem; one might call it "when to stop starting," or how far to go during the first—or any one—interview, when to stop for that day. An obvious factor is the time the doctor can give to this patient at the particular moment in view of his many other commitments. Many people, and especially beginner psychotherapists who have enjoyed some success, may think that—the doctor's time permitting—the more that can be achieved in one interview the better; in other words, that so long as a patient is producing new material, especially material accompanied by sincere and intense emotion, it is advisable to go on. The emergence of new emotional material is a sign that there is considerable pressure, or even

135

anxiety, in the patient's mind, and a continuation of the interview may lead to a desirable relief. This expectation often proves to be correct, but not always.

As I said, it is above all the beginner who is tempted to go on almost indefinitely with the "long interview." The beginner has enthusiasm, and often time to spare, and if the case seems to be developing well, why break off its organic development because of such an irrelevant, external reason as the clock? Why not follow the *dénouement* to its organic end? An experienced doctor is less likely to be seduced into this way of thinking. He is a professional and not an enthusiast; he has had his fair share of successes and failures, and one more or less does not make such a difference to him. Moreover, he usually has little time to spare.

An even more important factor is rather difficult to describe. Perhaps it might be called a sense of proportion. A "long interview" is a kind of give-and-take affair. The patient gives a great deal to his doctor, his confidence, some jealously guarded secrets, which may sometimes appear insignificant or even puerile to an outsider, but mean a great deal to him. If not enough happens to restore the balance, the patient is bound to feel despoiled, robbed or cheated. Afterwards he may have to devalue or withdraw what he gave to his doctor, or run away from him in indignation, humiliation, or even hatred.

It is exceedingly difficult to state exactly what it is that restores the balance, so that after the "long interview" the patient feels understood, relieved, or even enriched, instead of being despoiled or cheated. The difference is not what is called "correct interpretation," though correct interpretations form a part of it. Neither is it "reassurance," as we saw in the previous chapter. Perhaps the best that I can offer is to say that an experienced doctor has some idea "when to stop," and that the beginner should think twice before going on longer than an hour.

Our Case 18 well illustrates all my points. It happened at an enthusiastic period of our development; a number of the participating doctors had had successes in their psychotherapeutic experiments, and our spirits were high. This rather self-confident and self-assured atmosphere was so infectious that even the level-headed were occasionally carried away. One of them, Dr. P., otherwise a sceptical and critical practitioner, and very much an

advocate of good physical medicine first, an M.D. and M.R.C.P.,
reported one day as follows—

CASE 18

Mrs. J. rang me up for an interview. I did not know her; she said
she had heard of me through a mutual friend, but asked me not to
tell the friend she was coming to see me. A smallish, slightly fat
woman, looking fifty-five; told me she was forty-three. Came from
one of the colonies, has been here three weeks only. For about nine
months she has had severe giddiness. Two days before it started she had
teeth extracted but nothing abnormal had happened. For two years
she has had no periods. (No children, a number of abortions.) Has had
all sorts of medicines from previous doctor. I thought she might have
tinnitus, but she hears very well. She also has pains all over, as if she
had a fever. Was also terribly depressed, and cried a good deal. She
was very effusive. I intended to give her an hour, but it took three
hours. She is going back to the colony soon. She now feels her brain
is loose, and cannot move her head quickly because of it. She has
excellent appetite, excellent sleep. She originally came from Central
Europe, where she lost her husband through Hitler. Later she married
a man who has one child. She loves him very much, but not so much
as her first husband.

On examination I found slight propulsion of eyes, reflexes very
exaggerated, heart and lungs normal, some sensory dullness of hands
and feet, blood pressure 120/80. She said how difficult it was, she never
had orgasm with husband; she was now at an age when she wanted to
enjoy life and could not. She also told me she loved her parents very
much, but had had disturbing thoughts when she was young—she
wished her father dead. That frightened her very much, but it all
calmed down and only came back occasionally. Now she has similar
thoughts about husband. Suddenly she admitted she masturbated when
she was nine for a short time, then at thirty, and when she had teeth
out she started again. I told her giddiness was nothing organic; but if
she would like to see me again she could. She said she would probably
just ring me, and seemed quite happy.

She rang me up about four days ago, said she must see me urgently.
Was very excited when she came. (I mentioned in the first interview
that it was important to know her age, as she might have premature
menopause, and suggested she was fifty-three, which she confirmed.
She said her age was the only lie she had told me.) She said she had a
friend in the colony whom she had found gassing herself and whom
she revived. This friend had told her exactly the story that Mrs. J.
had told me when she came the first time. She said she wanted to get

advice for her friend, and that was the only way to get it. She was terribly nervous, fidgety. I did not know how to handle the situation. She said she was happy now she had told me. I told her she was more ill than I thought at first, and she replied, "You don't believe me." I said that she must think what she had told me before was terribly unpleasant and assured her that it was all in confidence. She started crying, and insisted it was true, it concerned her friend.

Of course I think what she said the first time was true, and the story about her friend untrue. I wonder now why she should have used this odd deception. Though it was very interesting to me, i.e. the result of this quick method. She admitted the physical symptoms were hers, but insisted the story was that of her friend. I said I would leave it to her; if she were in difficulties she could always come back to see me. She said that was very nice of me and went (without paying this time). How do you explain it? Something must have happened to make her so ashamed of what she told me.

Apart from the general conditions mentioned previously, there were a number of individual features in Mrs. J.'s case which inveigled Dr. P. into not stopping. The developing story was most interesting, the distress of the patient apparent, and the emerging material most promising. Almost certainly Dr. P. felt after the three-hour interview that he had done a really good job, and he was made uncertain only by subsequent events. Even after Mrs. J.'s second visit he was unable to see what had gone wrong.

So let us try to be wise after the event. Various "hunches," such as we had when discussing the case, are possible. It may be asked why it was so important to Mrs. J. that her friend should not know about her consulting Dr. P. Perhaps Mrs. J. had to live under pretences, her husband and friends not knowing her past, her real name or her real age; the two stories were really one; perhaps it was she who had attempted suicide or had felt near attempting it, and so on.

Apart from such "hunches," there are a few concrete points that may indicate a possible explanation. In the first place, Mrs. J. was made to admit that she had lied about her age. On the whole, it hardly ever pays to score against the patient in this way. For one thing, these inaccuracies rarely matter, and, for another, if they are demonstrated in the early stages of diagnosis or treatment, they create a strained and unpleasant atmosphere; and if the demonstration fails, the atmosphere is still worse. If the point is important and the treatment develops well, the patient will soon correct the lie, either by admission or by clear enough allusion.

The most important factor in my opinion, however, was Dr. P.'s failure "to stop." True, as he mentioned, Mrs. J. repeatedly begged him to be allowed to go on, asked him whether he could spare the time, etc. Nevertheless, he should have stopped her at a suitable moment and offered her another appointment, if necessary the next day. An inordinately long interview upsets the balance of give and take; the same material distributed over several interviews gives time for the patient to re-establish his equilibrium—if I may say so—by living between any two interviews. Or, in more familiar terms, the drug "doctor" must be administered in the right dosage. Obviously some patients cannot tolerate too concentrated a dose, but the intended therapeutic effect may be attained without serious risks if the drug is administered *in refracta dosi*.

Our next case history shows this problem from an entirely different angle. We shall see how the doctor "started," what he did, and what the results of his therapeutic intervention were. We shall also, incidentally, obtain a glimpse of why the doctor acted as he did when he decided to stop. This will bring us face to face with the problem of "when to stop," and we shall be able to follow the doctor and see how he solved this problem—interestingly there were several occasions to stop—and the ensuing consequences.

Dr. G. introduced his report, "In this case I did a real Smith— and it worked." In the same seminar there was another doctor— let us call him Dr. Smith—who in practically every case that came up for discussion advocated the use of rather forceful methods, and in particular the interpretation of as much of the patient's behaviour as possible. For a long time Dr. G. remained sceptical, and said so in no uncertain terms. Nevertheless, the possibility of doing something useful for his patients appealed to him, and he decided to experiment for himself. So he "did a Smith," as reported in our Case 19 in March 1953.*

CASE 19

The patient, Peter, a boiler coverer, aged 26, was a quiet, thin, pale, neat, inoffensive young fellow. Married three weeks before. Severe

* Part of this case history was published in the *British Medical Journal*, January 16, 1954.

headaches. No relief in tab. codein. Pain "behind eyes;" feels "something wrong with brain." Cannot go to sleep, and wife has to sit with him and hold his hand. Worries about "floods." For the last two months he could not go to the cinema; he gets lost in the film and suddenly "comes to," gets a "crowded-in feeling," feels panicky, screen seems to recede, and he has to rush out of the cinema. He also fears boilers now, and is jumpy when working on them. He has always found it hard to make friends and is content to be by himself.

No sex life before marriage. Satisfactory now for him, but wife has to be manually masturbated to achieve orgasm. "I feel funny telling you that." Feels content sitting in in-laws' house now, in spite of noise of numerous children, but is not so happy about going out. His wife has recently recovered from pulmonary tuberculosis and is at work again. The patient is very "fussy;" does all the housework himself, because he likes to do it, not of necessity. Gets a "kick" out of giving his wife breakfast in bed.

Family history—Mother died when he was three years old, and he and his two elder brothers were sent to an orphanage, where he stayed until fourteen. Father had tabes and was blind. When the patient left the orphanage he became the maid-of-all-work at home. It was he who did the shopping and cooking and cleaning. He led his father about all the time, not his brothers. (This I remember very well, as I used to treat his father, and knew the family set-up well.) His only hobby was motor-cycling, and he always took his father out on the motor-cycle. He thinks his father's blindness was due to war injuries and experiences. He himself often wondered what it was like to be blind, and often did a "silly thing"—drove his motor-cycle blind to see what it felt like. His father's mother was blind (he was told), and she was also the youngest in her family.

He dislikes his elder brother intensely, and the dislike is reciprocated. This brother always acted the big boss: he expected to be waited on, "took everything for granted," and expected the patient to wait on him like a slave. The brother does not drink or smoke and is a highly critical sort of chap. He even supervised the patient's courtship, told him when he should get home at night, and strongly advised him against marriage. The brother's marriage broke up after three weeks and was "annulled" (that was the word he had heard used). The patient was afraid of him, but now they are not on speaking terms and pass each other in the street.

Two weeks ago the patient was admitted to hospital for investigation because of the severity of the headaches. He was discharged after a few days, being told it was his "nerves."

Hospital Notes (seen by me)—"Came to hospital in taxi as he could not walk owing to severity of headaches. Admitted: ? sinusitis: ? migraine. Investigated, and no organic cause found. C.N.S. clear. Discharged. To be seen again next week. ? Psychiatrist."

March 13, 1953—He reported to me immediately after he left hospital, complaining that headaches were still persistent and that he could not get to sleep. "I don't know why I should be like this; after all, it is the first time in my life I have been free from financial worry—for example, paying off the motor-cycle—and my wife is over her T.B. and is working. Thus I can have little luxuries I could not afford before."

Immediate interpretation after taking history (this was what the doctor described as "doing a real Smith"): Assured not organic and nothing to do with father's blindness. "You have always been pushed around since childhood and always in an inferior position. The Cinderella of the family. You had no right to be all right. You always had to carry a burden and had no right to affection (which you really craved). Now you are suddenly free of your tasks (through which you were playing out your inferior position) and you are immediately obsessed with guilt. So you have to atone with a symptom, the obvious one being headache—behind eyes—associating yourself with your father, to whom you were attached (and perhaps unconsciously resented)."

"I thought of that myself."

March 16—Saw the patient again. He said he felt "marvellous." No headaches; knows it is not organic now, and understands symptoms are due to his previous life; sleeps through the night and goes off to sleep immediately; not frightened in a crowd, and is very grateful.

May 7—Patient has been back at work since March, is very happy with his wife, sleeps well, and has no complaints at all.

October 22—Man not seen for several months, only wife, who reported that he was fine. He occasionally gets headaches, which do not amount to anything, and he continues working. He is much easier to live with, and from the point of view of the wife he is a complete cure.

Now this is a really successful case. Peter was suffering from a very severe anxiety neurosis, amounting almost to a generalized phobia, complicated with headaches so severe that he not only had to go to a hospital as an emergency case, but had to be taken there in a taxi, as he was unable to walk. True, the doctor had known Peter and the whole family very well indeed, was familiar with many intimate details of their life, and so it was not difficult for him to establish the right sort of contact and to "start" at the right point in the doctor–patient relationship. This is another example of the importance of "mutual investment." The doctor, being in possession of a wealth of important information—as every well-established practitioner could be—did not feel the need to take a medical history but could "listen." The new pieces of intimate information fitted well into the picture he had formed of Peter, complemented it, and enabled him to "do a Smith." The result was excellent. General anxiety was relieved almost to disappearing, sleeplessness and headaches went, and the patient, who had been seriously ill and unable to work, went back to his job. Seven months after this single session the wife considered Peter as completely cured.

Was this now a good occasion to "stop?" I think that most psychiatrists would have proudly discharged Peter as cured. That was what the general practitioner thought too.

In May 1954, more than a year after the "Smith," the doctor reported again on Peter—

He came in to see me at the beginning of the week; he had been away from work for two days with severe headache. (The first time since the "Smith.") He was all right until he went to the pictures with his wife; they had to queue, and he suddenly got a headache, felt very bad and had to go home. He was much better when he saw me. He had not been to the pictures for a long time, does not like going; gets the same claustrophobic feeling that he used to have when he had to work in boilers. His wife is waiting to go into hospital for examination. She had T.B. and was cured. She had an hysterotomy done, but I cannot remember why. I wrote to the hospital saying she wanted a baby and could not manage it, and was it possible she was sterilized when they did the hysterotomy? They replied that they had no record of sterilization, but were taking her in for investigation.

I spoke to him, told him he did not want to go to the pictures, and the headache was his way of getting out of it. He himself suggested he was worrying over his wife; he said he had been absolutely well until recently. As regards the boiler work, he even goes out alone to other hospitals on jobs, which he has not done before. All he came to me for was the certificate for work—he intended going the next day. He came back the following morning, because he had forgotten the certificate, and the hospital did not allow him to start work without it. He said he was all right now, and he went off; no question of tablets; quite happy.

At first glance things did not seem to be too bad. True, there was a slight relapse; some claustrophobia again, but no need for tablets; two days off work, but that seemed to be all. It was perhaps all explicable by his worrying about not being able to have children because of the possible sterility of his wife. Moreover, the wife was under investigation and the facts would be known soon, so perhaps the best policy for the general practitioner was not to rush into action, but to wait and see.

On the other hand, it could be assumed with equal justification that Peter's visit to the surgery was a kind of mute request for more treatment; we know that it was difficult for him to make straight demands. Perhaps this was a rather better explanation, because it made his lapse of memory intelligible. Not having got what he came for, i.e. more treatment, he forgot his certificate, thus making it necessary to come again, when perhaps his doctor would be more responsive.

After some discussion, the seminar accepted the psychiatrist's opinion that the slip was significant, i.e. that Peter had come back to his doctor because he needed help in his troubles. We next learnt from Dr. G. that the wife's T.B. had been slight, with no cavitation at all, that she was now considered to have been healed, and that the specialist had no objection to her bearing children; further, that it was the wife who was anxious to have a child, while Peter did not seem to be much concerned. They had tried for some time, and as no pregnancy ensued, she had asked the doctor to find out whether the fault was in her. That is why she had been sent for investigation.

The seminar was now able to formulate what might have happened between Peter and his doctor. He had probably come with a dilemma, either of the possible solutions of which were equally unacceptable to him. If he could not give his wife a baby, he was impotent, he had himself to blame; if he gave her a baby, he would have to share everything with it, and so far he had not yet had enough himself; he had not yet recovered from the privations of his own childhood and adolescence; in a way he was still convalescing from the serious psychological deficiency disease of his early years. Peter's behaviour, both at the cinema and in the surgery, might be a symbolic expression of his insoluble problem. He went to the cinema, but turned and hurried home when he got to the door; he went to see the doctor but could not talk, i.e. express his anxieties, and had to go home.

We discussed next whether Dr. G. was right or wrong in his

assessment of the severity and urgency of the present situation. Opinions were somewhat divided. The doctors who liked doing minor psychotherapy and felt confident in their skill pleaded for immediate action; the others, who were less confident, advocated a policy of wait and see. The doctor's skill and confidence is obviously a most important factor in deciding "when to stop." Dr. G. described his attitude, "I do not think I could do the type of treatment Dr. F. does. (Dr. F. was one of the psychotherapeutically inclined.) The best I can do is to keep this sort of case going. If I cannot do that, I do not feel I can take it on at all. I have done enough prying with him. I went fairly deeply, from his point of view, and studied his problems. I do not feel I should go deeper than I did."

This was a weighty argument, but it was not allowed to decide the issue. It was pointed out that, a year before, Dr. G. had given his patient excellent treatment—say a pneumothorax—with very good results. Now the patient came back for a refill; why not give him one? Or, if he thought his skill might not be adequate, why not ask the help of a specialist?

This brought the discussion back to the main problem—on what grounds to assess the urgency of the situation. Should the small symptoms be taken seriously or lightly? Some doctors, the psychotherapeutically-confident ones, argued that the difference between the two attitudes was not so important, e.g. that it would have been sufficient for Dr. G. to say to his patient, "Hm, you forgot your certificate. Though you said you were keen to go back to work, something in you was not so certain." When we went further into this difference, it was realized that the issue was much more serious. What Dr. G. had done had meant reinforcing Peter's defences and repressions and allowing, or even slightly pushing, Peter back to work—nobody could tell for how long, it might be for a couple of years, or perhaps longer. What would happen during this time was anybody's guess. On the other hand, probing into his problem might precipitate a minor—or not so minor—breakdown, necessitating a considerable amount of help, either from the general practitioner or from a specialist.

The discussion ended on an interesting side-issue. One of us described what happened as follows: "Peter came to his doctor with the conscious facts of his problem, and the doctor reacted to them. The question is: should the doctor have reacted to them only, or also to the little voice which was whispering; 'Help, help'?" To this somewhat poetical, but searching question Dr. G. replied that he did not recognize the small voice. This explanation was not accepted; it was pointed out that Dr. G. had not only recognized it, but had responded to it, to the extent of remembering and reporting it to the group. But something in him had prevented him from taking it seriously there and then. Dr. G. was then asked whether he felt resentful when his patient came back, complaining of headaches, demonstrating that the therapy had not been entirely successful. He agreed that he had felt somewhat let down. This was a welcome opportunity to demonstrate the importance of "listening" to such slight emotional reactions in ourselves when dealing with our patients. This does not mean giving way to our emotional reactions, or even expressing them; but it does mean that we must "listen" to them, and then try to evaluate the information as part of the whole situation developing between the patient and us.

Next week Dr. G. reported—

Peter's wife came in to tell me that she went into hospital for the test for sterility, but they found she had a cold. They sent her home, and told her to go back in two months. I thought it was an opportunity to discuss things with her, and what the group suggested was borne out very strongly. The husband did not want it. He said, "Why bother to go?" She strongly wanted it. Now that she has been told to return in two months, he said, "No, let's wait for another year; it may be all right." I told her then that she had only just come out of hospital, that she had plenty of time to think about it, and not to decide anything at the moment. She was inclined not to go.

The reported episode seemed to show that the real problem was the husband's immaturity, which was intelligible enough in view of his appallingly barren childhood and adolescence. The question was how to help him to reach a sufficient degree of maturity before he was faced with the duties of becoming a father. For some time the group considered the idea of using the woman as a medium, analogous to the way in which therapeutic results can be achieved in immature, say enuretic, children by treating their mothers. Dr. G. considered the wife fairly normal and suitable for use as a therapeutic medium, but he did not like the idea of treating a patient who was not really in need of help.

He preferred to treat the husband directly, although he envisaged greater difficulties in doing so.

A fortnight later he reported again—

Everything really developed in the way suggested here. She came in. She did not seem to be keen about talking of him. I think she was rather protecting him. I said, "Would you ask him to come in for a chat," and he didn't turn up. He normally rushes. She herself said she thinks she will leave it now, seems to have gone in with him. I was being on her side a bit when perhaps I shouldn't.

What happened in the end was that the doctor agreed with the conscious wishes of his patient, although the patient warned him by the lapse of memory that not enough was being done about the real problem, the patient's immaturity. This agreement—not forcing Peter to grow up more quickly—was there in any case, so perhaps the complicated discussion in the seminar and the few interviews with husband and wife were much ado about very little. All this had caused the doctor some extra work, but had the game been worth the candle? The doctor replied—

Definitely, from my point of view. From the patient's point of view, nothing has really happened yet. On second thoughts, however, something has happened to the patient in his relation to me, there is no question. It touches him very, very much. Normally, if I said, "Come and see me," he would rush and like it. He always says when he sees me how marvellous it is that he has had no headaches. Now he just has not turned up; in other words, he is afraid, he senses what it is all about, that this great omnipotent figure, his doctor, may tell him something he cannot bear to hear.

Then we heard nothing until February 1955, i.e. eight months after the forgetting of the certificate and nearly two years after the disappearance of the headaches. The doctor reported—

Peter's wife is having a baby, but they are not very happy about it. Since my last report, about eight months ago, she has come occasionally, and finally I tried to talk to her. She said he thought it was best to put the examination off, and they did. I spoke to her in a very superficial sort of way, suggesting his possible fear of the baby; I didn't get very far. About two and a half months ago she came and said she was pregnant. She did not seem all that happy about it, and she has been in to see me more than usual, about physical things like tonsillitis. There is definite anxiety there. On the other hand, Peter has been well. He is quite happy about the baby now. At one time I got on the joking level with him; "You are going to be a daddy now . . ." etc. Nothing in his manner showed that he was not pleased.

We again asked ourselves whether the decision of eight months before, to wait, that is "to stop," had been wise. Had the doctor avoided unnecessary upsets by it, or had he missed an opportunity which might never return? Perhaps the answer will be given in some years' time by the development of the child born to this couple.

The last report is contained in a letter addressed to me in October 1955, two and a half years after the "long interview"—

The baby duly arrived into a not too hostile world in early September, with everybody superficially very happy. During the pregnancy I saw a fair amount of Peter's wife for the usual antenatal things. I used these occasions to bring out some of Peter's fears to her, which she readily understood.

Peter only rarely came in to see me—anxious to let me know that his odd resistance against his wife's examination was nothing serious.

In fact, one episode in which he was away from work for four days (the only time away from work in the past year) could have been the trigger for a longish illness—a head-on collision with a trolleybus (on his motor-bike). He had a large bruise on forehead and complained of headache (I think even you will allow him the comfort of a headache in these circumstances!). Suffice to say he was back at work in four days.

He seemed very happy about the baby, and his doctor was relieved that he could quell his own conscience and not delve deeper.

So, all in all, I feel that this is a really good result, especially when I compare him, originally an acute severe hysteric, with some of the cases who go backwards and forwards to our local psychiatrist for ten-minute talks, who in the long run don't appear to improve even superficially.

Or would you call this "The Case of the Frightened Doctor who rationalizes!"

I think the doctor's pride in his success is justified, and I even think his dig at psychiatrists understandable.

Apart from showing something of the way our discussion seminars work and our research proceeds, Peter's case history well illustrates the great responsibility thrown on the doctor when deciding "when to stop." It also shows that the solution of the question "when to stop" is determined, not only by the exigencies of the patient's actual situation, but also by the doctor's personality. It was clear to the group that some of the doctors would have treated Peter quite differently, but we have to admit that we do not yet know which method would have been the better. As mentioned in the first chapter, we see a number of new problems, but we are far from having all the answers. Research, both more intensive and extensive, is badly needed; and I must stress again, research by properly trained, observant and critical general practitioners.

In our next case we shall be able to study both our problems "how to start" and "when to stop" from a new angle. The doctor "came to the end of his resources" and in the autumn of 1952 asked the Tavistock Clinic for advice. As mentioned, we instituted a kind of emergency service for such occasions on the condition that the doctor was willing to continue the treatment of his patient. As this patient (Case 20, Mrs. N.) was one of the first referred under this scheme, the doctor's initial report is over-conscientiously long and had to be somewhat shortened.—

CASE 20

Headaches for twelve years. They started after she weaned her six-month-old baby, and have troubled her off and on ever since. Rare free intervals of at most two months. They would come on about ten minutes after getting up, would last all day and then pass off in the evening. If she took tablets to ward them off, the headaches would come on later in the day.

She describes the headaches as extremely severe, and as taking all the pleasure out of life. The pain is over the eyes, and she has the feeling of a tight band round her head, which gets very hot. An X-ray of the sinuses showed no trouble. She has bad nights. She gets a queer sensation all over her, as if someone were tickling her from head to foot. And in the evening she gets the jitters and can't keep still. Fidgets and kicks. She has seen three or four doctors. One had her eyes tested, another said it was nerves and gave her phenobarbitone, and another said she was anaemic and gave her iron.

Her father was a chauffeur-gardener, changed his work frequently, so they moved house a good deal. She describes him as a moody man, rather cantankerous, given to prolonged sulks about very little. Her mother was always afraid of saying anything to upset him. Patient got on well with him, better than her mother. She is the second of four sisters. Got on well with them and with her mother too.

Her school life was happy and uneventful. After leaving at sixteen she wanted to study dancing, but her father didn't think it was a good idea, so she went into an office and did shorthand and typing. She didn't resent her wishes being thwarted, though she never cared for office work. She doesn't mind it now, because she only does two days a week.

She married at twenty-one a man ten years older than herself. Had a lot of boy-friends before marriage, but nothing serious. She wanted to marry her husband, not just to get out of the office.

When war broke out she had one child a few months old. In 1940 they were evacuated to a village while her husband stayed in London on essential war work and came down to see her at intervals. He was blown up by a bomb, but not badly hurt. His temperament changed for a time, and he was very difficult to cope with. He was off work for some time, and then was sent back to her for another fortnight's rest. He would not take any interest in anything, even in the baby, which she thought very peculiar. It was at that time the headaches started, she doesn't know more exactly when.

Her marriage has been very happy. She says the first few years were the happiest years of her life, and she always thought it was so good it couldn't last. Never had any other love affairs.

She was very much afraid of being pregnant a second time, and for some months wouldn't let her husband near her. When at last she allowed intercourse, she was much worried about pregnancy. In 1945 she came back to London and went to a birth control clinic, and after that her fears left her. She would not mind another child, except that they are not living in their own house. She had always longed for a house of her own, and never had it. But the woman who shares their house is very nice, and they get on well. It was chiefly because of not having a house of their own that she went out to work after marriage. She wanted to get out of the house. The housing situation does not bother the husband, and she wishes it did more, so he would make some sort of effort to move.

She went away for a fortnight's holiday recently. The headaches were absent for the first week, and then came on after a game of badminton, and she had them every day for the second week.

She is a pleasant, rather good-looking young woman, who gives no impression of great suffering. She is always nicely dressed, and I can't get anything out of her which would explain her headaches. She persists that with minor troubles, such as housing, which is not so bad after all, her life is quite happy and satisfactory. I should be very pleased to spend time on her if I could be told what to do. At present I have come to the end of my resources, which is why I am sending her to the Tavistock Clinic.

Our procedure was that the patient was tested by a psychologist*—either a Rorschach or a Thematic Apperception Test was used—seen by a psychiatrist, and both, without seeing each other's reports, reported their findings to the seminar.

The psychologist reported—

Mrs. N. is a cheerful-looking woman with the lively, expressive face of the hysteric. In her manner she appeared quite "normal." She put up a show of co-operation in the test, though she needed a fair amount of prompting.

This is a very difficult T.A.T. to interpret clinically because there is nothing very pathological in it. Her stories are nearly all conventional and could have been given by any normal person who is in a state of conscious or semi-conscious conflict over an important decision and feels guilt in relation to this problem.

There is a dominant problem expressed throughout the T.A.T., namely, whether she should remain in a certain situation which is causing her dissatisfaction, or whether she should break away and go

---

* It was decided to include in the book some of the reports of psychological tests in order to show the work of the seminar also from this angle. These reports may be somewhat startling to people who are unfamiliar with them. They may think, on the one hand, that it is improbable that a psychologist can obtain so much and so intimate information about a patient's illness, consequently, the whole might strike them as being mainly unfounded guesswork. Others might feel that if this kind of penetration can be achieved by a simple psychological test, why bother about psychiatric interviews?

We have met both these reactions in our seminars. Under the impact of further experience, however, these exaggerated initial opinions calmed down and people gradually recognized that, though these projective psychological tests are very valuable helps (as X-rays are, for example) and occasionally one can even confidently base a diagnosis on them, as a rule the psychiatric interview, in spite of its many shortcomings and limitations, is still our mainstay, at any rate for the time being.

I do not wish to discuss here the principles and techniques of the two projective tests that were used in our work, and have to refer readers to the literature. Suffice it to mention that the two tests we used were:—

(a) The well-known Rorschach Test in its original form, though the patient's responses were interpreted according to more recent views and techniques.

(b) A Thematic Apperception Test. The form used was that devised by Mr. Phillipson, Senior Psychologist, Tavistock Clinic, who calls it Object Relations Test. It consists, in addition to a blank card, of three series of four pictures, each portraying, in rather vague shading, one person, two person, three person and group situations. Patients are shown these pictures and asked to bring them to life in their imagination and compose a brief story describing how the social situation came about, what is happening and how it turns out in the end. The test is designed to show how the patient sees different social situations and what rôle he tends to take within them. The test material and the technique of administration and interpretation have been recently published in book form.

to something unknown but more exciting. A theme of this type appears in eight of the thirteen stories. . . .

It is difficult to know at what level to interpret this. One can say that the character structure is hysterical, that in her behaviour in the interview she was denying that the anxieties expressed in the test were real, that she is showing a severe degree of guilt and self-punishment, that men are seen as overpowering sexual figures towards whom she fears to submit; but, beyond those very general features, there is no internal consistency in the themes that would point to an underlying character disorder.

My feeling by the end of the test was that she was expressing a conflict which was very near the surface and was probably operating in her real-life circumstances. I felt that she had probably become involved in a conflict of loyalties between her husband and some other man, and that her headaches were a direct expression of her self-punishment in this situation. One story is of the woman who is seen by her daughter making love to a man who is not her husband. She ends up, in the naïve way of the hysteric, with, "I know my daughter would resent anything like that." This gains in significance when at the end of the test she said that her daughter can always tell when she has got one of her headaches.

I may have completely misjudged this case, but, if a person with an hysterical though reasonably healthy personality had become involved in a conflict such as is described above, this is the sort of T.A.T. record I would expect. I was left very much with the impression that she was at least partly conscious of the problem, but was unwilling to admit this to me.

Lastly the psychiatrist's report, also somewhat verbose, like that of the practitioner's, due to the same kind of over-conscientiousness—

There is very little to add to Dr. C.'s case history, except to repeat that Mrs. N. has had her headaches for about twelve years. They are quite irregular. Drugs do not help much, and all sorts of physical examinations produce negative results. Occasionally she is free from the headaches, but that is rather rare.

Any excitement tends to bring them on, and it makes no difference whether it is pleasant or unpleasant. The same is true about somewhat energetic physical exercise, like badminton or square-dancing. Walking, on the other hand, tends to ease the headaches. When she has them she must look different, as her daughter, aged thirteen, knows without asking whether mother has a headache or not. Mrs. N. herself feels depressed and irritable at such times; she flops and cannot stand any noise.

She is rather a precious woman, almost amounting to mannerism, with a kind of childish face, appealing manners, making a very "proper" impression. According to her, everything is perfectly all right in her life, except that she has not got her own house and she has to live with other people. In fact she has a self-contained top flat where nobody interferes with her. All this might be a reminder of her childhood experiences, where for the first ten years or so the family accompanied the father, who was a chauffeur-gardener living in servants' quarters "amongst other people, not in their own house."

A further clue might be that father and mother, both over seventy, live now in their own house on their old age pension and on the capital that father saved up. They are all right, but father is usually worried about his uncertain financial situation. In fact, according to Mrs. N., they are quite comfortably off.

I used this as a lever to get behind the absolutely smooth surface that she presents to the interviewer. I interpreted tentatively that perhaps she too may be worrying about not quite important things. She responded to it by telling me that she is kind of slave-driver to herself. She has to finish things, "the jobs are always ahead of me," she has to "race around" to cope with her duties. Although her part-time job is quite easy and pleasant, she always has a bad night on Wednesdays, because she goes to work on Thursdays and Fridays.

It was rather difficult to get this much out of her, as all the time she tried to muddle me up, and, so to speak, put me off the scent by quoting things against any possible connection between her character and the headaches. After I pointed out to her that it is highly important to her to convince everybody, including herself, that everything is all right, she began to talk about her "jitters." When she can be still and at peace, she either relaxes and dozes off, no matter where she is—in the cinema or in the theatre—or just the contrary, she gets a spasm of restlessness, and must either get out to take a long walk or calm herself down with aspirins. These spasms occur, not only in theatres or cinemas, but also more frequently during the night at home, when she has to get out of bed and walk about, make tea, or take some drug.

At long last she was able to tell me something about her sexual life, which, however, I think was rather a rosy picture. According to her everything is all right, everything is highly satisfactory to both of them, but it happens only roughly once a fortnight, the main reason being that she is usually tired and is asleep when her husband comes to bed. Lastly, when she knew that she would have to leave in a couple of minutes, she mentioned that in the country, when she was evacuated, she "knew" a few men who were very good friends to her. I do not think there were any sexual affairs, but I suspect rather intense love play, not amounting to intercourse.

Diagnosis: On the surface there is a very well integrated over-compensation, everything is perfectly all right. This very likely can be maintained only by a strong inside pressure and, in my opinion, the headaches are a kind of manometer to show the actual pressure. Another means to keep the balance is her being a slave-driver, occupied all the time, in order to get a house of her own with no dangerous people in it. When not occupied, especially under stimulating conditions, such as theatre, cinema, dancing, bed, she either gets bad headaches, or falls asleep, or has the jitters, which means she has to run away. I can only guess that the danger is sexual excitement, but have no material to prove it.

To sum up, I consider her case as a mixture of obsessional over-compensation and hysterical conversion.

It is very difficult to decide what to recommend as therapeutic procedure to the doctor. There are several possibilities—

(1) To let her go on in her strenuously balanced state, admitting that one cannot help her and taking the blame for it while trying to keep up her spirits with sympathy.

(2) The doctor could try to ease somewhat her slave-driving, keeping the whole therapy on a fairly rational level, a kind of sympathetic re-education to a better way of life.

(3) If my last assumption is correct, one could try to bring out her repressed sexual fantasies and work out with her some way how to satisfy them better than with hysterical conversion.

An added reason why I quote all three reports here is that they give some idea of the help a psychiatric clinic can give the general practitioner. As just mentioned, all three reports are somewhat verbose; now, after more than three years of experimentation, all three of us can do better. Better reports, however, would inevitably have meant later cases with a shorter follow-up period. Dr. C. ended his report, "I have come to the end of my resources." The clinic reports explained to him why this happened. Mrs. N. had a fairly strong, fairly well integrated ego which developed an efficient system of defences, consisting of a mixture of obsessional and hysterical mechanisms which presented an almost impenetrable front. They also showed, however, the most likely successful point of attack—Mrs. N.'s intense sexual fantasies possibly based on some sort of guilt-laden experiences. The

history of the treatment will show how far this diagnostic prediction proved to be correct.

The reports came up for discussion in November 1952, and
Dr. C. decided to accept the most ambitious of the recommendations put to him and try to bring out the patient's heterosexual
desires and fantasies. But, as there was a possibility that the
syndrome might be caused merely by premenstrual tension, he
decided first to give a fair trial to progesterone—a proposition
accepted but not approved by the psychiatrist. As this brought no
results, it was given up in January, 1953.

Dr. C. then saw the patient regularly twice a week for about
three months, all told about twenty times. He several times
reported to the group about the progress of the treatment. Here
I shall quote only his retrospective report of these events, dated
November 7, 1955—

Bad-tempered and quarrelsome with elder sister up to her marriage.
Suppresses her anger now, e.g. at man in office who makes passes at
her—and at the other girls.

Many aggression and frustration dreams, such as being chased with
knives and guns, or by wild animals; trying to find things or to go
somewhere and being stopped. Dissatisfied with her position as clerk,
and with unambitious husband. Sorry he was not accepted for army—
he might have got high rank. He can't be spurred on—but she says
nothing.

Since adolescence reserved with boys and parents—and now with
husband and daughter of twelve. Easier with very young children.

When evacuated she was the youngest woman in village. Inhabitants
talked about her. Was excited and repelled by other women's love
affairs. Had a sexual affair with a Pole (officer!) at the end of this time.
Really in love with him. "I lost control for the first time in my life."
"Seethed with rage inwardly" at husband's neglect when he came on
leave.

Remembered that the headaches started after an old sweetheart
wrote her four or five passionate letters. Wanted her to elope with him
but she didn't care for him much. But the letters upset her greatly.
Made her blush, even if she was alone. She told him to stop it.

In April 1953, the question arose between Dr. C. and his
patient whether they had reached a good point to "stop." On the
one hand the headaches had disappeared, on the other Mrs. N.
apparently lost interest in the treatment. Although somewhat
repetitive, I shall quote the doctor's report to the seminar—

This was the woman who always suffered from headaches if she failed in anything. She was very frustrated about her husband, who was not a bit ambitious but was very content to jog along as he was. She must always have possessions as good as or better than those of her friends, and she wanted to advance in the world and be better off financially at the end of each year. I had suggested to her that she should satisfy her own ambitions by working on her own, e.g. setting up in a bookshop and working for herself, instead of working part-time for someone else, as she did now. She thought it was quite a good idea and said she would think it over, but since then she has not been to see me regularly.

We find here the same problem as with Peter, though in a different form. The presenting symptoms, the headaches, disappeared in both cases and life became easier and happier for both. In both cases there remained unsolved a number of neurotic symptoms and problems, though in the doctor's judgment none of them was very serious. The difference was that in Peter's case the doctor—after a long and intimate acquaintance—did all the therapeutic work in one concentrated interview and then stopped, while in Mrs. N.'s case the therapy was prolonged and the patient's co-operation eventually flagged. Should the general practitioner agree to "stop" or press his patient to continue? After some discussion, Dr. C. decided to accept his patient's "offer" to stop. An additional reason for his acquiescence was the apprehension expressed by several members of the group that by probing further he might endanger Mrs. N.'s somewhat precariously balanced marriage.

The next report is dated December 1953, i.e. about eight months after the end of the treatment. Mrs. N. had not been seen for seven months, but about a month previously she had come back—

Her headaches are now a thing of the past. She still has some other troubles, restlessness, cannot sit still anywhere, must get up in the night to make tea, etc. She either falls asleep in the cinema or wants to run out. She still has dexedrine. Still very ambitious.

When questioned what, in his opinion, the next step ought to be, Dr. C. replied, "She is not seriously ill, is managing all right, no headaches. She has certain disabilities, such as restlessness, but not sufficient to justify seeing her for a couple of hours a week."

In June, 1954, Mrs. N. was mentioned again—

We discussed last time whether we should go any further or not. I have not seen her for some months. Her headaches and other symptoms were better, and she is trying to better herself in life, get more money to buy another car, etc. Everything was going on as usual. She has never been to me for tablets.

The last report, dated October 1955, contained no further news—

Mrs. N. has not reported again. Ceased to work in my neighbourhood in July 1954, but lives not far away, and could easily get in touch with me if she wanted to. Met her in the street in June 1954. She was her usual bland, smiling self, and said she was much better.

In Mrs. N.'s case we witnessed a favourable turn of events. The doctor, though blocked at first by the patient's efficient defences, was able to make use of the help given by the clinic, did an honest piece of work and achieved some success. This did not amount to a complete cure, but the patient's life was made incomparably easier. Parallel with this, the patient's co-operation became unreliable. A number of symptoms remained unresolved, even untouched, but the doctor thought it would cost him and his patient too much work and effort to try to change them too. In addition, there was the danger of the marriage breaking down. So, in agreement with his patient, he decided to stop—perhaps correctly. Unfortunately, the patient has not seen her doctor since June 1954, and so we do not know whether the reason why she did not come again was that she felt better, or that she felt dissatisfied, either with Dr. C. and had transferred to another doctor, or with medicine in general and preferred to be left alone. But perhaps I am too cautious, and the most likely explanation is that the patient has been fairly well.

CHAPTER XIII

The Special Psychological Atmosphere of General Practice

IN the two previous chapters we discussed at some length two aspects of psychotherapy in general practice, "how to start" and "when to stop." We did so at length because these two problems play an incomparably greater rôle in general practice than in psychiatry or, in fact, in any of the other branches of medicine.

When the patient arrives at a psychiatric outpatients' department or in a Harley Street consulting-room, he has gone far beyond starting. The decision to start was taken either by himself or by his general practitioner; the psychiatrist has had no share in it. What he does is to try to follow the patient on the way, and if possible to catch up with him. This catching up with the patient is called the technique of the psychiatric interview, which will not be dealt with in this book. What I wish to emphasize here is that the technique of the psychiatric interview and that to be adopted by the general practitioner when he decides to "start" in many respects differ widely. Admittedly a number of features are common to both, but to say that the general practitioner must come to us psychiatrists to learn "how to start" would be entirely unjustified. Apart from the fact that our technique for the routine psychiatric interview is far from being as securely founded, as well tested out, and as standardized as that for the routine clinical examination, we psychiatrists have very little experience indeed with patients in the "unorganized" phase of their illnesses. It is in this phase that the decision "to start" has the greatest importance. The way the start is made may have a crucial influence on the "organization" of the patient's illness.

The situation is somewhat better for us psychiatrists with regard to the second problem, "when to stop." This arises in every psychotherapeutic case, and has to be decided upon in time by the therapist. The similarity, however, does not go much further. This is because, for the patient of a general practitioner, stopping has a meaning entirely different from that which it has for the patient of a psychiatrist. The latter has only one kind of relationship with his patient. True, it is a rich and highly involved relationship, but it is of one kind. If it is discontinued, no matter whether by the patient or by the therapist, what can be described, in spite of all its complications, as the single thread between them is broken. There is a finality about it that is lacking in the case of the patient of a general practitioner. The relationship between the latter and his patient has numerous threads, and the truer the general practitioner is to his vocation, the stronger and the more numerous they are. So the practitioner can take considered risks with his patients, risks which cannot be taken by a psychiatrist. Even if the openly psychotherapeutic relationship is broken off, the patient may, and indeed does, come back to his doctor with a cold, or indigestion, or a whitlow, or a bruised finger, or to have his child inoculated, and so on *ad infinitum*.

Whereas the psychiatrist hardly ever comes up against the problem of "how to start," and the problem of "when to stop" is for him a major decision having serious and even final consequences, for the general practitioner both problems are, so to speak, part and parcel of his routine work. They may crop up at any time in his practice, and he has to make decisions on the spur of the moment. True, he usually does not examine the consequences of his decisions very critically; as often as not expediency is his only, or his most important, criterion. His feeling of guilt, arising from awareness that perhaps he may not be doing the right thing, is one reason why he so meekly accepts the psychiatrist's claim to know most of the answers to psychotherapy in general practice. The other reason is the perpetuation of the teacher–pupil relationship, which we discussed in Chapter IX. The follow-up reports of our research seminars enabled us to study closely the special relationship between the general practitioner and his patients and its effect on our two interlinked problems. Let us see what we can learn from them.

A good start will perhaps be the case of Peter (Case 19). At one stage of the treatment, when Peter did not respond to Dr. G.'s invitation and did not appear at the surgery, the treatment was continued without ado through Peter's wife, using her antenatal examinations for that purpose. The results were quite acceptable, and in spite of Peter's initial resistance to having a child, "the baby arrived into a not too hostile world," as Dr. G. put it. It is fair to say that no psychiatrist would think of continuing the treatment of a patient who refused to attend by using his wife's antenatal visits for that purpose. Even discussion of a broken-off treatment with a wife (or husband) is on the whole contra-indicated in psychiatric practice—except perhaps in the case of a severely psychotic patient. What is inadvisable, impossible, or unthinkable for a psychiatrist can be perfectly plain sailing for a general practitioner. Many doctors may even be surprised at my making heavy weather of such a self-evident proposition. What could be more natural than that a woman having a baby should consult the family doctor, and that the two should talk about the husband, in whom both are sincerely interested and who is a problem at the moment? It is just as natural that the husband should know and accept this—and almost certainly will benefit by it in the long run, if the doctor is skilful enough.

Psychiatrists have some ideas about what is likely to happen in these circumstances. They may even have quite good ideas, but their *first-hand knowledge* about what can and should be done in these cases is somewhat meagre, and it certainly *does not entitle them to play the rôle of omniscient mentors*. Here again we are confronted with the need of proper research, conducted jointly by general practitioners and psychiatrists on an equal partnership basis.

As our next illustration, may I revert to the case of Miss M., Case 10 in Chapter VI. We saw "how the doctor started" by rather impetuously breaking down the patient's defences and obtaining confirmatory evidence for his diagnosis that Miss M.'s real problem was her unhappy love affair, and the worries and fears caused by it. Perhaps the patient's defences were too strong, or perhaps the doctor's technique was too inconsiderate; the fact remains that Miss M. consistently refused Dr. R.'s psychothera-peutic overtures. The last report we had was in February 1954, when she was still having the affair with the Armenian, which, according to Dr. R.'s diagnosis, was the chief cause of her many minor respiratory ailments.

Now let us continue the story. Dr. R. reported at the end of December 1954—

I last reported on this patient in February 1954. She returned on November 11th, 1954, complaining of "bouts of nausea and retching," associated with vague abdominal pain. This had been present for just over a year, but had been much worse for the last two or three months, particularly just before a period was due. The menses were rather irregular, and preceded by pains for a week. Physical examination of tongue, pulse, abdomen, etc., was negative. (Vaginal examination was not done.) While I was examining her abdomen, I asked her what she associated nausea with, and she replied that when younger she had always felt sick when excited; this made her pause, as though she had just thought of something, and she then said that this nausea and retching had started just after she had begun to have sexual intercourse with her boy-friend (the Armenian). She then told me, with some difficulty, that he had gone home, and she had come to realize that he did not really love her, but only "used her for what he could get." She felt very bitter and upset about this, and I was duly sympathetic, but said that this was what we had discussed when I saw her in February. After a long interview, she said that things seemed clearer to her. We discussed what happened now when she felt sexually roused (she did not know the word "masturbation," and after a simple explanation she said no, she didn't do that. She hadn't been out with boys, and didn't get roused. She said that she had no more worries now, except her "spots" (acne). I suggested that that might help to keep the boys away if that was what she wanted in order to prevent further upsetting love affairs. She smiled, almost as though she knew what I meant, and said that perhaps later she would be less frightened of "men," and would go out again with them. I prescribed Belladenal tablets and asked her to come and see me in two weeks' time.

On November 29th, 1954, she reported that she felt much better. After two days on the tablets, all symptoms stopped, and in addition to that, when she next had a period it was on the right day, and there was no pain before or during it. I offered her another appointment, but she said she would come and see me if there was need in the future.

A fortnight later I was called to see a young man, a newcomer to London, at the same address as Miss M. (it being a boarding-house). He had an acute virus infection (type of 'flu), and at the time of my second visit he referred to "my girl-friend who phoned to ask you to come and see me" . . . his "girl-friend" is Miss M.!

A few days later I saw Miss M. again—with classical 'flu—and when she came to see me for her final certificate she brought her boy-friend with her to introduce him to me. They are now engaged to be married!

Had Miss M. been treated by a psychiatrist whose approach had been the same or similar to that of Dr. R., any of the many breaks would almost certainly have been final. Having Dr. R. as her general practitioner, she was able to return to him again and again in spite of her overt refusal of the psychotherapeutic help offered. It may be suggested, perhaps correctly, that a skilled psychiatrist would have used less forceful methods, and would thus have avoided hurting her feelings and arousing strong indignation, resentment and resistance in her. Be this as it may, we must admit that the tempo of the treatment would very probably have been slower, necessitating many more man-hours to achieve the same result. That is what I mean by saying that *the general practitioner may take considered risks*, as his patient has other sorts of relationship with him apart from the psychotherapeutic relationship. I may mention incidentally that part of the psychotherapeutic work was done while Dr. R. was palpating the patient's abdomen. This is a perfectly normal situation for a general practitioner, but I rather doubt how many psychiatrists would be able to use it in a similar way. I may add also that many general practitioners—as disclosed in our discussions—carefully separate their psychological from their physical work; only the physical examination is done while the patient is undressed, the psychological examination is postponed until the patient is fully dressed again. We shall revert in a later chapter to this difference in technique.

Another interesting aspect of this case is Dr. R.'s firm stand. Once he got his bearings, he "started" at once whenever the patient appeared, no matter what the presenting symptom happened to be. This firm stand remained unshaken in spite of the patient's consistent refusals. Undoubtedly Dr. R.'s confidence in his diagnosis helped Miss M. to endure fairly well her abandonment by the Armenian, followed by several months of loneliness, and to admit eventually that her doctor had been right after all. One may even suggest that the fact that Dr. R. saw through her defences, and, so to speak, was on the side of her healthy self, helped her considerably to overcome her difficulties.

The epilogue contained in a follow-up report dated November 1955 seems to confirm this view. To the end Miss M. remained absolutely true to herself. She gave her doctor the satisfaction of fitting her with a cap—in view of her history a very important propitiation—but did not let him know about her marriage. She disappeared again, but has not yet registered with another doctor. It is difficult to say how much of this very marked ambivalence is due to her character and individuality, and how much of it is a response to Dr. R.'s technique. But, whatever the answer may be, it is certain that without Dr. R.'s help things would have been much more difficult for her.

Our next case (Case 21) again demonstrates how much greater the scale of a general practitioner's "responses" to his patient's "offers" can be. This enables him in many cases to weather situations which would be entirely beyond the technical possibilities of a psychiatrist.

Dr. M., after trying his mettle for some months and encountering serious difficulties, in September 1952 referred his patient, Mrs. Q. to our emergency service, as follows—

CASE 21

Mrs. Q., age 23, married, has attacks of trembling. She often has pain in her right lower abdomen, thinks then that she might have appendicitis, thinks compulsorily of the impending operation (though intellectually she is aware that she is not likely to have appendicitis) and has then an attack of trembling.

Characterologically, the girl is a hysteric, but I found it very difficult to pierce her defences anywhere. She acknowledges interpretations as correct, but is quite unmoved by them.

She is very strongly attached to her mother, and has not been able to give up an infantile rôle towards her (mother runs the home, Mrs. Q. only has five shillings pocket-money, she had to come back from furnished rooms to her mother's overcrowded house, etc.). With this reluctance to give up mother as sole love-object she has also retained a penis-wish, and is quite unable to be a woman. She is frigid, is afraid of having babies, even dreads dancing.

She used to be a bed-wetter, nail-biter, masturbated manually, and remembers vividly "doctor-games" with her siblings. (When she told me that, it was the only time she showed any emotion.)

She has a vivid fantasy life, but is unable to tell about the contents of her day-dreams.

She hates her father, by whom she feels rejected. She sees her father very much as her rival for mother's love.

Listening to her, one has the impression that, not only has she got stuck emotionally in the early phase of the oedipal period, but that sometimes she regresses to anal levels (over-cleanliness, concern about money, sadistic behaviour towards her husband).

She has an illicit love-affair with a former boy-friend of hers, and is quite unconcerned about possible consequences. She is generally so concerned with her deep anxieties that reality difficulties leave her quite undisturbed. Today is all that matters, and tomorrow can look after itself. She told me once how she is in the habit of buying her whole monthly sweet ration* and eating it in one go. I explained that on above lines to her, and, though she quite agreed, I felt that this, as many other interpretations, did not go through her armour at all.

I have been seeing her since February of this year, and she has had approximately seven sessions. She appeared to improve so far as her hysterical symptoms went, but her character defences were not touched. She then stopped coming, but she came back to me a few days ago and told me that the trembling attacks had come back worse than ever; I feel that I am not getting very far with her.

Do you think she might benefit more in an expertly guided group? I think she might, if she were prepared to face the rough-and-tumble of a group world. I should be grateful for your opinion.

This report, too, belongs to the early days of our project, and I am certain that Dr. M. would write a different report today. On the other hand, it well illustrates the atmosphere in which Mrs. Q.'s treatment was carried out. Dr. M., though a true general practitioner, was obviously well versed in psycho-analytic literature and was using its terminology with ease and, let us say, gusto. Almost certainly he used his knowledge of psycho-analytic concepts with the same gusto towards his patient, in the form of firing interpretations at her.

The case came up for discussion early in October. The psychologist did a Thematic Apperception Test†, and I shall quote his written report. (This is couched in technical terms, and in fairness I have to add that he presented his findings to the seminar in a less technical language and illustrated them with the patient's actual responses.)

Initial contact negative: really unco-operative, though a show of co-operation is built up when she feels she is getting attention.

---

* Chocolates and sweets were rationed in England at the time of the report.
† See footnote in Chapter XII, p. 150.

Aggressive, negative feelings displaced on to the pictures: "not proper pictures," "a mess," "not distinct." She blames these inadequacies for her poor performance, just as she unconsciously blames the psychologist for not giving her what she wants quickly and without condition.

She shows in behaviour and comment her continual need for support, and puts up a consistent picture of helplessness. Interpretation of her behaviour produces little or no dynamic effect, only a show of acceptance which is belied by immediate self-centred comment or behaviour. Her final comment was to express uncertainty whether she wanted help anyway.

Her responses to the pictures are brief, bitty, descriptive. There is no real story, no interaction of personalities, and no work-through of any problem. There are many illogical interpretations and sequences, and several extremely unusual concrete perceptions.

It is extremely difficult to piece together any coherent personality picture—perhaps because there isn't one. She views the world very much in terms of her infantile needs, and responds with poor control and considerable projection when these needs are not gratified.

Near the surface is a generally obsessional relation with people and with the world; she views the world fairly crudely in terms of the incongruities and contradictions inside herself. Heterosexual relationships figure little in the stories; she needs attention from men, is afraid that her sexual life may be seen and disapproved, and in general shows great indecision and ambivalence in her relations with men.

The deeper picture suggests efforts to defend against quite severe depression resulting from infantile aggression in face of frustration of oral needs. A dominant theme is loss of support and affection, rejection by parents, lack of comfort and amenities. Direct oral demands intrude, often rather illogically. Her concern with tidiness and cleanliness is at once an expression of anger and contempt for parents who do not provide and gratify her wishes, and an attempt at control. Obsessional effort is, with her, a rather weak defence. Basically she is angry with the breast for frustrating her, and there is a good deal of paranoid projection. This paranoid projection is carried over into her sexual fantasies, which she fears might be pried into and discovered. This suggests that the fantasy relations which determine her heterosexual life are mainly of an infantile oral character.

In situations which present a direct emotional challenge from other people, control is poor. On the surface there will be a show of compassion and concern (probably with religious fervour), underneath childlike rejection temper tantrums, crude tearing aggression (basically against women?), fantasies of power and control by the side of some (futile?) depression. She is not able to keep separate the internal and external world, viewing external reality very much in terms of her fantasies. Her capacity for change is very little: there is so much aggression underneath, so few effective defences, and so little capacity for real affection.

The psychiatrist reported as follows—

The case itself is quite simple. She is an immature, narcissistic, hysterical woman, very much tied ambivalently to her mother, and still more ambivalently to her father. Her attitude is, "I am a baby, everybody must look after me, and in return I shall be nice and kind and accommodating to everybody." As far as I could make out, her abdominal pains are not very perturbing and, though she would accept some easy treatment for them, for the time being she is not willing to envisage anything at all that might put a strain on her.

The circumstances of her life are rather awful, but highly characteristic. She and her husband live in one room in her mother's house, the room is cluttered up with furniture that they bought in the hope of getting a house. The husband pays so much a week to Mrs. Q.'s mother, and the mother looks after them, prepares the dinner and does the washing. Mrs. Q. does not even clean her own room properly, as it is so difficult to move all the stored furniture. The only thing she does is some odd dress repairs, and occasionally she helps mother with the ironing. She has no money, and is quite content to get some pocket money from mother out of the money paid by her own husband.

Her husband wants children, but she is terribly afraid of the pain, and cannot even envisage having any. Her husband is a baker and must go to sleep very early, and so their sexual life is much less intense than she would like it to be. Again she puts up with it and cannot even think that she might, for instance, seduce her husband and make love to him.

All this is obviously well known to Dr. M. too. The question is what to do with this patient, and I deliberately concentrated the whole interview on that point.

With the charming *belle indifférence des hysteriques*, Mrs. Q. agreed to all my findings. What I tried to show her is that she is just drifting, and, as she is afraid where she might drift, she closes her eyes and if possible goes to sleep. Somehow she knows that in ten or fifteen years' time she will be terribly sorry for all that, but this knowledge perturbs her very little now.

The problem is: what should and what can a general practitioner do under these circumstances? He can decide, instead of the patient, that this kind of life is no good, that the patient *must* take full responsibility for herself and her family and *must* take her fair share in life. This will obviously arouse the resistance of the patient, and the result will be a bitter fight between her and her doctor.

The other possibility is to allow the patient to continue her life as it is now, but this puts a very heavy burden of guilt on the doctor, who, so to speak, tolerates with open eyes that a young and otherwise healthy woman of good possibilities throws away her life for very little immediate gain.

The real cause of the whole problem is the patient's fear of pain, which she must avoid at all costs. Pressing treatment upon her means exposing her to the traumatic situation and very likely she would respond to it by running away, so my recommendation is to put this problem frankly, firmly and *repeatedly* to the patient, always showing that nothing can be done unless she asks for it. That is what I have done, but I am quite certain that the impact of this will wear off very soon, and that the doctor will have to start almost from scratch.

The two reports were not in agreement. The psychiatrist was in no doubt about the severity of the problems, but did not regard the case as entirely hopeless. He did not contemplate taking the patient over, but encouraged the general practitioner to carry on patiently, taking one small step at a time and being prepared for long, empty intervals. In fact, this prognosis made her case more suitable for treatment by a general practitioner than by a psychiatrist hampered by a rigid time-table. The psychologist's report was very serious indeed. He found no coherent personality, hardly any existing controls over her primitive demands, very poor contact with reality, very little capacity for change, and so on. We were rather puzzled by the discrepancy, as reports from these two sources usually agreed well, confirming and complementing each other. After some discussion, it was decided to ask a second psychologist to do a Rorschach test with Mrs. Q. It was hoped that some of the discrepancy might be cleared up by a different test.

The second test was reported to the seminar a fortnight later. As the report is rather long, and as it agrees in all main points with the result of the previous test, I shall quote only the diagnostic summary.

The defences shown in this record are clearly not adequate for the maintenance of mental health, but they are sufficiently stable to keep her going in her present immature hysterical condition so long as she is not forced into a situation where the defences will be threatened.

She is managing to control her anxieties by living in a fantasy world where all the ogres can be passed off as teddy-bears, and thus is able to ward off her latent psychotic depressive problems. There are very few other strengths and very little apparent capacity for insight. It is characteristic of her that the more pressure is brought to bear in the Rorschach, the more psychotic-like her responses get. After seeing her, I was left with the strong feeling that to penetrate her defences would be dangerous, and that she is far better left as she is.

Thus the discrepancy remained unsolved, and we were uncertain whether it would be wise for the doctor to embark on a rather doubtful therapeutic venture. A week later Dr. M. reported that Mrs. Q.'s maternal grandmother had died in the meanwhile. This meant that the grandfather, who was crippled, had had to move to his daughter's (Mrs. Q.'s mother's) house. Thus the patient and her husband were crowded out and had to look for accommodation. For the time being, as was to be expected, Mrs. Q. had refused any approach by Dr. M. to come to grips with her problems. It was decided to leave things as they were but—in spite of the two test reports—not to give up hope that the independent life forced on the patient by external events would bring home to her the need for proper psychological help.

Our expectations proved to be correct, and Mrs. Q. asked for treatment early in 1953. We learnt from Dr. M.'s periodical reports that Mrs. Q. went every day to her mother's house to rest there for several hours, that she told her mother literally everything that happened to her, including the topics brought up during the treatment, that she could never give anything to any man, whether husband, boy-friend or doctor. The first breach in this almost impenetrable defence system was made when Dr. M. succeeded in bringing it home to Mrs. Q. that she indulged in daydreams and fantasies while she was resting in her mother's house. The patient admitted that she did not tell her mother about the contents of her daydreams. It soon became clear that the contents of her fantasies were crude and aggressive sexual experiences. In a short time she spoke freely about these daydreams, about Dr. M. as her love-partner, and especially about her urge to take men away from their women (her husband was married before, and both her boy-friend and Dr. M. are married). These violent transference reactions were duly interpreted.

In October 1953, she thought that she might be pregnant; Dr. M., who normally does a good deal of antenatal care and midwifery, did not carry out a P.V. as he thought it too early. Mrs. Q. in her resentment went to another doctor in the neighbourhood, who in one important respect closely resembled Dr. M. She came back shamefacedly; the opportunity was used to bring out the similarity between her oscillation between her husband and the boy-friend and her running away from Dr. M. to the other doctor.

Although the pregnancy was a false alarm and the periods returned, to Mrs. Q.'s great disappointment, she continued with the treatment. Soon, however, she started to come late for the interviews, and her interest began to flag. Regular attendance was discontinued at the end of 1953, and Dr. M. saw Mrs. Q. only irregularly as an ordinary patient.

I shall now quote two letters by Dr. M. about Mrs. Q. in August and November 1955.

By Christmas 1953 she had considerably matured, went out to do a job, made her flat into a nice little home, and early in 1954 became pregnant.

She had no sickness during her pregnancy, particularly no vomiting, attended me for ante-natal care, insisted on having the baby at home (in her maternal home), and was very insistent on my delivering the baby. Her blood-pressure rose a little during the final stages of the pregnancy.

The delivery, which I attended, was one of the easiest I have seen for years. She was very co-operative, wanted to see the baby at once, and had done all the caring and planning in a mature way.

She had regarded her husband prior to her treatment with much disdain. A few minutes after the birth of the baby, when the midwife wanted to show the baby to the family, she said, "Let my husband hold the baby first, please."

The main feature in the counselling sessions was the discussion and interpretation of her transference, where she did a lot of testing out. Once she even ran to another doctor, and came back, guilt-laden; she even now makes me into the father of her baby ("the baby has hair like you, Dr. M."). This has been brought so much into consciousness and accepted by her that she can cope with it by just being a faithful patient.

What strikes me so in this and similarly treated cases is that, after the completion of one's psychotherapeutic work, the patient is *not* independent, but that some new, and perhaps more mature, form of dependence arises which is satisfactory to both patient and doctor. Mrs. Q. apparently is no longer in love with me, but I have become, much more than I was ever before, the doctor of the whole of the family, and I am called a "friend of the family." Instead of there being a separation, a cut, as I imagine occurs after psychoanalysis, the patient and I are still bound together by tenuous, not strictly speaking *medical* bands. In another case the patient is also in love with me, and would like to deviate it into a relationship where I could become a "friend of the family," or something not overtly sexually determined, but still outside the strict realm of doctor–patient relationship, where one has to be ill to see the doctor. Perhaps this means that the patient has grown away from an infantile dependency on the doctor, but still needs him for something. I do not quite know what this something is.

Even if we disregard the two agreeing psychological tests, Mrs. Q. was a serious case with very doubtful prognosis. In fact the patient broke off treatment at least twice—in April and November, 1952. For most psychiatrists this much would have been sufficient reason not to make any more serious efforts, even if the previous history had been less appalling and the patient's immaturity less impressive. In fact the psychiatrist would not have been called on to make a decision, as Mrs. Q. would certainly not have returned to him.

This case shows once more how different are the relations between the general practitioner and his patients on the one hand and the specialist and his patients on the other. Events which could prove fatal in specialist practice can be taken by the general practitioner in his stride. When the psychotherapeutic relationship is broken off, he changes back into a doctor; then he becomes a psychotherapist again, then changes back into a doctor, and then into an obstetrician—having all sorts of intimate contacts with his patient which would be impossible to a psychiatrist—and finally turns into a "friend of the family." During all this he has helped an impossibly immature, severely hysterical neurotic to grow up into an efficient woman, a wife and, very likely, quite an acceptable mother. All this has been achieved in less than two years—from February 1952 to November 1953, and in about fifty sessions. Without the treatment Mrs. Q. *and* her children would have been a constant drag and irritation on their doctor. It will not be very difficult to calculate how much time the doctor saved, say in ten years, by those fifty sessions. But it will be more difficult to calculate the saving in wear and tear, both to the patient and to the doctor, achieved by the avoidance of the frustrations, disappointments and irritations during those hypothetical ten years.

The incomparably wider scale of possible forms of relationship between general practitioner and patient has an important special aspect. We met it in practically every one of our cases, but we have not been able to study it systematically. The doctor can "give" something to his patient, something good and useful. This something is the medicine, the "bottle" traditional in England. By this I do not mean *placebos*. *Placebos* were first ridiculed and then reduced nearly to disappearance in our cases under discussion. The usual, merciless question was: What was the doctor's purpose in prescribing the bottle? Was it the best possible therapy at that moment and in that case?

If one looks at "prescribing a bottle" from this angle, a number of fundamental problems emerge. Let me quote a few. The doctor has a crowded surgery and cannot give a patient sufficient time, though it is obvious that he needs something. One possible way out is to offer him another appointment at a mutually convenient time *and* to give him a bottle, so calculated that it will just about be finished by then. Thus two birds are killed with one stone; the patient will have an additional reason to keep the appointment, and the doctor an easy, natural opening question: did the medicine help? Alternatively, if for some reason or other the progress of the treatment has become blocked, and further probing is either unsuccessful or inadvisable for the time being, a well-calculated amount of medicine will bring the patient back at a time when the atmosphere may be more favourable. Again, if the practitioner is uncertain whether the time has come to stop, arranging for the patient to come back for a new prescription or a check-up enables him to keep an eye on developments and to "start" again if events demand or suggest it.

Sending a patient for various examinations is another method often used to maintain contact. The report is sent to the doctor, and sooner or later the patient comes back to ask about the result, thus giving the doctor another opportunity. These techniques were mentioned in various cases referred to in this book; moreover, every doctor knows and uses them. What is not usually mentioned, however, is that the unexpected happens fairly often. An innocent drug, given as a contact-maintainer, causes a chronic symptom to disappear; though the bottle has been used up, the patient does not come back; a patient does not reappear to learn the result of an important X-ray, and so on.

Why is it that these techniques sometimes achieve what we expect from them, sometimes astonish us by achieving much more, and sometimes fail us painfully? This is undoubtedly an important field for research, but I have to confess that we can only point to it, but cannot yet contribute anything. Once again we must point to the need for more and properly planned research, the more so as any real understanding of these problems would certainly profoundly influence the nation's painfully high drug bill and unnecessarily overworked specialist services.

CHAPTER XIV

The General Practitioner as Psychotherapist

A. Two Illustrative Cases

HAVING discussed, but by no means solved, the many problems of "how to start" and "when to stop," and seen how many more strings a general practitioner has to his bow than his specialists, it is time to study him at work as a psychotherapist. A number of difficulties face us here. The first is common to all descriptions of psychotherapy. The mind is multidimensional to an impossible degree, whereas any description is limited to one dimension. Language can describe only one sequence of events at a time; if several occur simultaneously, language has to jump to and fro among the parallel lines, creating difficulties, if not confusion, for the listener. A further, almost insurmountable complication is caused by the fact that mental events not only take place simultaneously along parallel lines, but influence each other profoundly. That is one, perhaps the chief, reason why there are so few good psychotherapeutic case histories. The majority are confusingly complicated and long-winded. I am afraid that, in spite of my efforts to the contrary, mine may be of the same kind.

A second difficulty is caused by our being very much only beginners. General practitioners' psychotherapy has hitherto been a well-meant, haphazard, empirical skill, hardly tested out, and a long way from being safely standardized. This, though to a much lesser extent, is true of all types of psychotherapy—including psychoanalysis, which latter has been the subject of most study—but it is nowhere so true as in our field. Consequently the doctor had to be allowed great freedom in dealing with his cases according to his individuality. As we had set out to study "the most frequently used drug in general practice," our task would have been impossible if we had imposed rigid conditions on our drug, the doctor. So it was decided, not without some misgivings on the part of one or two of the participants, to adopt a sink or swim policy. Every doctor was allowed, and even encouraged, to use his whole personality freely. This resulted in a great diversity in the techniques adopted.

To give a representative picture of our work, this chapter would have to include at least two cases of each of the fourteen doctors who made up our research seminar. This is unfortunately impossible, and perhaps even undesirable. So it was decided to report only two cases in this chapter. In addition, another, a very difficult case, will be discussed in the next. In selecting these three cases I had in mind giving examples of good work, acceptable to us in the seminar both as regards the method used and the result achieved. These, taken in conjunction with the other cases described in the course of this book, will show what, in our opinion, a general practitioner can be expected to undertake.

That does not mean that *every* general practitioner should do as much. That would be foolish. Some doctors, over and above their normal practice, like undertaking minor surgery, and others antenatal cases and midwifery; others again are interested in children, or in anaesthetics, and so on. None is interested in every one of these branches of medicine. On the whole the same will be true of psychotherapy.

Looking now at my choice of cases, all three of them, though they were not intended to be so, were treated by those of our group whom I have described as "psychotherapeutically minded." This could have been expected. If anyone undertook research on obstetrics in general practice, the material would inevitably come from obstetrically-minded doctors. Conversely, this means that not everyone who attended our seminar could have undertaken or was interested in undertaking, this kind of treatment. In fact a considerable number of the participants were interested, but not all.

The last difficulty I have to mention is that I wished simultaneously to demonstrate how our seminars worked. This involves frequent interruption of the case histories to report our discussion of the various problems as they arose. I hope that by this method the case histories have gained in liveliness, as our discussions brought to light the many clashing opinions, criticisms and preoccupations that prevailed among us, as well as our many problems and uncertainties.

In June 1953, Dr. H. reported as follows on our Case 22, Mr. V. aged 30, whom she saw about eight times (twice weekly) and who improved considerably—

CASE 22

In the first place, the wife had visited me and told me that her husband was moody, depressed, had bad abdominal pains, pains in head and neck. He often became violent and threw things at her; she was frightened of him, and was sometimes on the point of running away because of his behaviour. She was advised by the psychiatrist who treated her husband at R. Hospital to be fitted with a cap for birth control, and since this has been done she thinks relations between them have been much better, but he still cannot get rid of his depression.

The husband was subsequently seen by me. He was first seen in 1949 at R. Hospital (a teaching hospital), suffering from an anxiety state. He was then referred to B. Hospital, where he stayed for four months. Since 1950 he has been seen on and off by the psychiatrists at R. Hospital, who do not seem to do very much, except to keep him going with tablets.

Dr. H. supplemented her description by reading a letter from R. Hospital, to which was attached a report from B. Hospital:

From: R. Hospital.

To: Dr. H. June 1st, 1953.

Dear Dr. H.,

<u>*re Mr. V.*</u>

This patient attended here first of all in December 1949, improved greatly, and was discharged two years later. During this time he was an inpatient in B. Hospital, and I am enclosing photostatic copies of his inpatient notes. When last seen he had experienced a recurrence of his original symptoms and also his pityriasis capitis had recurred. If there is any further information you require I shall be pleased to give it to you.

Yours sincerely,
Chief Assistant,
Dept. of Psychological Medicine.

B. Hospital: Medical Report on Mr. V. Aged 26, married.
Admitted: 28.12.49, via R. Hospital.
Discharged: 14.3.50.
Occupation: Painter and Decorator.

Complaint: Fearfulness, cannot stand crowds, is afraid of being hurt. Bad dreams, disturbed sleep, sweats, tremors.

Family History: Parents alive and well. Two brothers and four sisters. Eldest of the family (one other sister older, died).

Father, *aet*. 53; painter and decorator. Gets on well with father. "He is a man of aggressive nature, sticks to his point of view. Not like me, he is afraid of nothing." Quick tempered. Very popular, mixes well.

Mother, *aet*. 53. Quiet, peaceful nature, "although she can be roused." She runs the home efficiently, seems to have had more to do with the upbringing of the family than the father. Not anxious. There is roughly two to three years between each sibling. All get on well together. No family feuds. "We were all always treated alike."

Personal History: Normal infancy. No ill health. Rather nervous as a child, scared of violence, but cannot remember any specific instances of this that he witnessed. Not scared of the dark or animals, etc. Used to play with his brothers and sisters, make-believe games, etc. School from four to fourteen. Liked school, but not very bright, although reached the top class. Mixed well with others, until *aet*. ten to twelve; others began career of delinquency, he then left them, and was for a time unpopular. At this time did not mind defending himself if attacked, although avoiding fights if possible.

Work: Canteen assistant, six months; left because of insufficient pay. Lift boy, eighteen months, left because of war; evacuated. Liked the country life, stayed at the job until call-up.

Whilst in the country helped mother in house, made several friends, used to go to dances, etc. Several girl friends, none serious. Married four years ago after ten months' courtship. One daughter, *aet*. 2 yrs. 9 months. Sexual intercourse satisfactory, once–twice weekly. Good adjustment to wife. Happily married. Live in two rooms at top of a house. Inadequate, does not like the accommodation; on housing list. Wife also works. He now works with father as painter and decorator. Smokes ten cigarettes daily, drinks very little.

History of present illness: Called up in 1942. Trained in this country for infantry. Sent overseas seven months later to Middle East. Did not mind call-up, looked forward to it. Was excited about thought of going overseas. After being in M.E. some time, was sent to one of the Greek islands held by British troops after capture from Italians. It was invaded by Germans after a period of heavy bombing and he was captured, taken P.O.W. Whilst P.O.W.

was in several camps, in most of which he was badly treated. On release and return to U.K. started working as decorator and painter; married in 1946. Found he could not mix as before, was scared of crowds, felt there was going to be a fight. Found he was scared of "men with rugged features" lest they should attack him. Feared that lamp-posts would fall on top of him, or that knives would cut him, etc. Became moody and irritable, had frequent bad dreams; not necessarily of battle experiences, e.g. of seeing bodies in a trough being beaten to a pulp. Attended his local doctor, who ordered him a sedative. Recently felt much worse, went back to doctor, had not seen him for some time and advised to attend psychiatric outpatients' department at R., when admission to B. was arranged.

Mental state: He is tense and anxious, looks fearful, speaks in a quiet voice, which is often tremulous. His manner gives the impression of being a trifle theatrical; thus when asked what he was complaining of he stated: "I am afraid." Often on the point of tears, especially when war experiences are mentioned. Appears of average intelligence, no evidence of psychosis. General impression given is one of timidity and inadequacy, of genuine fear and anxiety, which is dramatically presented.

Physical findings: N.A.D.

Diagnosis and general impression: A very immature hysterical personality showing at present anxiety feature.

Treatment and progress: 24.1.50. Abreacted great fear reliving battle experiences on Greek island under pentothal, and expressing guilt feelings about his having killed Germans who had "wives and children." Felt much better on coming round, expressed relief. Was reassured and comforted. . . .

27.1.50. Feels much better. Not so scared. Told how he hated fighting and killing Germans. "Some of them were older men, like my Dad." Any uncovering therapy in this man is contraindicated; he responds well to supportive treatment with reinforcement of his strong repressions, which suffered a blow in the fighting of the war.

8.2.50. Feels well, but is rather worried about slight domestic trouble—wife thinks his mother ignores her, and he is anxious about the possibility of unpleasantness. Encouraged to tackle his mother. As soon as a course of action was mapped out for him, he felt and looked much better.

3.3.50. Much better. No fears now; "It all seems silly." Fit for discharge end of next week.

Diagnosis final: Anxiety state in a basically hysterical personality.

Condition on discharge: Improved.

Prognosis: Good for present anxiety state, poor for the basic inadequacy.

(Signed) Psychiatrist.

Dr. H. was rather scathing in her comments both on the letter and on the report. The first amounted to hardly more than a few polite, empty phrases, and was of no help whatever to the general practitioner; the latter was pompous, inaccurate, and in many important points faulty and incomplete. She reinforced her criticism by giving us further details of Mr. V.'s history—

When the patient first came to see me he was very anxious, tense, shy, could hardly speak, but he gradually opened up. At first he spoke of his aches and pains, was convinced there was something wrong, although all investigations had proved negative. He comes of a very large family, eldest of seven children. When he was three years old his elder sister died of peritonitis, and he has always been afraid of having to have a similar operation. He had a terrible childhood, took over all the responsibility which his sister would have had had she lived, such as looking after the younger children, doing shopping, etc., and he became mother's confidant. He also felt responsible for all his brothers and sisters (one of his brothers was a bed-wetter). They all lived in two rooms, and he felt ashamed of his mother every time she was pregnant. When he was at B. Hospital he was told his illness was connected with his experiences as a prisoner of war, but he could not understand this, as he had been so glad to get away from home, which he hated, and he was afraid of fighting, so it was a relief to him when he was taken prisoner.

Apparently his illness began when he returned from the war. Although the family had moved into a better flat, he hated being back with them, and tried to escape by marrying. However, he and his wife for the first year had to live with his parents, and this proved too much for him. He was terrified of father and still is. Father was a boxer, a very strong man, always ready for a row and a fight, and patient tried to protect his brothers and sisters from him. He feels he must always be loyal to his father although he is often in the wrong, and at work (they are both in the same trade—painter and decorator) if father does anything badly he feels he must cover up for him. He says he is sorry for his mother, and wants to make up to her for father's ways. He was always terrified to masturbate, as mother had told him that he would be mentally ill if he did so. He tried to restrain himself, and masturbated rarely.

Patient says he feels so much better now, because he has been able to discuss masturbation with someone for the first time in his life. He can go out now, sleeps well, takes no drugs, works better, has no pains. He has a really satisfactory relationship with his wife now. From the parents' flat they moved first to rather unsuitable accommodation. Three months ago, however, they got a council flat. He visited his family for the first time for three weeks, and was glad to find they could manage quite well without him. He can now play with his child, aged six, whom he never had patience with before. She was a bed-wetter, but in the last fortnight this has completely stopped.

The striking discrepancy between the hospital and the doctor's reports is almost certainly due to the difference in technique. The first is a typical result of "medical history-taking." *The doctor taking the history asked a lot of questions and he got the answers—but nothing else.* The answers were pieced together, a diagnostic tag attached to them—anxiety state in a basically immature and hysterical personality—pentothal abreaction was tried, and the results necessarily interpreted in the light of the diagnosis. As the relief from abreaction soon disappeared, the patient was put on the inevitable phenobarbitone tablets and eventually referred back for further treatment to his doctor—in practically the same state as he was in before going to R. Hospital. A not uncommon outcome.

Dr. H., however, had by that time learnt "how to listen." Without asking questions, she obtained from her patient important information which not only shed new light on the structure of the neurosis but was followed by considerable improvement.

In the discussion on this report it was pointed out that the psychiatrist at B. Hospital was almost certainly on the right track: he had correctly noted that under pentothal the patient mentioned how he hated killing Germans who "had wives and children" and resembled his father. Influenced by his impression that any uncovering therapy was contra-indicated in this man, the psychiatrist had not wished to go deeper, even when the patient relapsed. Obviously, his father was in the centre of the patient's neurotic conflicts and masturbation only a secondary symptom. Possibly it was only another aspect of the same conflict that Mr. V. had the urge to rescue and protect his mother from the bad, aggressive father.

It was felt that the success already achieved was probably only temporary, and that Dr. H. should be prepared for some storms

and should certainly not terminate the case hurriedly. In particular, she should be careful not to be carried away by the
patient's need to paint prematurely a beautiful picture of his
improving state.

A fortnight later we learnt—

Mr. V. has on the whole maintained the improvement, but he came
to the surgery on Monday complaining again of abdominal pains,
headaches, depression. Apparently he had had a row with his boss over
a time-table, and with his workmates over the question of wages. In
the latter case he felt obliged to take up the question with his employer
on behalf of his workmates, although it was not necessary for him to
do this. In our discussion he realized that he was repeating the situation
as it had been at home with his father (boss) and brothers and sisters
(workmates). Then he said he knew he had hung some paper on a wall
the wrong way and he dreaded it lest the occupier of the house noticed
it and told his boss. He said he was going to find another job, because
he was fed up with his present one. He did not go to work on Monday,
but he felt very guilty about it. I pointed out to him that he wanted
to throw up his job because he was afraid his boss would find out
about the paper being hung wrongly. I told him further that he could
come and see me again on Monday or Tuesday evening, but he did
not come either time. I wonder whether I should go and see him.

The storm was definitely there, and some of us had second
thoughts about whether the psychiatrist at B. Hospital had been
right after all. On the other hand, it was possible that the patient
was testing how good a doctor Dr. H. was. In the end she was
advised not to go and see him if she did not want to get further
involved in the case; but, if she was particularly interested and
willing to risk the consequences, she should do so, but should be
careful how she handled him.

Dr. H. decided to visit the patient at his home, and the treatment continued. We heard periodically about him, but I propose
to quote only the retrospective, summing-up report made in
June 1954, i.e. about a year after the general practitioner started
psychotherapy. Although inevitably this second report repeats a
good deal of what was mentioned in the first, it will be given
here in full, as it shows how the same facts assume a new importance with the progress of the treatment.

Mr. V. is a great success. He was a prisoner of war in Germany and
was very badly treated there. Came home in 1946–47 and could not

settle. He had severe abdominal pains, and he was in B. Hospital for more than two months. In 1949–50 the diagnosis was an anxiety state in a basically poor personality and the prognosis good for the present anxiety state and poor for basic inadequacy. He was constantly taking himself to R. Hospital to the casualty department, and getting filled up with phenobarbitone and medinal. The psychiatrist wrote to me, "This combination seems to suit him very well." Then I started some psychological treatment with him. I found out that the whole trouble did not originate in the war (as the hospital thought) but went back to his childhood and relationship to his father, who was a boxer and decorator. Previously Mr. V. has been constantly changing jobs and taking drugs. Now he has had the same job since Christmas, and has advanced to being a foreman. He is remarkably well, has recently seen me once a month only, does not take any drugs, has no pains. The child, who used to wet the bed, is now perfectly well, and the wife, who was ill, is well, too.

I went fairly deep with him. He gets more and more confidence because he was able to achieve more than his father. He is a better decorator now than his father, and he can stand it. When he is with father he can relax now, and is not frightened.

He was the eldest of many children. One thing which played a great part—he was terribly annoyed with all the babies which mother had one after the other; then had great anxieties about the sister, older than he, who died of peritonitis following appendicitis. I found out that his abdominal pains went back to that event. His sister died when he was four or five, and he could never forget that; whenever he has something wrong it is appendicitis or peritonitis. He was bullied and punished by his father very much, constantly had to look after the other children and to play the nursemaid, was not allowed to grow up and live a life of his own. He was badly maltreated; it is true, he always provoked it. We discussed all this in great detail. He hated it in B. Hospital and the abreactions he had there. I went through what the pentothal meant to him, his feelings of being killed and overwhelmed. I got him to go to the dentist for the first time last week, and he had a tooth out with an injection. Of course, he had been very much afraid of that. He came repeatedly about it, and he knows he can come. He had also backaches and headaches. He always got a pain if he had seen his parents or was involved with his family or with the boss at work. He saw the connection that the boss at work more or less represented father. He begins to see it more and more.

The seminar, especially the psychotherapeutically-minded general practitioners, congratulated Dr. H. on the successful treatment. The psychiatrist, too, joined in and admitted that originally he had had grave doubts as to whether anything could be done in this difficult case by a general practitioner not fully trained in psychotherapy.

We spent some time discussing the factors that were probably responsible for the success. The first was Dr. H.'s capacity to listen and to allow the patient to make use of her. The fact that she was a woman probably helped. Mr. V. would certainly have had greater difficulty with a man. In any case, two highly skilled men—the psychiatrists at R. and B. Hospitals—had rejected him, as his father had done, and in so doing had perhaps prepared the ground for an understanding, motherly woman like Dr. H. Finally, Mr. V., though not a dull man, was not an intellectual. The insight gained into the mechanisms that produced his pains, troubles and anxieties must have given him considerable satisfaction, and the intellectual achievement of being able to control them had given him confidence and pride; these things might not have impressed a more sophisticated mind. However that may be, Mr. V., after being given up by psychiatrists with a poor prognosis, was cured by the psychotherapy of a general practitioner. In case the word "cured" is objected to, I propose to quote the follow-up report dated November 1955, nearly a year and a half after the termination of the treatment.—

Mr. V. is keeping very well. He is now working as a foreman for a big firm of decorators. He has not changed his job for over a year, and has had no time off work. He rarely comes to the surgery (about once in every three months) with a minor complaint. I generally have a little chat with him, and he leaves without a prescription. His wife is pregnant now—this is a planned pregnancy—and he is very pleased about it.

Our second case in this chapter, Case 23, will show the psychotherapeutic work in greater detail. It will also illustrate the criticisms which the doctor's technique evoked, and which of these were confirmed by events and which were not. In so doing it will demonstrate not unsatisfactorily the extent to which our technique is securely based and at what points further experience and research are badly needed. Let me reiterate that the reports of this case—as of all the others quoted in this book—are based on a shorthand record. The criticisms were made at the time and in the terms reported here.

Miss S., aged 22, about three years ago, "offered" dyspeptic symptoms to her previous doctor; these were "accepted," and patient and doctor settled down to an agreed, chronic, but not incapacitating illness. The patient then moved to a new district. Dr. R. reported to our seminar in February 1953—

CASE 23

Miss S. came on November 20th, registering as a new patient. Very young, hair done in ribbons; she looked anxious. Said she had had a lot of indigestion for the last two and a half to three years. In July her previous doctor told her she might be getting a peptic ulcer, and must keep on a strict diet. She came to ask for more alkaline tablets from me. This was in the middle of a busy evening surgery, so I arranged to see her again. As she was getting up to go, I asked her if she was worrying about anything, and she said she had some examinations coming up, but she need not talk about it. She is a student, has a grant for an art school for a year, then for another year is going to do a diploma in teaching. Then she said there was something else, her boy-friend, but she would tell me about it later.

She came again on December 4th. She said that from the age of five to eight she used to get bilious attacks, but she grew out of them. She was unhappy at school, which she started when she was five, and she changed schools at eight. She was not happy, because she was shy. She has been happy at college; she likes it, but is not very enthusiastic about it. She has no real desire to paint, it is her mother who wants her to do it. Mother, aged fifty-four, remarried a few years ago. Very unhappy woman. Stepfather and mother do not get on well. Mother does not like the patient to get on with her stepfather. Patient's own father left his wife when patient was five; mother said he was a drunkard. I asked whether she missed her father much, she said she did now. I said, "By that you mean you would like to talk over your difficulties with your father?" She said, "Yes." She told me about her boy-friend, a penniless student, living on a scholarship. Known him for four years, they had been thinking of getting engaged soon, despite the financial difficulties, but mother does not like him. I asked her whether she had been intimate with him and she said no, but I later found this was not true.

It was easy for the psychiatrist to repeat his truism: if one asks questions, one gets answers—and hardly anything else. It would have been better to wait. The question induced the patient to give an untruthful answer, which might be difficult for her to remedy later.

Dr. R. was not to be beaten. He continued—

Later on, I said, "When did you have intercourse?" She remembered what she had told me, and blushed. I remarked on it, and said it did not matter. She has one brother, whom she loves very much. I examined her; there was nothing abnormal, except some tenderness, which she said was her gastric ulcer, and which I said was nonsense. I gave her a talk about the effects of emotions on physical conditions and told her there was no point in her dieting. I asked her how her indigestion was, and she said she had not had any.

On December 8th, second interview, she told me mother was very domineering, wanted to live her life through the patient. They had the same tastes, but she was always fighting her mother like mad. She threatened she would leave home, but mother said how much she had done for the children, had married the stepfather for the sake of security for the children. One night they had a row, mother walked the streets for half the night, then came back, and wrote a letter which she left by patient's bed. It was a terrible letter, which patient tore up as soon as she had read it. In the letter the mother demanded things which were not possible, she wanted patient to be with her all the time. We talked about guilt feelings she had towards mother. I gave her an appointment for a week later, but three days after she rang and said she must come to see me, as she was in a turmoil. Mother had come to town for the weekend. She had arrived in the afternoon, and the girl said she was already weary of being with her. She said, "I would not care if I never saw my mother again," then cried for about ten minutes at having said this awful thing. We had a long discussion about guilt feelings and hatred of mother, and at the end she said she felt much better. I advised her to have her cousin (who lives with her) with her as much as possible over the weekend, so she would not be left too much alone with her mother.

She came again on December 15th. The weekend with mother was extraordinary, because, following some of the things I had suggested, she had managed mother quite well, and it was the first time mother had not managed her. Then we talked about her boy-friend. She did not have full intercourse, but as near it as did not matter, and she was very guilty about it. She was going home for Christmas.

She phoned after Christmas, said she had something to show me. Came on January 22nd, and showed me her engagement ring. She had had a long discussion with her boy-friend about the future, had considered the various problems, and the result was they got engaged, with their eyes wide open. Mother, much to her amazement, had taken it well. Then she said since Christmas she had been able to meet people and talk to them without feeling shy and blushing. I said, "You don't feel ashamed any more," and she said, "Yes, that's it," and I said, "You have nothing to be ashamed of, and you can face things in an adult way."

She had stopped wearing her hair in ribbons, and had some make-up on. I saw her again on February 5th. She felt much better, but had been thinking a lot about her father, had been feeling worry for the way mother must have treated him. I put it to her that if she put her mind to her present problems it might be better. Then she talked about work, wished she could be in X., where her fiancé was studying, that they could be married, that she could work, and that he could go on with his studies. That is as far as we have got. She laughs about indigestion now, says, "Fancy me taking all those tablets for years." She could have been saved three years of that.

For doctors inexperienced in this kind of work, it must appear surprising, almost unbelievable, that Miss S. could be cured of her dyspepsia so quickly, almost as if by a miracle. A complaint that had persisted for about three years must, after all, be serious, and the previous doctor must have been impressed by it, as he had warned the patient of a possible peptic ulcer. This is another example of the danger of thinking of an organic diagnosis first; after a few more years of "agreement" between doctor and patient on a possible physical illness, the latter may really develop.

It is true, on the other hand, that Dr. R.—in accordance with his nature—used rather forceful methods to bring about the change from physical to psychological illness. After firmly establishing himself as a benevolent and understanding father-substitute, he rejected and ridiculed any possibility of an organic illness, and used his whole weight to convert Miss S. to his own psycho-somatic faith. He actually "preached a sermon" on the subject in the first "long interview;" it was a good opportunity to convert Miss S., as he had demolished her first defences and she had had no time to organize herself again. This is an instructive example of "apostolic" fervour in the doctor, driving him to do his best to impart to his patient his conviction of what an illness ought to be.

In the discussion after this report these two aspects were barely mentioned; they were nothing new to the seminar. But we spent considerable time on Dr. R.'s rather forceful offer of himself as a father-substitute to his patient. He had actually gone much further than simply accepting the rôle of the sympathetic and all-understanding father; he had deliberately turned against the mother and sided with his daughter–patient against her. This—as many childhood histories of subsequent neurotics show—is a not undangerous step. Moreover, Dr. R. had in so many words "advised" his patient not to have guilt feelings for hating her mother, and not to be ashamed of having had sexual experiences. The results so far were certainly very good and encouraging.

The attitude of the seminar was divided. One doctor recommended that Dr. R., having achieved so much, should diminish the intensity and frequency of the sessions, withdraw and gradually fade out. Another, Dr. S., who likes to be the wise doctor who knows best, was for continuing the rôle adopted. He thought that the patient would feel safe now, would be freer to do things having Dr. R.'s approval and would mature thereby. Then we had a little tussle. Dr. R. protested against calling his approach approval or disapproval. Dr. S. also declined to accept this description of his approach; he wanted it to be called "supporting" the patient in her decision. We shall return to this point in the chapter on the apostolic function.

There was, however, general agreement on two points. One was that Miss S., like her mother, was perfectly capable of "managing" things and people, and, now that she had Dr. R.'s example behind her, there was a considerable degree of probability that she would start "managing" her fiancé as Dr. R. "managed" her. The other point was that the doctor, spurred on by his success, might become over-ambitious and in his rôle of ideal father might try to tidy up the very complicated mother-daughter relationship, which would be much more than should be reasonably undertaken within the limits of general practice.

Dr. R. agreed with both points, and added to his report—

At the last interview she said she felt father was probably still alive, and she would like to meet him. I pointed out that she had built up an idealized picture of him, and he might not come up to her expectations.

It was a real surprise to the seminar to learn at the next meeting how near the truth our predictions had been. Dr. R. reported—

I saw Miss S. on Friday night and again yesterday (i.e. Tuesday). On Friday she was very much concerned, because she had had a row with her landlady and had given notice. Her fiancé had visited her last weekend, and had used her friend's room. The landlady had suggested to her that her mother would not like to know she was with her boy-friend so late at night. Then she said, "Besides, you have left the landing light on all night, wasting electricity." Patient told her she was tired of her grumbling, was going to leave, and they had a row. She started telling me quite calmly, and then cried. I asked what her landlady was like, and she said, "A spinster, sixty years of age, very domineering." I suggested she had really been having a row with her mother again, and she said, "Yes, she is just like my mother." We had a long talk. She remembered she had not got on with a teacher at school because she was domineering like her mother, and she has difficulties with a woman at her present college because she is similar. Whenever she comes up against women in authority she cannot get on with them. Then she said she did not know where to go, where to stay, so I referred her to another patient of mine, whom I knew had rooms vacant. She came again last night. She had taken the room, and thinks she is going to like it there. Her two friends, whom she lived with before, are going to leave the old house too, and they are all going to live together again when they can find accommodation. She said that over the weekend she and her fiancé had decided to marry in the summer, and that she will work in X. while her fiancé continues studying. Then she said she felt rather indecisive, is not sure whether she is marrying him because she loves him or as a solution to her problems. I asked if it was a good idea to marry as a solution to problems and she said it was not, but she could not see how she could back out of it without upsetting him. Then she said she did not think she did not want to marry him because she did not love him, but she was in a state of conflict about it. We did not get very far. She surprised me at the end of the interview by saying she felt much happier about things now, but I don't really know what went on in that interview.

The whole situation had definitely changed. All the "offers" of physical illness had vanished. Dr. R. added—

She asked me if rheumatism had anything to do with emotional troubles. She always had it, but she had not had it now for two months.

Instead of "offering" physical complaints, Miss S. presented her doctor with a number of psychological problems, which he accepted. A new "agreement" about what the real problems were had been entered into, and patient and doctor had settled down to work out a solution. The two difficulties predicted last week appeared fairly and squarely in the last two interviews—

(*a*) The complicated relationship between a somewhat inhibited but basically rebellious and "managing" daughter and any domineering mother-figure.

(b) The yearning for a good, understanding and helpful father to support her in the fight against mother.

What was the right thing for a general practitioner to do in this situation? As we saw, Dr. R. fell in with Miss S.'s wishes, and played to the best of his ability the rôle of understanding and powerful father. Was this a sensible therapy, and, if so, how much of it should be given? At what point was the doctor to "stop?" Let me recall our point of departure: the doctor as a drug. This case is a good example of how important this drug is, and how little we know about its pharmacology.

The seminar quickly realized that Dr. R. could not "fade out" as one of us had recommended a week earlier, partly because the patient was not allowing him to do so—she was, in fact, "managing" him all right—and partly because he did not wish to fade out. The success he had already achieved was too tempting, and he obviously wanted more of it. This is an extremely important aspect of the general psychology of many doctors; they want to be, in fact must be, "good doctors," and Dr. R. was perhaps the most convinced representative of this class in our group. We could follow the development of this kind of situation in several of his cases. He helped his patient, the patient improved but wanted more help, to which Dr. R. had no choice but to respond with more help, leading to more improvement, and so on. In a number of cases it was possible to put a stop to this spiral at a favourable point, but in some it led to exaggerated expectations in the patient or in the doctor or in both which could not be satisfied and the treatment ended in bitter disappointment.

This was the problem that we had to solve. Would it be wise to decide to "stop," now that the presenting symptoms of dyspepsia and slight rheumatic pains had disappeared and the two most pressing psychological problems, establishing a *modus vivendi* with mother and deciding what to do about marriage, seemed to be on the way to solution? Dr. R. would have to remain in the background, of course, and to be available when necessary, but this would mean reducing himself from a therapeutic to a maintenance dose.

Another alternative would be to continue with the rôle of the powerful father supporting the daughter against the mother, but this might lead to more serious difficulties and complications than that of finding Miss S. new lodgings in an emergency. A third alternative would be to make Miss S. conscious of how much she needed a powerful father-figure, and how readily she involved Dr. R. in her problems. This might help her but, as we know how desperate she was when her father left the family when she was five, it might stir up in her urges more intense than could be coped with within the limits set by general practice.

Gradually the seminar realized that "behaving like a father but not bringing it out into the open is a different thing from not behaving quite like a father, being somewhat out of it, but allowing the patient to feel towards you as if you were father." They are two different therapeutic atmospheres. "Or, in other words, sensing what the patient wants from the doctor and fulfilling expectations and being a father to a fairly limited degree —that is one thing. The other thing is not being the father, but making the patient aware that she expects something like that from her doctor, and that he can fulfil it to a certain extent but never completely. How much of it, and in what form it should be conveyed to the patient—that is one of the main problems of general practitioner psychotherapy."

After that it was not very difficult to sum up the situation. Dr. R. was acting as an understanding, forgiving and powerful father. It was uncertain to what extent the patient should be made fully conscious of this, but it was certain that Dr. R. must become fully conscious of his rôle. That, in fact, was the help he got from the seminar. The danger was that if he continued to act the father rôle, he would not have much control over the relationship between Miss S. and himself, because he would not be on his guard against the kind of expectations that would be stirred up in her. It was very probable, for instance, that in her row with the landlady the expectation of getting help from Dr. R. or even of forcing him to help her, had played a considerable rôle. Further, it should not be forgotten that the row had started about her boy-friend's sleeping next door to Miss S., to which the land-lady objected but which Dr. R. approved, or was made to approve. Dr. R. was urged to be on his guard against further involvement which might easily become excessive.

A week later we learnt from Dr. R.—

Miss S. came on February 16th, talked a lot about ambivalent attitude towards fiancé and why she was indecisive about marrying him. She suggested she was afraid of rousing mother's wrath by marrying him—

if mother would give her blessing, she would go ahead. I asked if there was anything else she was frightened of. She said all sorts of things, finding a home, financial difficulties, and so on.

February 23rd: the three girls have found a new flat together. Although not quite in my district, she is going to stay on my list. She said she had not much to say, her work was going on better, her thoughts were going round and round about the uncertainty of marriage. First she said she felt guilty about taking up my time, that her problems were those any girl would have before getting married. I told her it was not waste of time if it was helpful to her. Then she asked if we would be able to deal with all her problems before she went to X. if we continued talking once a week. I said possibly she was wondering about going to X. and leaving me, she might feel that leaving me was a repetition of leaving her father. She said yes, it was. We talked around that for a short time, then she went off and said she felt quite happy.

It was very interesting to watch the growth of the "managing" side in Miss S. She was not quite steady yet, but was taking on more and more responsibility. She was beginning to feel uneasy about taking up the doctor's time, and to realize at the same time that, even with his willing help, she would not be able to solve all her problems before deciding whether to get married now or later. So we all came to the conclusion that the greatest part of the psychotherapeutic work to be undertaken by a general practitioner had now been done in this case and that the rest would not take up more than a few sessions. We repeated that perhaps this was the type of case that might be satisfactorily tackled by a general practitioner, namely, a fairly healthy personality faced by an acute problem which turned out to be too difficult because of some neurotic conflicts inherent in the mental structure. The patient, being unable to achieve a solution, retreated into illness; if one of his offers happens to be acceptable to his doctor, the danger arises that all the patient's energies will be tied down to combating the "agreed" illness. In this case, this unfavourable outcome had been successfully prevented by Dr. R.'s intervention, his fatherly help had enabled the patient to get on her feet again, and perhaps the rest could look after itself.

The next report came in mid-March—

Miss S. came back to see me on March 9th. She had been home for the weekend, had had long talks with mother, who had agreed that marriage was the right thing for the girl and her fiancé. The girl was very surprised that things had gone so well, and that her brother, who ordinarily did not take much notice of her, supported her against mother about getting married. She said she was much happier, and she looked it—she had had a "perm" and looked very well groomed. She said she was going to X. for the weekend, and that she felt she could now manage on her own. She asked if I wanted to see her again, and I said there should be no need for her to see me again but, if ever she felt she wanted to come, I would see her. She thanked me, and went off. They hope to get married in September. She phoned me this morning, said she would like to come and talk to me about something that happened in X., but on the whole she was very pleased with things. I am going to see her tomorrow evening.

Although things had been developing well, it was growing more and more obvious that Miss S. needed Dr. R. as a good father and could not allow him to fade out.

At the end of May we heard about Miss S. again—

An extraordinary thing has happened. She has heard that her father, who disappeared when she was six, has reappeared, and is living with his brother in Y., and she wants to go and see him. She asked me whether she should do that; we talked about it. She said she would like to see him out of curiosity, but feels she will probably hate him. After discussion, we decided that she would write to her uncle and ask whether her father wanted to see her. If she does see him, I think she will be awfully upset; she has built up an ideal picture of him, and she says he cannot possibly be as nice as she hopes. Can one do anything?

The unanimous answer was that the only thing Dr. R. could do was to discuss the possible disappointment.

He replied, "I did that last night. She is going to write, and is coming to see me next week. But everything was splendid until this happened."

In spite of the justified apprehensions, things turned out fairly well. At the end of June we heard from Dr. R.—

Miss S. phoned me, and came on June 22nd to say goodbye. She was going home for the summer, and was going to marry her fiancé. He had recently passed his examinations, and had won a £50 travelling scholarship, with which they were going to have a honeymoon in Paris. She looked very different. I remarked on it to her, and she said she had been amazed to find what a great effect the mind has on the body, and once she realized it and accepted it she was able to see things in a different light. She found discussing things with me very helpful. Since she had broken away from mother she felt much freer and happier. She talked about father, whom she had rediscovered. She had heard from her uncle that her father was not very interested in seeing her, but she thinks for all that that she will meet him with her fiancé in the summer, but she is not going to be disturbed or upset if he does not show interest. She has quite a reasonably adult attitude towards things now. She is going to send me a piece of her wedding-cake.

This was a definite success. We learned that since November 1953, when she registered with Dr. R., Miss S. had had twenty "long interviews," each lasting for about an hour. In the first fortnight she had been seen four times, and subsequently with gradually diminishing frequency. What we did not know, however, was whether what she had got from her doctor would be enough in the long run; that is, whether her basic problems had been sufficiently dealt with to enable her to develop on her own, or whether she would need further help later. Dr. R. closed the discussion—

In the last interview she said, "I suppose I can expect to have tummy trouble if I get upset about anything in the future, but I will know what to do—talk over my troubles with my husband—or doctor— if I can."

No doubt, Miss S.'s conversion to the "psychosomatic faith," i.e. Dr. R.'s faith, was complete, and perhaps it would prove lasting. It was very probable that in an emergency it would help her considerably not to slide back into developing dyspeptic or rheumatic "illness" again.

At the end of September 1954 we heard from Dr. R.—

Have received a piece of wedding-cake from Miss S.; she wrote they are very happy; she has made a good relationship with her father, who gave her a big wedding present.

CHAPTER XV

The General Practitioner as Psychotherapist

B. A Difficult Case

OUR next case to be reported was difficult indeed, for a number of reasons. First, the case itself was difficult: severe depressions in a basically hysterical man, on the borderline between neurosis and psychosis, on the point of being admitted to a mental hospital as a voluntary patient. On top of it the treatment was started by the general practitioner without previous discussion in the seminar, at a critical phase of our development.

The seminar had by that time achieved some progress. A minority of the participants were in an exuberant and defiant mood, feeling that we general practitioners—if only we put our backs into it—could do about as good psychotherapy as the psychiatrists, if not even better. The others, the majority, felt out of their depth, envying their "courageous and talented" psychotherapeutically-minded colleagues, while ambivalently and mistrustfully looking up to the psychiatrist to lead them and wanting him to take full responsibility for pointing out "where to stop" with their patients. Some of the latter group in fact gave up psychotherapy for a period at that time.

Dr. H. belonged to the smaller, psychotherapeutic group. Any doctor attending the course who undertook psychotherapy could ask one of the consultants on the staff of the Tavistock Clinic for regular supervision of his cases. The leader of the seminar did not undertake any supervisory work, as it was felt this might have given the doctor working with him a kind of privileged position. Although the consultants for short periods dropped in to take part in our discussions, they kept away from us as a rule. It was foreseeable that this loose arrangement might lead to complications, but we decided to take the risk rather than tie down every-body in a rigid "co-operation."

It was in this atmosphere that a triangular crisis occurred, involving the patient, Dr. H. and the supervising consultant, Dr. X. In no time the seminar and its leader found themselves on the brink of becoming involved too. As at that time we had already gained some knowledge about the "collusion of anonymity," the "dilution of responsibility," and the "perpetuation of the teacher–pupil relationship" (which were discussed in the previous chapters, VII–IX), the leader succeeded with some effort in keeping himself and the seminar out of the clash caused by the crisis. He was thus able to use his not-involved position to help the general practitioner to shoulder the whole responsibility, and to take full charge of the case—irrespective of her feelings of resentment and insecurity on the one hand, and a tendency to be over-critical on the other. It was a difficult task for everyone concerned, and I am grateful to the protagonists in this drama for their permission to print this account.

There are several reasons why I wanted to include this case history. Its difficulty was such that it marks about the limit of a general practitioner's possibilities. I am fully aware that some people will say that a case such as this should not on any account be undertaken by a general practitioner. I have no quarrel with this view as on several occasions during the treatment I was highly uncertain myself. Fortunately—with some, though not very great, help by fate—the treatment succeeded, and I think this fact is worth recording.

I must qualify what I have just said. Not every general practitioner could even think of accepting such a case. Dr. H. had a special flair for psychotherapy and in a way she had "green fingers." The feeling that she possessed these qualities made her bold, though never irresponsible. She undertook the treatment of cases which would have been a serious test for any trained psychotherapist. She naturally had her share of failures as well as successes.

This history also well illustrates the great help that a seminar of our kind can give a general practitioner if he gets in trouble with his patient. I am certain that all concerned will agree that if Dr. H. had not been able to discuss her technical difficulties and personal involvement at our seminars she would not have succeeded in circumnavigating the rocks among which both she and Mr. P. were driven by her bold decision to accept him for treatment.

And lastly this history shows also something of the difficulties and hazards of the consultant–general practitioner relationship. In fact it demonstrates so well all the features of this relationship discussed in previous chapters that it would have been difficult, if not impossible, for me to find a substitute. All of us made mistakes at one time or another during this treatment, and I wish to express my appreciation of the fact that no-one objected to this history, including his part in it, being published.

I wish to remind the reader that all the details of this case were taken from a practically verbatim shorthand record of the discussions.

Dr. H. reported for the first time on January 6th, 1954, on Mr. P.—

CASE 24

Mr. P. had acute depression over Christmas and pestered me terribly. I discussed his case with Dr. X. on Monday and he has agreed to see him. But his secretary phoned me to say he cannot see the patient until February 3rd. What shall I do—his case is urgent?

Mr. P. is 34, married, has two children (girls). He came in July for the first time. He had a nervous breakdown three or four months before. His previous doctor had asked a consultant psychiatrist to make a domiciliary visit and patient was admitted to C. Hospital for three weeks. He had only tablets and talks, got well and was discharged. He broke down again a fortnight after his discharge. Then he came to me because he heard I did psychological treatment. I saw him regularly, at first once a week, then twice a week. For two periods when he had acute depression I saw him every day, in each case for not quite a week. He is a civil servant in the clerical grade and during these six months he managed to keep up with his work. At Christmas he broke down completely and has not been back to work since.

He has only one leg, lost the other at Dunkirk and has an artificial limb. He has severe anxiety attacks, fear of death and terrible guilt feelings about the past. Married after the war, has been constantly unfaithful to his wife. He always has to go with women who are below him, has them for one day, then throws them up. Has also guilt feeling, about masturbation and about the habit he has of peeping into cars to watch people making love, then going home to masturbate. Also gets excited when seeing films or reading love stories. Never got real satisfaction from wife.

He comes from a lower-middle-class family. Father a soldier, very strict. Patient's ambition was to work himself up; was always afraid people would find out he came from a lower class. Did not have a very good education. Just before the war tried to join the Navy, was rejected, so he became a soldier, intending to make it his career, but loss of leg prevented this.

He had about twenty operations on his leg; he has guilt feelings about being alive, says the others were killed, so he should be dead, too. He had a difficult childhood, parents constantly quarrelling; when there was a row, parents would not speak to each other for days on end. He was terrified of both of them.

We discussed his parents and his feelings about them, he began to understand quite a lot. Then his wife arranged that his parents should come for Christmas and that was the starting-point of his breakdown. There were scenes again and parents did not speak to each other. He took the blame for everything that happened. He came to me on Christmas Day, crying like a child, not knowing what to do. Since then the wife has come and the rest of the family too. I have had to give certificates for him to stay away from work, and tablets.

Patient has a dread of E.C.T.—he has seen other people having it—and everybody tells him he should have it. His wife also says he should go to a proper doctor and get proper treatment. People where he works tell him to go to a hospital where his depression could be treated. Dr. X. feels it is a too strong negative transference and it will be impossible for me to deal with it because I am the family doctor as well.

He is terrified of committing suicide. At one time he could not travel in trains; he can now. He has feelings he is fainting, headaches, humming in ears, all the usual symptoms. As a child, patient nearly lost left arm through a bad vaccination; he also had severe burns on both legs. He is much worse at the office, better at home. The severe breakdown early in 1953 was brought on because he was downgraded in his job. He is a very efficient clerical worker and his superior always tells him he is the best man in the office. The Ministry found out that he had not been properly trained as a civil servant (he got the job through the hospital where his leg was amputated) so they downgraded him and put another man in his place. He had been quite well till then, though he was not happy, his marriage has never been satisfactory.

His wife has been very much depressed all these years. She comes from A. and always wants to go back there to her parents. They left A. and came to London because patient was fed up with his wife always being with her parents.

All of us were impressed by the severity of the case, and by Dr. H.'s temerity in undertaking this treatment, but—as explained above—this happened at a critical period of our development, so I decided not to interfere, but to leave it to Dr. H. and her supervisor Dr. X. to sort things out. Dr. H. added—

Mr. P. always wants to test me out and to force me to send him back to hospital for treatment, which means E.C.T. When he came at Christmas he said he was quite prepared to go to hospital because I would be fed up with him. His wife urged me to do something.

After some preliminary discussion we arrived at asking ourselves three questions: First, whether it had been wise or not to accept this case for treatment. Second, what had gone wrong between Mr. P. and Dr. H. that caused him to get so much worse that he had to disturb his family and Dr. H. to such an extent. Third, whether the "negative transference" or the "negative therapeutic reaction" was a sign, as Dr. X. seemed to think, that the general practitioner should stop therapy.

For a time it was impossible to get the seminar to discuss at all the first question. When, at long last, I succeeded in pinning the participants down they simply refused to examine the problem. The only point that was admitted as valid was that general practitioners were hard-pressed for time and therefore could not undertake time-consuming patients. I had to leave it at that because, as mentioned above, this happened at a critical stage of our training. The only thing that I could get accepted was that if a doctor accepted a case such as Mr. P.'s he must be prepared for some crises. The question was whether the general practitioner could deal with such crises in his surgery. If not, he should not take the case on.

As the next step the doctors were able to see that to tolerate crises of this kind is not only a question of time but also of the doctor's ability to bear irritation, frustration and even anxiety caused in him by the patient. This was admitted by the doctors, but they pointed out that the consultant's function was, or ought to be, to relieve the doctor's irritation and anxiety. The consultant, by his specialist knowledge, could see more, and would be able to clear up difficulties; a better understanding should dissipate anxieties and frustrations caused by a crisis. An ambivalently rosy and optimistic picture—which I thought better to leave alone.

We then speedily agreed that there were three possible ways in which Mr. P.'s treatment could be continued—

(1) To get help and advice from a consultant.

(2) To ask the consultant to take over the patient, sort out the actual difficulty and then hand him back to the general practitioner—both courses well known and constantly resorted to in medical practice.

(3) There is the possibility that the general practitioner might come to understand the cause of the crisis with a consequent diminution of irritation and anxiety to tolerable levels.

Dr. H.—half willingly and half unwillingly—volunteered for the third possibility, but said, "The whole thing was provoked by his parents' visit. My impression was he felt guilty about them. The only way for him to deal with his guilt was to be declared ill, physically or mentally, and to get his punishment." This was not accepted. It was pointed out that possibly two topics were presented by the patient to his doctor—

(1) His parents arrived and that was too much.

(2) His diffidence in Dr. H.'s method of treatment.

When a patient presents two topics, it depends to a large extent on the doctor which topic is worked through. Perhaps Dr. H. was apprehensive about openly discussing the dissatisfaction the patient felt with her and *pushed the emphasis unduly on the parents.*

Dr. H. admitted this as possible. She was then asked how in the six months of treatment she had dealt with the patient's mistrust of, and dissatisfaction with, his doctor, i.e. with his "negative transference." Possibly not enough attention had been paid to that topic. Dr. H. first rejected this idea, "I was always hoping for something but it was always the opposite. He always told everyone he preferred this treatment."

She was reminded that Mr. P. had a compulsion to raise expectations in women in order to let them down. Dr. H. then added an important detail to her report: "He very often put me on the same level with his wife, and said he could not have a woman who was on his wife's level. His mother was very much the castrating, punishing person, and he has sometimes told me that I remind him of his mother in appearance."

It could then be shown to Dr. H. that—

the present crisis is not so much about mother, but mother is an excellent way of expressing it—the crisis is with Dr. H. The whole idea of Christmas, too, the birth of a son to a mother who was sweet and not castrating, belonged to the patient's actual conflict. Perhaps by her interpretation Dr. H. *stopped him expressing his aggressiveness to her and pushed him into a depression.*

Instead of being put off by being shown that she had missed something, Dr. H.—as was her custom—became more interested, and she now realized that Mr. P. was rather an important patient to her. Many people knew him, his office, where his colleagues took so much interest in him, was in her district—a resounding failure of the treatment might endanger her reputation, which she could ill afford as she was just building up her practice. Once the ice was broken she remembered—

What I found interesting was that he did not mention me at all in his application form to the Clinic. Where it says "Introduced to the Clinic by . . ." he left out my name.

Then still more details of this kind were revealed—

Since Christmas he has not come by himself, either his wife has come with him, or lately he has brought his little girl, and he has come during the surgery hour instead of afterwards, and has had to wait. He is looking forward to coming to see the specialist. In the meantime he is coming to see me, says he could not exist without coming to see me.

The atmosphere of the seminar had become much easier by now. We recognized again that ambivalent, i.e. aggressive and appreciative, feelings could be present simultaneously both in the patient and in his doctor, not completely repressed and not completely admitted either; and that this might lead to serious crises because, causing unpleasant tensions, they are pushed into the background of the mind, somehow out of the reach of the responsible part of ourselves.

Further details were then disclosed and gradually the idea emerged in us that Mr. P. might not be so weak after all. Quite possibly he got not only his family and his colleagues anxious about his illness and treatment, but also Dr. H., and through her Dr. X., her supervisor, as well. We did not have time to start to discuss this latter complication closely connected with our third question, namely, why Dr. X. thought Mr. P.'s case unsuitable for treatment by a general practitioner. However, I undertook to get in touch with Dr. X. with a view to arranging that he should see Mr. P. as an emergency case, to enable Dr. H. to carry on with the treatment.*

A fortnight later we heard that Dr. X. had seen Mr. P., but that Dr. H. had neither received a report nor had she seen Dr. X. for the supervisions during that time. Attention was drawn to the discrepancy between Dr. H.'s pressing need for help a fortnight earlier and her present nonchalance, and it was suggested that the reason might be that she had needed some therapy for the irritation and anxiety caused in her by Mr. P.'s failure to get better. She had achieved that two busy consultants, Dr. X. and myself, as the leader of the course, had to arrange an emergency consultation for her sake, perhaps her irritation had been appeased by this and the rest apparently was not important.

Upon our enquiry whether the treatment was continuing, Dr. H. reported—

After the seminar I was not sure whether I wanted to give him up or continue. He then saw Dr. X. and came to see me the following day. After the appointment with Dr. X. was arranged he was much better, his depression disappeared, he went back to work. After the interview he was very well. He enjoyed being tested, found it very interesting. Very much impressed by Dr. X. They discussed E.C.T., and Dr. X. told him, as I had, that E.C.T. would not be deep enough treatment for him, and offered him group treatment. What impressed him most was that Dr. X. offered to write to his (Mr. P.'s) superior about it. He told his boss the following day that he had seen a psychiatrist and the psychiatrist would be writing to him, and it pleased the boss very much. Everybody in the office envies him that he was to have treatment at the Clinic—at last something real is being done for him. I am going on seeing him once a week for an hour. I feel this was really helpful. I saw him last Thursday and arranged for him to come tomorrow, but he came on Monday at 12 o'clock. Before he always complained of headaches, but now it was his heart. His brother-in-law had died suddenly from coronary thrombosis and now he had

---

* When the draft of this chapter was discussed, Dr. H.—I think correctly—criticized the wisdom of my intervention. Admittedly we had had to face a crisis then and she herself had asked at the time for help, still, it would have been wiser if I had been able to remain true to my own teachings and to refuse the rôle of the helpful mentor. Now she felt that things had really started to go wrong between Dr. X. and herself after my intervention. The most interesting point for me is that until the day of the discussion I had no doubt that my intervention was certainly a very sensible, and perhaps the only sensible, way out of an *impasse*. I am not so sure about it now.

pains round his heart; he realizes now he always transfers illnesses on to himself. I am seeing him again tomorrow.

It is in this way that the "dilution of responsibility" begins. Dr. H., prompted by her aptitude and her somewhat optimistic ambitions, had accepted a difficult case for treatment. She wanted to do a better job than a psychiatrist, and in fact achieved some success. In her desire to be a "good doctor" she neglected to pay proper attention to her patient's "negative transference," i.e. his mistrust of powerful women, his urge to humiliate them, and his fears of retaliation connected with these sentiments. A crisis developed, and instead of clarifying the dynamisms causing it, possibly through her anxious reporting she involved Dr. X. in the crisis too. Meanwhile, with the help of the seminar discussion she sorted out the situation to a large extent, but omitted to inform Dr. X. The reasons for the omission are not difficult to guess; embarrassment about her recent inadequacy, some friction nearly always present in a supervisor–supervisee relationship, resentment that Dr. X. had not prevented her from making a mountain out of a molehill, and last but not least, the general defiant, disrespectful and disparaging mood of the seminar against psychiatrists. According to Dr. H., this last reason—though true for the group in general—did not apply to her relationship with Dr. X. Dr. X., no doubt impressed by the disproportion between the severity of the patient's illness and Dr. H.'s not quite adequate psychological skill, as revealed by the crisis, decided to have Mr. P. taken over by the Clinic. Unfortunately, he omitted, for obvious reasons, to inform Dr. H. of his motives.

At the seminar we witnessed Dr. H. impotently grumbling at the psychiatrist's decision; she said, "I cannot go back on his recommendation, the patient has set his heart on it." She was scathingly critical that Mr. P. was put on the waiting-list, with no firm promise when he may start treatment, and in the indefinitely long period of waiting, abandoned to the mercy of fortune and to the deficient skill of his general practitioner. Despite her apparent acceptance of Dr. X.'s recommendations, Dr. H. was continuing with the treatment as if nothing had happened. All the elements of the "collusion of anonymity" were present: a difficult case, an annoyed, grumbling and rebellious general practitioner, and a consultant mistrusting the general practitioner's adequacy on apparently good grounds.

The first task of the seminar, in my opinion, was to explode the anonymity. One of the two doctors involved had to be made to take full charge of the case and, instead of criticizing the other, to accept full responsibility for the patient's future. So I pointed out to Dr. H.—

If a patient is seen urgently at your request and no letter is received, it does not matter who the specialist is, it is up to the general practitioner to take the necessary steps to get what he needs. You are responsible for the welfare of this man. Dr. X. is only your expert assistant. You cannot say you did not give medicine to a patient who needed it because your secretary forgot to remind you. The responsibility for the case as long as he is under your treatment is yours.

In spite of our past—we had been then working together for more than two years—this was too much for the seminar to accept. All sorts of arguments were put forward: Dr. X. was, after all, a specialist of repute; it was impossible simply to disregard his considered opinion; it was his fault that Dr. H. had not received a proper report; what could a poor general practitioner in a difficulty do, other than consult a specialist? should Dr. H. rebuke the consultant? and so on.

All this and much more was simply not allowed to stand. I pointed out, "Dr. X. said something like this, 'This man will be taken over into a group, until then carry on.' We do not even know whether Dr. H. agrees with it or not." The atmosphere gradually calmed down and I thought the time was perhaps ripe for an interpretation of what the events might have meant to Mr. P., why he had improved, and also what all this meant to Dr. H. I pointed out that it was highly probable that now that she had been superseded by Dr. X. she was no longer the good woman; she had been deposed. That would be consistent with the patient's neurotic pattern—he picked women up only to drop them.

We do not know whether it is a good thing or a bad thing for his future that it has happened again. Maybe Dr. X. does not even know about this pattern.

One of the participants then added—

The patient's improvement was probably due to the fact that he was able to manipulate the consultation with Dr. X. against Dr. H.

I rounded off my interpretation as follows—

Very likely—perhaps you remember the discussion we had a fortnight ago—the parents were the ones who upset the patient and they were pushed into the foreground, but the real trouble was with Dr. H. Dr. X.'s action causing Dr. H. to be demoted fits in very well. Dr. H. was punished and the patient got away with his usual pattern. The whole relationship between patient and doctor was not dealt with at all.

This interpretation apparently went home, as Dr. H. admitted—

I realized how much I panicked only after we discussed it here; I should have gone on and not stirred all this up, should not have sent him here. I did it because they were talking against me in his office and my reputation could be too easily damaged. Next time I must have a bit more courage and not send the patient up so quickly. I think it would be much better if the psychiatrist had said to the patient, "I will discuss it with your doctor," and had not told him straight away that he was being put on the group waiting-list, and that he would write to his boss. It means taking the patient out of my hands. It will be difficult to go back and say, "I am going to treat you." I have learnt a lot from this.

The grumbling, and the blaming of the consultant were still there, but the storm had largely spent itself and the atmosphere was practically clear. Dr. H. saw the part she had herself played in the crisis, and was able to ask herself whether what we had threshed out in the seminar should not be brought up and discussed with Mr. P. She was somewhat mercilessly reminded that once again she had tried to involve a consultant, this time the leader of the seminar, in the treatment. She good-humouredly accepted the rebuke and we agreed that she must be the judge of how much tension the patient would be able to bear and must make her decision accordingly.

A fortnight later, on February 10th, we were told by Dr. H.—

I certainly did the wrong thing in sending Mr. P. to the Clinic, I lost my confidence. It has come out in the subsequent sessions that he resented being sent here very much. He thought my aim was to let another psychiatrist see him so that between us we could certify him. This whole affair turned out to be the breaking-point. Now he really opens up, he really tells me what is going on, which he never did before. There is a strong positive transference, or rather it varies, he comes out with both. I tried to explain what had happened, that he had provoked me to send him away; that this is what he does to women, seduces them and then provokes them to drop him. For instance, he makes a date with a woman outside a cinema, then lets her wait half an hour, even watches her waiting, so he is sure she will be angry and break it off with him. He understood that he manœuvred me into the same situation.

This was good progress indeed. The opportunity was used to demonstrate the importance of the interplay between patient and doctor. If this interaction is understood on both sides, the treatment can proceed—as it was now doing in this case. It is true the patient tried to repeat his compulsory pattern with women in relation to his doctor. In general, if the doctor understands the pattern and can demonstrate it convincingly to his patient, the rigidity of the repetition loosens up and something else may happen. In Mr. P.'s case the something different was that the woman whom he let down did not break off with him, but understood him, and so he could continue with her.

A week later, on February 17th, we heard from Dr. H.—

I have got to the stage where we can talk openly about his fantasies. The transference is coming out more clearly. He has sexual dreams about me, and he can accept all this because I can bring it back to his childhood experiences. For instance, he slept in his mother's bed and up to this day does not know whether he had sexual play with her or not. On the other hand, his parents often punished him cruelly and he always expects punishment from me. In one of his fantasies he imagined he wanted to be transferred to a better job and to go back to A. where he came from. The moment he discussed it with his wife she immediately took it up and was very pleased about it. Now he imagines he could not leave me. On the other hand he wanted to test me. If I had said it was a good thing to go I should have again pushed him off. That was last week. On Monday he phoned and said he had been invited to a snooker match and asked whether he should go. I said I must leave it to him. He went. Yesterday at lunch-time his wife rang asking me to go and see him, she said he was as bad as ever, really desperate. Now, after the event, I think he wanted me to say "come later" when he phoned about the snooker match. Anyhow, I went. It took me twenty minutes, then he was perfectly all right again. He put me to the test again, said he must have shock treatment, why must he go on with me month after month. I explained it to him. The moment he cancelled the appointment with me he felt guilty, lost the snooker match. I think I got him all right again.

This was another crisis, but this time weathered by the general practitioner without outside help.

Parallel with these events, another series of events occurred between the general practitioner and the consultant. Here the seminar and its leader had to admit failure. The consultant apparently was convinced that Mr. P.'s case was unsuitable for a general practitioner without proper training in psychotherapy. His reasons could have been that the patient was too severely neurotic; that Dr. H.'s skill was not adequate to the hazards caused by the patient's uncanny skill in involving everyone around him in complicated transference patterns; that the kind of psychotherapy by general practitioners with which we were experimenting was dangerously irresponsible and ambitious, and so on. A real effort was required to overcome the difficulty created by this open disagreement between the aims of the seminar and the views of Dr. X. The most useful way out of the labyrinth of conflicting respects, loyalties and dependencies was to point out time and again that only one doctor could be in charge of any one patient. He who carries out the treatment is the one who must make decisions and then must bear the responsibility. The criterion of the soundness of a decision is whether or not it creates better therapeutic prospects for the patient. Thus, whenever Dr. H. tried to keep the back door open, she was consistently called on to decide which in her opinion was better for Mr. P.—group therapy with its long waiting-list, or immediate help by herself—and to act accordingly. In the end this led to her breaking off the supervision sessions with Dr. X. and she had to find another supervisor to help her.

This period—from Christmas when the crisis broke out to about mid-March when Dr. H. was able to settle down with another supervisor—was anything but easy either for Dr. H. or for the seminar, or for its leader, or—for that matter—for Dr. X. Somehow all of us rode the storm. I think everyone benefited from these experiences; all of us, including the leader of the seminar, achieved a more mature appreciation of the possibilities and limitations of our therapeutic power.

In April we heard of another crisis with Mr. P., Dr. H. reminded us that—

According to Dr. X., this patient would probably have a lot of depression, and might be too difficult to deal with in general practice. After that I carried on with him and we got on well, although he had depressions on and off. However, for the last fortnight he has been severely depressed. All the time now he has had fantasies and dreams about me, and it is all centred round having intercourse with me. I cannot get him out of it this time. There's one thing I must mention. He had sexual games amounting almost to intercourse with his mother when he was nine; e.g. he woke up in the night and found himself on top of his mother; he says she awoke his sexuality, but when he tried to do it again she just laughed at him. He tried again with his sister when he was eleven and she thirteen; she told their father and he got a good hiding. When he was eleven or twelve his mother had a serious breakdown and was ill for two years at home following the death of her father. This all came out, and he has now realized that this set the pattern for what he tries to do with women. I stand for mother; but, he says, I am not his mother, I am an unmarried woman, and why could it not be reality. Another change has taken place; formerly he always tried to force me to send him for E.C.T.—now he is absolutely disinterested in everything. He sleeps badly now, will not eat, and is developing all sorts of organic symptoms; he has pain in his heart, feels sick. He asks me why I don't send him for an X-ray as there is something wrong with him. The last time I saw him was on Monday. He came at one o'clock in a dreadful state, quite sure there was something wrong with him. He had been to work in the morning, but said he could carry on no longer.

As every experienced doctor—no matter whether general practitioner or specialist—knows, the childhood history that emerged in this case is not so rare as one would desire. Severely disturbed and dissatisfied adults like Mr. P.'s mother may make use of their defenceless children to vent their repressed emotions. Afterwards, under the weight of their guilt feelings, they have to ridicule the foolish child who took seriously what happened and expects it to continue. The case is also typical in that after being rejected by mother the boy tried his luck with his sister—which also ended in disaster. No wonder that the boy when grown to manhood had an irresistible urge to seduce women in order to reject them afterwards, thus doing to others in his unappeased resentment what was done to him. The fact that the emotional mechanisms determining his behaviour remained unconscious made this repetitive pattern uncontrollable.

The first reaction of the seminar to the report was shock and anxiety. A number of doctors were in favour of referring the patient immediately for E.C.T. The argument advanced was his recurrent depression, but perhaps the real reason was the shocked apprehension provoked by Mr. P.'s appalling childhood history.

Other doctors recalled Dr. X.'s opinion and began to waver—
perhaps this kind of treatment was really too ambitious for a
general practitioner. I must admit that I, too, had some pangs of
doubt. Nevertheless, I maintained that before making up our
minds we must know all the possibilities. What was there besides
E.C.T. or handing him over to the Tavistock Clinic for group
therapy?

Dr. H. continued—

He also asked me last time to send him to a man. I explained to him
that that is the same situation as E.C.T., in other words, sending him
to father for punishment, as happened in his childhood. I feel I should
carry on. If only I can get him to see that his depression is just a
repetition. . . .

One doctor then diagnosed the emergency correctly. He
said—

Obviously if we send this man now, after he had admitted his sexual
desire for Dr. H., to E.C.T. or to a man psychiatrist, it would be
repeating and reinforcing his pattern caused by the traumas in his childhood. Could we give instead supportive treatment to Dr. H.?

I then reminded the seminar and Dr. H.—

There may be some repetition in your case, too. It is not the first time
that we see you getting hold of a very interesting and difficult case,
making excellent progress with the treatment, and then getting into a
crisis. Perhaps the crisis is in you and not only in the patient?

An amusing episode occurred here. A number of male doctors
reported that they found it advisable, if they had to deal with a
sexually aggressive woman patient, to have either a nurse, their
wives, or someone else, sitting in their surgery, or at any rate in
the next room. When I pointed out that men doctors were
apparently more afraid that a patient might attack them sexually
than women doctors, Dr. H. replied that she was not afraid in
the least, and another woman doctor amusedly enquired whether
a woman doctor could be struck off the register if she had an
affair with one of her patients.

It turned out that the doctor–patient relationship in Mr. P.'s
case included an element of sexual attack in a fairly transparent
symbolic form. Mr. P., whenever a new physical symptom
appeared, insistently demanded that Dr. H. should examine him.
She, however, consistently refused any physical examination, but

offered to send him to any consultant of his choice. Dr. H.'s reasons were that she did not want to overburden the already overtly sexual transference relationship between the patient and herself by asking him to undress for a physical examination.

The question whether a doctor involved in a close psychotherapeutic relationship with his patient should or should not examine him physically has all the time been one of the favourites of the seminar. It is an inexhaustible theme with innumerable variations: doctor and patient can be of the same or of the opposite sex; their ages can be about the same or wide apart; the examination may extend above or below the waist; there may be a non-psychotherapeutic past in which such examinations were a matter of course, or the relationship may have started with psychotherapy; the doctor may be the family doctor and why should it be in order to examine A but not B for a similar complaint, and so on and on. As it is impossible to lay down general rules, this topic became one of the most frequent red herrings used in our seminar. After we had summed up the situation that, at this intense stage of the treatment, any physical examination would amount to a symbolic sexual attack on him, while refusing to examine him would mean rejecting and ridiculing him as his mother had done, all we could do was to leave it to Dr. H. to decide with her patient which of the two would be the lesser evil. In any case there was a third possibility—referring him to a hospital for examination.

After that, with some prompting by me, the seminar returned to what—in my opinion—was the crucial question, why it was that crises occurred more often with Dr. H. than with any of the other participants. Various explanations were suggested. Dr. H. accepted very difficult cases; she went deeply into her patient's problems; true, as a beginner she had more time to do so than the other doctors in the seminar; and so on—none of these explanations very revealing.

Dr. H. then repeated why she was worried—

Mr. P. for the first time does not eat, cannot sleep. He used to feel relieved after his session, but this is lost now. He is disinterested and he does not feel better after seeing me. He is not openly suicidal, but what worries me is that he has had a number of accidents in his life.

I then summed up by asking—

Whose anxiety should have first consideration? If Dr. H. sends her patient to hospital her anxiety has been dealt with but the patient has managed to get another repetition of his trauma. Sometimes we doctors have to decide whether a mother's or her child's life has to be saved; apparently sometimes we also have to decide whether a general practitioner or a patient should be saved.

I was not surprised that this was not received at all well. Nearly all the doctors sided with Dr. H. and it was felt that she had had her innings, that she must admit that she had lost and that the best course was to accept Dr. X.'s offer and refer Mr. P. for group treatment. It was agreed, however, that Dr. H. should first make enquiries about the possible length of waiting time and that in the meanwhile she should continue as before.

A week later Dr. H. reported—

I saw him again on Thursday after our last meeting. I tried to show him that he was very dependent on me at the moment and that he has regressed really to being a baby who is completely dependent on mother, and that I have not quite satisfied him. This made him come out with the real basis of the whole depression. He and his wife had both got a questionnaire from C. Hospital enquiring how he had been since his discharge. He did not know what to do about it, and was in great conflict. At first his fantasy was that the psychiatrist stood for his father who was wondering about him and wanted to say "Come back to me." We discussed it. He postponed answering the questionnaire for a long time. One day he answered it, and wrote back that his doctor was giving him psychological treatment which he found more helpful than the treatment he got in the hospital. He was very pleased at having sent the letter off, but in the last fortnight he has felt very guilty about having shut the door on his father-psychiatrist; he had always felt he could go back, but now he feels he cannot any more. At the same time he bought himself a bird which was lame, as he is. He tried to nurse this bird for a few weeks, but was persuaded by his wife to get rid of it and to buy another one. I explained the similarity to shutting the door on father and that helped him very much. I showed him he fantasises the psychiatrist as a good father who protects him, but really he is not his father, and he is just a patient to him, and it was just an official questionnaire.

I also brought E.C.T. in, the father who hurts. I also brought in that he was longing for father, because father protected him in his childhood when he had to face something unpleasant, such as dentist, hospital, or school. Father took him to hospital for months to have burns treated. Mr. P. then asked me whether his father took him because of fatherly love or because he felt guilty as he was responsible for the burns.

Apparently another crisis had passed away. The problem around which this last crisis seems to be centred was Mr. P.'s conflicting loyalties between the powerful father who could hurt him (beating, E.C.T.) but was interested in him and protected him (being taken to hospital, sending a questionnaire), and a mother who stimulated him but perhaps did not love him enough. With very little help Dr. H. saw all these currents and decided— once again—to carry on, and to cancel her request for an emergency vacancy on the Clinic's treatment list. On the other hand, we got a glimpse of the possible cause of the recurrent crises—in Dr. H. She could give excellent service to her patients so long as she could feel that they needed and appreciated her; if a patient turned against her or threatened to prefer someone else, her confidence was shaken and her grip on events, her therapeutic acumen, became less strong.

The next report is from the end of May, more than a month after the last crisis—

You remember I reported a crisis about two months ago. After that I went quite deep, and explored the situation with regard to the relationship between him and myself, that I had become the mother. In the last two months there has been a sudden change. He has been remarkably well, no more physical complaints. He suggested himself that he should come only once a week. He has taken on a lot of extra activities. He is Chairman of the Tenants' Committee. He does umpiring for cricket. . . .

He still has ups and downs. He has quite a few anxiety feelings, but he can understand and cope with them. Before, he either collapsed or came pleading to me, but now he can really cope with life. He is going on holiday next week, which would have been impossible six months ago. I have never examined that man.

The "two months" mentioned in Dr. H.'s report shows how great her relief was that after all she had been able to steer her patient's ship through the rocks. In fact the two months were only six weeks. Of course all of us felt greatly relieved. After rejoicing with Dr. H., some of the doctors brought up an important point. Would Dr. H. be able to extricate herself from this intense transference relationship? Would it be possible for her to revert to the rôle of family doctor or would she have to go on for ever being the "good mother?" Would she inflict another trauma upon Mr. P. if this intense relationship became too much for her and she had to wean her patient?

My views were more hopeful. After all, mothers have to go on being mothers all their lives. True, children grow up and become more or less independent, but in the depths of their minds, they remain children for ever. Why should Dr. H. not deputise for a while for the "good mother" whom Mr. P. never had? And there was another point. Every child demands attention from the very first. There are two ways of responding to a child's demands. Parents, prompted by their own repressed urges, may respond in an openly sexual way and subject the child to a form and intensity of stimulation which he has not asked for and which is much too much for him. Something like this had happened between Mr. P. and his mother. He had approached her wanting love, and his mother responded by grossly sexual behaviour.

In the therapeutic relationship between Mr. P. and Dr. H. something entirely different occurred. For the first time in his life a woman responded to his plea by giving attention on a not sensual, not grossly sexual level. Moreover, however hard he tried, he could not induce her to go beyond that level. This enabled him to modify his ideas at least about *one* woman, and perhaps about women in general. Perhaps it would be possible for him to develop from that point and to build up a picture of a woman who does not demand too much, who is willing to give him according to his needs. This might be a basis for a more mature attitude to life. In any case Dr. H. had been warned.

True, my picture was optimistic, but for once reality surpassed the optimistic prediction. A month later, at the end of June, we heard—

Mr. P. went on holiday for three weeks for the first time since he has been coming to me. He sent me a postcard saying he was very well. He came back yesterday and to my surprise he is extremely well. While he was away he went to A., where he used to live and where his wife's family is. For years his wife has wanted to go back to A. and he wanted to escape. Now he has decided to go back. He used to work for the Ministry of —— and he got a transfer from A. to London because the family situation there became unbearable. That started his whole depression. While he was in A. this time he went to see his former superior officer, who said he was longing to have him back and would give him immediate promotion. Mr. P. also made arrangements with the A. Council to build him a house. Moreover, he has found a man who has a prefab., and wants to exchange it with someone who has accommodation in London; Mr. P. is going to arrange the exchange with this man and have the prefab. until the house is built. He was perfectly well, said he hasn't had a single anxiety attack, no hatred against in-laws, no depression, felt perfectly happy. His wife has completely changed since he has given in about going back to A. His only doubt is whether he can leave me. He will be moving in September, said he hoped he would be able to continue seeing me to discuss things until he goes. I agreed and suggested a longer interval and he said he would come in a fortnight.

But still more was to come. At the end of September Dr. H. reported—

Mr. P.'s case has really finished now. He went to A. about a fortnight ago and he was very well. He managed to get himself a very good job. He got away from me quite easily. The interesting thing was that last time he came he told me that his wife was pregnant and that he made her pregnant more or less without her knowing it. He had always wished for a boy—they have two girls. At first she was a bit upset, but now she has accepted it, as they are going home. He has a job now in the same Ministry, exactly what he wanted.

Dr. H. certainly deserved our congratulations and the hopes we expressed that Mr. P.'s improvement would be permanent. One of the participants added, "If only it would be a boy."

Sometimes everything happens in the right way, as we learned from the follow-up report, in November 1955—

I never heard directly from Mr. P. since he went to A. last year A friend of his told me that he is very well, has a good job and that he has a little son now who was born about six months ago.

During the lifetime of the seminar, i.e. in more than three years, four such "difficult" cases were treated. These cases were: a border-line schizophrenic who, after very promising initial improvement, had to be given up because of her ever-increasing inordinate demands on her doctor; a severely disturbed anxiety hysteria whose case may be classified as a qualified success; a middle-aged woman with a deeply ingrained character neurosis of the obsessional-domineering type, who at times had to resort to complicated and highly involved confabulation in order to mislead her doctor to keep him on tenterhooks, in my opinion she too should be considered at least as greatly improved. And lastly Mr. P.

Now, looking back at the events, it appears that some features were common to all four. Above all the intensity of suffering and, connected with it, the wellnigh irresistible clamour for help which induced the doctors to undertake treatment—even against their better judgment. In all four cases crises occurred one after the other; the dynamic background of the crises showed individual differences, but all of them had in common that the patient felt his doctor to be not sympathetic and not helpful enough and had to express this criticism in the form of increased suffering, creating thereby strong guilt feelings in the doctor and an urge to do more for the patient. It was only with great difficulty that the doctor in charge could be convinced that showing "more sympathy" and trying "to do more" would be of no avail as it would only set up an endless vicious circle. We succeeded in some directions in stopping this spiral but failed in others.

When, in January 1956, we discussed the draft of this chapter, the seminar agreed that all four cases had been extremely difficult, that the doctors had just managed, so to speak, by the skin of their teeth to get on with the treatment and almost certainly would not have been able to do so without the help of the seminar. A further important point was that the doctors who had treated these four cases were unanimous that they would not undertake them now when they knew what this undertaking would mean; and they were equally unanimous that they were very glad to have had this experience as they had learnt so much from it. Surprisingly, some of the other doctors said that they would not mind trying their mettle if a suitable case should turn up.

My opinion, for what it is worth, is that a general practitioner should think twice before undertaking the treatment of such difficult patients and should certainly not undertake it unaided, on his own.

PART III

General Conclusions

CHAPTER XVI

The Apostolic Function: I

ALTHOUGH the various phenomena of the "doctor's apostolic function" are unequivocal and easily observable by anyone, for the writer this chapter was fraught with greater difficulties than the rest. The difficulties were caused, not by the intricacies of the subject, but by consideration for the doctors involved. As mentioned several times, all the cases quoted in this book were observed by general practitioners who took part in our research seminars. When planning the book we agreed that each report chosen for publication would be submitted for approval, both to the practitioner in charge of the case and to the whole seminar.

By far the greatest part of the phenomena which constitute the "apostolic function" are expressions of the doctor's individual ways of dealing with his patients, or, in other words, his personality. It is not surprising that the doctor was generally the last to become aware of his own peculiarities, and in particular the last to welcome them in black and white. Often one or other of these peculiarities became plain to the whole seminar while the doctor concerned was still completely unaware of them, or still sincerely convinced that a particular action of his—i.e. one of his stock "responses"—was either the only possible, the only natural, or the only sensible way of dealing with the problem at issue.* It even happened that when some case, convincing to the rest of us, was quoted as an example, no matter whether by one of the participants or by the leader of the seminar, the doctor in question remained unconvinced. Thus, it was not at all easy to choose illustrative material which was both convincing to outsiders and convincing and acceptable to the doctor involved.

* That the leader of the seminar was no exception to this rule is shown, for instance, by his behaviour during one crisis of our "difficult case" as described in the footnote to page 199.

Apostolic mission or function means in the first place that every doctor has a vague, but almost unshakably firm, idea of how a patient ought to behave when ill. Although this idea is anything but explicit and concrete, it is immensely powerful, and influences, as we have found, practically every detail of the doctor's work with his patients. *It was almost as if every doctor had revealed knowledge of what was right and what was wrong for patients to expect and to endure, and further, as if he had a sacred duty to convert to his faith all the ignorant and unbelieving among his patients.* It was this which suggested the name of "apostolic function."

It is easy to recognize the working of the apostolic function when the problem is mixed, that is one in which both medical and moral issues are involved. For instance, one day a doctor reported to the seminar that a rather flashily dressed girl came to his surgery and asked for a certificate which would entitle her to a fortnight's extra holiday. Such requests as we all know, are by no means uncommon. The doctor flatly refused to comply, and capped his refusal with a short moral sermon. In the discussion another doctor expressed the opinion that the moral sermon was out of place; he would have advised appealing to the girl's sense of social responsibility by pointing out every citizen's rights and duties under the National Health Service. A third (admittedly trained in psychology) found fault with both recommendations and suggested that before doing anything—i.e. before responding either positively or negatively to the patient's "offer"—the doctor should have tried to find out why the patient wanted to get more than her fair share in this way. That is, as he explained, before refusing or agreeing to the request, the doctor should have tried at least to arrive at a differential diagnosis between neurotic malingering and callous malingering for gain. There was also some feeling that the doctor should perhaps shut one eye in some cases, especially if he knew the patient to be normally a decent sort. This would lead us to an important aspect of the apostolic function, to be discussed in Chapter XVIII, which we have called the "mutual investment company" between doctor and patient.

As we see, in this case there are a number of possible "responses" to the patient's "offer." All those quoted are in one way or another reasonable enough. The important thing is that it is almost entirely the doctor's personality which determines which sensible response he will choose. If asked, he will readily quote impressive reasons for his choice, but these on closer examination reveal themselves to be secondary rationalizations. Behind them it is easy—at any rate for an outside observer—to perceive the doctor's firm convictions about what a patient is entitled to expect from his doctor. Moreover, the aim—and very often the effect— of the response is to induce the patient to adopt the doctor's standards, i.e. to convert him to believe in, and make him live up to them.

In the case just quoted the problem is not fully medical, and the moral implications make the working of the "apostolic function" easily observable. But even in apparently purely medical cases, it is as a rule very difficult for the doctor to avoid showing his hand, that is to say, disclosing what in his opinion is right and proper for a patient to do in a given situation. The result is that the patient has either to accept his doctor's "faith and commandments" and be converted, at any rate superficially, or to reject them and settle down to chronic haggling or, as a last resort, to change to another doctor whose "faiths and command-ments" are more congenial.

This description is admittedly and intentionally lopsided, and thus unfair. Against it any doctor can point to the great variety of his relationships with various patients in his practice. I readily accept this. Naturally the doctor–patient relationship is always and invariably the result of a compromise between the patient's "offers" and demands and the doctor's responses to them. In this chapter, for the sake of easier presentation, I propose to leave out of consideration the patient's part and to concentrate on the doctor's contributions and their effects; the patient's contributions to the patient–doctor relationships will be discussed in Chapters XVIII and XIX.

So, after accepting the fact that every doctor is elastic and adaptable enough to allow a great variety of relationships to develop between himself and his patients, I propose in this chapter to discuss the limitations of this elasticity, the individual factors that determine its boundaries, and the fashion in which these limitations affect the doctor's "practice," having regard to nearly every shade of meaning of this rich word, such as (to quote the Concise Oxford Dictionary) "habitual action," "repeated exer-cise in an art," "habit," "professional work," "scheming," etc.

Instances in general practice when the doctor openly tries to convert his patients to adopt his standards are legion. An often-quoted example concerns night calls. Every doctor agreed that when the National Health Service began the number of night calls suddenly increased. Since then it has dropped back to manageable proportions, mainly because of the apostolic function of the whole medical profession acting in concert. As a curiosity I should like to record here the method by which one doctor coped with the situation. He pointed out to his patients that if everybody expected him to pay a night call for every little ailment, next day he would be too tired to be able to cope properly with the serious problems of his practice. According to this doctor, this apostolic method worked well.

Another example is the attitude of doctors towards telephone calls in general. A woman doctor reported to the seminar that she told all her patients that she kept a certain hour of the day free during which they could telephone and tell her about any problem they had. In her experience this was an excellent arrangement; the patients appreciated it; they did not ring her up at other times, and, moreover, they did not crowd into her surgery with minor requests and problems. She was severely criticized by a number of male doctors, who said that it was unwise in principle to give answers to patients over the telephone, which should be used only for short, factual reports, such as what the patient's temperature was; whether he had had further pains, how he had slept, etc.; and any other communication in either direction should be made only by word of mouth in personal contact. It was also pointed out that leisurely telephone chat took up much too much valuable time.

I do not wish to take sides in this controversy, but I wish to point out that patients were able to accept either system and make good use of it. Moreover, it is clear that in each case it was chosen by the doctor, who, because he thought it a good system, converted his patients to adapting themselves to it. This is yet another instance of the apostolic function. Obviously both systems have wider implications. One implies a kindly, material attitude, somehow conveying to the patient that in any of his petty troubles he may expect at least warm sympathy, and often some immediate help as well. The other might be called a realistic, fair, and sensible paternal attitude, expecting the patient to cope with his fears and suffering up to a certain point, and to ask for help only if it is essential, when he may be confident that help and sympathy will be forthcoming.

There are innumerable other fields in general medical practice where the apostolic function is easily observable. I cannot enumerate them all; the most I can do is to give a few more examples of how fundamentally it influences the treatment of a patient. Case 25 was reported by Dr. S. in July 1954 as follows—

CASE 25

Mrs. T. (family consisting of mother, father, three children). In 1949 I came to the conclusion that this woman was rather neurotic. I tried to find out what her trouble really was; as a result she left my practice, and I did not see her for a year. Then she asked me to take her back, which I did. Again I had a lot of trouble with the family, children always ill with all sorts of infectious diseases. During this period mother had the third child, which she did not want, worried me all the time to help her to get rid of it. She suffered continually from an allergic catarrhal condition, running nose and eyes. I gave her antihistamine drugs and she was all right, but then she came with other symptoms. Again I tried to find out what disturbed her emotionally. She talked quite freely, and disclosed that she was not happy with her husband. But she did not come any more, and she again took the whole family off my list. That happened four or five months ago. She has just phoned me again, "Can I come back on your list?" I said, "Why did you leave? We parted good friends when I saw you last time." She said she left only because the other doctor was near at hand. In fact the patient lives only about five minutes' walk from me, about as far as from the other doctor. I asked her why she did not stay with the other doctor, and she said she could not settle down with him. I said I was sorry, but I had no vacancies. She asked, "Is it a fact or an excuse?" I said I had no vacancies for the time being, but, if she phoned in three months, I would tell her whether I could take her on or not. I did not mind losing the family, although it means five people. Twice she left me and for the same reason—that I tried to probe into her complaints.

There are several points in this fairly common history which well merit discussion. First, one might ask whether it is advisable for a doctor who has functioned for a long time as a support to turn into an inquisitive investigator, and, if so, how to choose the right time for it. Then, what sort of technique should one adopt to make this transition acceptable to the patient, that is, to avoid upsetting him or even putting him off? Some aspects of these problems were discussed in Chapters XI and XII, "How to start" and "When to stop." The ways the doctor chooses to cope with these technical problems will, as we have seen, greatly influence subsequent events. Here we are concerned only with the third question, that is, the working of the apostolic function which prompted Dr. S. to put off his patient when she asked to be taken on again, in a way punishing her for her misdeeds and demanding from her that she come back as a repentant sinner.

We must bear in mind, however, that, whatever attitude the doctor adopts, it will influence for ever his relationship to this patient. What this influence will be, whether it will be conducive to better therapeutic results or to the opposite, is an important problem; some of its implications have already been discussed in previous chapters. What we are concerned with here is the fact that this kind of event is of great emotional importance to doctors, as was shown by the heated discussion in the seminar. One doctor, for instance, declared that he made it an absolute rule not to accept any patient who had previously removed himself from his list. When he was reminded that this amounted to a severe punishment for the patient, he replied that his feelings were aroused in such cases and he had no objection to punishing the patient to that extent. I must add that this doctor is sensitive and sympathetic, and not in the least the harsh individual that his "rule" might perhaps suggest. His attitude was supported by others, several of whom pointed out that Mrs. T. had left her doctor twice before and would possibly prove to be a chronic recidivist in this respect.

Another doctor's opinion was that the patient should be taken back without further ado, and yet another suggested that the patient should be asked to come to the surgery for a talk, during which it might be possible to raise the question why she had twice left the doctor when he tried to probe into her emotional problems. A third doctor pointed out that all this coming and going was probably a recurrent crisis, a symptom of the patient's personality, which ought to be understood and treated, not forcibly changed by educational methods.

I should like to mention a few more characteristic individual ways—discussed at the same seminar—in which doctors face this particular problem. One doctor, for instance, said that if patients left him, it meant that they were no longer satisfied with him; consequently he did not feel justified in taking them back. If the reasons for leaving him had been discussible, the patient would have discussed them before taking action. Thus, if a patient left of his own free will, the doctor felt that it must be for a very serious reason indeed and consequently that he had been intentionally hurt.

Another doctor agreed with this, and added that when a patient left him he felt he suffered a sort of humiliation. Previously he had felt guilt as well, besides great anger with the patient. Now, after attending our seminars, he did not feel so guilty, but just thought that his personality and that of the patient did not fit. Nevertheless, he maintained that it was sensible to punish the patient, so if a patient wished to return to him he charged him one and a half guineas for the first appointment, and if the patient refused to pay him immediately he refused to see him again. Yet another doctor reported of his partner that he had always taken pleasure in seeing a patient come back and then saying to him, "This is not the way to run a general practice. Once you have gone, you have gone," and finish with him.

These examples show that a complicated conflict of emotions has to be dealt with in one way or another by the doctor concerned. He cannot help feeling that he has been let down and humiliated, that it has been rubbed into him that he is not such a good doctor as he ought to be, or feels himself to be. Although we readily admit our imperfections to ourselves, it is a different matter when the implication comes from someone else, particularly a patient. That is the first group of emotions arising out of the situation. Broadly speaking there are two ways of dealing with it. One is to project the cause of our resentment on the patient, stamp him as ungrateful and unappreciative, and punish him for it in some way—that is the second group of emotions. Then there is a kind of turning-the-other-cheek attitude—the third group—acknowledging that one is not so good as one ought to be and taking the patient back meekly whenever he chooses to come. Apart from all this, there is the financial side of the matter, and, last but not least, there is the general attitude among doctors that we have, after all, been trained to help people, and ought to be gratified if our help is required again.

This conflict of emotions exists for every doctor. Every doctor has to find a solution which will satisfy the emotions most important and most acceptable to him and at the same time frustrate or repress the less important and less acceptable ones. This response, then, will be his individual routine, not absolutely rigid, still setting discernible limits to his elasticity. The doctor is hardly ever called on to state explicitly the motives behind his "normal" routine. When he is called on to do so—as happened in our discussions—the result is a mixture of puzzled embarrassment, of almost transparent rationalization, of excuses and attempts to explain things away, of aggressive criticism of any other routine suggested, and, last but not least, of reluctantly becoming aware of his own limitations and the motives behind them.

To round off the case of Mrs. T., Dr. S. reported in May 1955—

A few months ago she came back on my list, after my making her wait for a vacancy, and I must say she has behaved very well since then. I used to have to go very often to see the children. Now I have seen the mother once only, and one of the children once after an operation. Even the antihistamine tablets which she has had for some years from me are usually asked for over the telephone.

Clearly a peaceful situation has been restored, and perhaps to the satisfaction of everyone concerned. But—there is no mention of any emotional problems in the follow-up report, and it is fair to assume that the price of peace was a tacit agreement to let sleeping dogs lie. In other words, this time it was the patient who "converted" the doctor to give up his attempts at probing into her emotional problems and to accept—at any rate for the time being, but possibly for good—the rôle of a mere support. Some people will say this was a good solution and that it was a great pity that the patient had been put through unnecessary upheavals by the doctor's unwarranted and unprofitable psychological curiosity. We must admit that the doctor was not successful, perhaps because his technical skill was not adequate in this particular case. This lack of success, however, should not distract our attention from the working of the apostolic function.

Another important sphere in which the apostolic function can be studied is the question of examining the patient psychologically. This problem was incidentally involved in the previous case, Case 25. When a doctor examines the eye reflexes or the heart-sounds, he knows he is not going to do much harm, but he does not feel on such safe ground when he is called upon to enquire into the intimate details of the relationship between husband and wife, or into any other "psychological" problem. There are many reasons for his diffidence. One is lack of skill. As pointed out many times, medical training does not offer the future doctor sufficient experience in this skill, though it is a necessary skill in dealing with at least a quarter of his patients, if not more. It is his everyday practice that compels him to learn this skill at his own cost and peril—and at that of his patients. The other reason is, as discussed in Chapter XI, that physical examination belongs to the sphere of one-person biology. In this field it is nearly true to say that the patient can be examined as if he were a mere object, like a car is examined to find out whether the carburettor is getting enough petrol. It can, with some exaggeration, be said that a physical diagnosis does not demand much more than this, while in a psychological examination the doctor has to establish a personal relationship with his patient, which means entering an absolutely different field, with different methods and different personal involvement.

A third group of reasons for diffidence might be called respect for the patient's intimate life. When a patient consults us about pains in the precordial region, or about obstinate indigestion, are we justified in enquiring into the details of his sexual régime or of his emotional life? We have come up against this problem several times in the previous chapters. As on so many other occasions, we are dealing here with a half-truth. In a case of indigestion no doctor would hesitate to carry out a rectal examination, or even a sigmoidoscopy, if he suspected a pathological process in the lower intestines. Does this not amount to a violation of the patient's privacy? The answer must be an unconditional yes, but we can add that an objective and sympathetic approach by the doctor will enable the patient to accept the unpleasant intervention; and, if the doctor has acquired the necessary skill, these and similar examinations can be carried out without causing much embarrassment or pain to patient—or doctor.

The same is true of psychological examinations. An objective and sympathetic approach prepares the patient for it, and if the doctor has acquired sufficient skill he will be able to conduct the examination without causing much embarrassment or pain. But he must be convinced that the examination is desirable or necessary. In several cases quoted in this book we saw a number of different shades in the doctor's positive or negative attitude towards psychological examinations.

There is a further complication. When one of our fellow-beings is physically ill—though we shall certainly be sympathetic —we may remain detached and different from him (or her), because we are in good health and are not suffering from diabetes or virus pneumonia, or rheumatoid arthritis, or whatever it may be. But if a patient is unhappy about his share in this world, or has a problem with his sexual partner, we doctors cannot help feeling personally involved, because we all have problems of a similar nature, with which we cope either well or not so well. Somehow, when we examine our patient, we cannot escape examining ourselves, which is tantamount to disclosing our own ideas and wishes about what ought to be done in the particular situation.

This last factor far outweighs the others in importance; in fact it provides the explanation for the persistence of the first two— lack of psychological skill, and its counterpart, the possession of skill limited to treating patients "objectively" while avoiding any subjective two-sided relationship with them. These two are due to our traditional medical training, maintained by our teaching hospitals and accepted by students. Teachers and students—for good reasons—tacitly agree to avoid situations which might lead to an examination of their personal problems and their individual solutions—even though only by themselves.

The most frequently used method for excluding external pressure or internal need for this examination is to proclaim one's individual solutions to be the best or most sensible, and then, fired by apostolic zeal, to "practise" medicine in such a way as to convert all unbelievers to our "faith." It was really surprising to discover how many doctors quote in their "practice" their own ways of solving one or other of their personal problems and as a result expect the patient to take these solutions as models. Among many other cases, that of the company director (Case 6) is a tragic instance of this "practice." A successful conversion with a happy ending occurred in Miss S.'s story (Case 23). Mrs. C. (Case 1) was also successfully converted, but only temporarily, as her subsequent history in the Appendix shows.

This is an extremely important factor. Avoidance of self-examination and apostolic fervour are, as a rule, interlinked and reinforce each other. I wish to stress again that apostolic zeal—

like reassurance—is not in itself wrong; on the contrary, it is a highly powerful drug, with great potentialities. As with re-assurance, the trouble with apostolic zeal is that it is usually prescribed wholesale, without any attempt at a differential diagnosis. One of the chief ways of improving the doctor's psychotherapeutic skill is to make him aware of his compelling apostolic function and so to enable him not to "practise" it automatically in every case.

There are many fields in present-day medicine where science is of little help to the practitioner, and he has to rely chiefly on his common sense, which is just another word for apostolic function. These fields are easily recognizable by the uneasiness and em-barrassment with which doctors discuss them.

One of these fields may be called "visiting the sick," especially if the sick is a private patient. By "the sick" I mean chronic invalids who are beyond the power of medical cure. Many are very grateful for, and appreciative of, the little comfort and hope that they get from their doctor's visits. This, however, only increases the doctor's uneasiness, as he knows only too well that his "professional" skill and knowledge can be of little use. He earns gratitude, appreciation, and even money, for what he con-siders to be mostly a sham. "Objectively" this assessment of his services is correct, but not psychologically. As psychological values are not openly recognized in medical training, the doctor has to use his common sense in devising his own standards. In other words, he has to convert his patient to accepting the doctor's individual standards for visiting the sick as the only sensible ones.

Another field, a more dangerous one, is the doctor as "com-forter." Nowadays, with more and more of us becoming isolated and lonely, people have hardly anyone to whom they can take their troubles. It is undeniable that fewer and fewer people take them to their priests. The only person who is always available, especially since the beginning of the National Health Service, is the doctor. In many people any emotional stress is accompanied by, or possibly is tantamount to, bodily sensations. So they come to their doctor and complain. In a very great number of cases the complaining itself is the important thing, the symptoms, at any rate in the "unorganized" stage of an illness, are objectively irrelevant, and usually there are no signs to be found. Here again the doctor is at the mercy of his common sense, for his training taught him only how to treat "real" physical illnesses. More often than not, in his embarrassment, he will prescribe a bottle— on highly insufficient indications—thus inflating the national drug bill. Still, some people get better on such bottles, though nobody —least of all their doctor—knows why. On the other hand, as we saw in several of our case histories, the first bottle may set people off to "organize" their illnesses in a therapeutically in- accessible form. Again nobody—least of all the doctor prescribing the bottle—knows how many. But, as a "long interview" would need psychological skill, that is examining one's own solutions, it is easier to convert the patient to belief in bottles and proprie- tary medicines, especially as the whole population has had some considerable previous training in believing in them.

Then there is a third field, a most interesting one, of which unfortunately we know very little. This is the doctor as "father- confessor." I have to apologize for borrowing so many terms from theology; my excuse is that they describe exactly what I have in mind. Falling ill, and especially being ill, is felt by many conscientious people as defaulting, demanding unfair advantages. They feel guilty about getting more attention than seems fair to them, about not working, about living on someone else, and so on. Then there is the type who is all out to get more than his fair share, to whom any semblance of an illness is more than welcome, who goes out of his way to "catch" diseases. Both these types feel guilty, though for different reasons, and it is extremely difficult to get them better if the doctor cannot do something about their guilt feelings. This means that the doctor must enable these people to talk freely to him about their apprehensions and guilt feelings; that is, he must act rather like a father-confessor, even to the extent of giving absolution. Medical text-books mention these situations only incidentally, so again common sense, i.e. his apostolic function, must come to the doctor's help.

Two other interesting types of patients belong to the same field. Both are over-anxious. One is terrified of developing some illness and comes frequently to the doctor for reassurance that he is all right, only to return with the same or a new apprehension a short time later. The other type cannot allow himself to be weak, still less ill. To him illness is an irremediable humiliation, a weakness which can never be made good. The "complaining" people cost the nation legions of bottles a year, and the two last types cost legions of futile specialist examinations. But what else can a doctor do? He can find nothing wrong with the patient, whose anxiety persists, so why not reassure him by a "second opinion?" After some months, if the condition remains the same, another second opinion, or a third opinion, will be needed. We have met the dilution of responsibility, the collusion of anonymity, and their consequences in Chapters VII–IX.

All this has an important effect on the patient. If in trouble, he expects from his doctor a physical examination and a bottle. If this is of no help, he expects to be sent to a specialist, who will use some complicated and mysterious piece of apparatus. What he does not expect is a "long interview," a proper psychological examination; and a suggestion that he should see a psychiatrist may be a severe shock to him. By their apostolic function doctors train the population from childhood what to expect and what not to expect when they go to the doctor's. This training, though very efficient, is not unalterable. We have taught our patients not to be unduly embarrassed when showing us their bodies; it should not be very difficult to teach them that often their psychological problems have to be shown, too. The first step towards achieving this aim is, of course, to train the doctors.

To return to the general reluctance to probe into a patient's personal, i.e. psychological, problems, we found—as expected—that probing into questions of sexuality roused the greatest reluctance. In many instances doctors reported about couples who had been well known to them for years, couples to whom they had for long been close personal friends as well as trusted medical advisers, couples whom they had always regarded as unquestionably happily married, but in fact turned out—to the doctor's great surprise—to have been living an utterly miserable life of strife and discord all the time. This painful discovery was so frequent that if a doctor started reporting about a happy couple one partner of which came to see him, the whole seminar started smiling condescendingly and knowingly. Doubtless the couple had their share in the collusion of silence, but so had the doctor. After the report we were nearly always left wondering whether it had been good policy and good medical "practice" for the doctor to accept the collusion of silence, and how much friction, unhappiness, and suffering could have been prevented by a frank discussion of the marital problems at the right time.

The difficulty facing the doctor, however, is nowhere so great as in the field of sexuality. When dealing with any problem relating to this field he cannot escape disclosing his own views and convictions about what is right and wrong for anyone—i.e. for himself—to expect and to demand. Is adult sexual life with proper satisfaction essential? Or, though advisable, not very important? Or, though quite pleasant, really unimportant or even negligible? In any case involving marital relations, such questions are implicit and must be answered. Unfortunately we know but little about them, and the little we know is generally omitted from medical text-books, so again the doctor's only ally is his common sense, i.e. his apostolic function.

Lastly there is the immense question, which is similarly left to be dealt with by common sense, of how much pain, suffering and renunciation are part and parcel of human existence, and as such must be tolerated. When is it the doctor's duty to intervene either to relieve suffering—e.g. by morphia—or to impose renunciations—e.g. by prescribing strict diets for ulcer patients or a sober and bland life for people with heart trouble or hypertension? Obviously his advice will be coloured by his views about how much pleasure and excitement makes life worth living, what is the amount of suffering and privation that changes life from an empty, superficially agreeable, shell into something real. Here, too, we find a free field for unfettered apostolic zeal.

Equally uncertain is our knowledge about the effects of the form the apostolic function should take, or, to use our other metaphor, about the form in which the doctor should administer himself. Should he be a kind of authoritative guardian, who knows best what is good for his wards, who need give no explanation, but expects loyal obedience? Should he act as mentor, offering his expert knowledge and ready to teach his patient how to adjust himself to changed conditions, how to adopt a new, more useful attitude? Should he be a detached scientist, describing objectively the advantages and drawbacks of the various therapeutic and dietetic possibilities and allowing his patient complete freedom of choice, but also imposing upon him the responsibility for the choice? Should he act the kind protective parent who must spare his poor child-patient any bad tidings or painful responsibility? Or should he be an advocate of "truth above all," firmly believing that nothing can be worse than doubt, and acting accordingly?

The answer, of course, is that the doctor must judge what is best for each patient. Judge he certainly must, but who can tell him the criteria relevant to his judgment? It is left to his common sense, i.e. his apostolic function. In fact it is not so much the patient's needs but the doctor's individuality that determines the form in which the doctor administers himself. The various forms just described characterize the habitual behaviour of certain doctors rather than that of certain patients.

Another endless problem is whether or not the patient should express his appreciation of the doctor's services and, if so, in what form. This is closely connected with the endless problem of fees. Is it therapeutically better or worse if a patient is dependent on, or independent of, his doctor? If he feels superior because he is paying the doctor, or inferior because the doctor is above financial matters? Any answer to these questions, as old and respectable as medicine itself, rests only on common sense.

The situation would be entirely different if we knew more about these important side-effects of our drug, the doctor. To mention a few which we have already referred to in this chapter: When looking after an invalid, i.e. when "visiting the sick," should his rôle be that of a shamefaced exploiter *malgré lui*, a not-quite-honest consoler-comforter, a detached scientific observer, or what? In sexual matters should he be an ardent fighter for the happiness of every individual, or the guardian of the sanctity of marriage? In either case, should he persist in his attitude at any price, or, if not, at what price? How much expression of gratitude from patients suffering from chronic, incapacitating illnesses should he expect and accept in words, presents, or money? And how much criticism, resentment, or even hatred should he tolerate when his therapy is unsuccessful?

All these and many more problems contribute to what we have called the pharmacology of the drug "doctor." What is desirable is that we should know roughly as much about this drug as we know about, let us say, digitalis. We know that each year's crop is different, but that the crops can be standardized fairly well; that many patients have individual idiosyncrasies to digitalis, which have to be watched; that there is a great difference between preventive, therapeutic and maintenance doses. This knowledge has been acquired by painstaking research; the same is needed for our drug.

CHAPTER XVII

The Apostolic Function: II

AN especially important aspect of the apostolic function is the doctor's urge to prove to the patient, to the whole world, and above all to himself, that he is good, kind, knowledgeable, and helpful. We doctors are only too painfully aware that this is a highly idealized picture. We have our moods and our idiosyncrasies, and consequently we are not always as kind and sympathetic as we should like to be; our knowledge is incomplete and patchy; and, even with the best will in the world, there are some patients whom we cannot help, if only for the reason that there are, and will always be, conditions that are incurable.

Still, most doctors, especially the young and conscientious, feel a strong need to relieve all human suffering so far as is possible within their powers. Unfortunately, in psychological, just as in physical medicine relieving suffering at all costs may lead to calamity. We had to learn, for instance, that in vague abdominal cases suspected of appendicitis it is inadvisable to give morphia, because the relief of pain may mask relevant developments, and the doctor may be lulled into a false security. Something similar is true of many cases in psychological medicine. The fact is far from being generally recognized. On the whole, whenever there is some sign of mental suffering or anxiety, the first thing that the doctor does is to attempt "to reassure" the patient, hoping to relieve the suffering. Good examples of this hopeful attitude are Cases 15 and 17. The results are the same as in physical medicine. If the doctor succeeds in relieving the pain, the symptoms may become masked, may even completely disappear, and both doctor and patient may remain in the dark about the real cause of the illness, while more often than not the pathological process progresses, eventually making any therapy most difficult, or even hopeless.

It is easy to advise the doctor, "no treatment before diagnosis," that is, to give the patient no reassurance before knowing what is wrong with him. The doctor accepts this advice intellectually, but cannot follow it because of his own emotions, i.e. his need to behave according to his apostolic function. Witnessing anxiety or mental pain without doing anything is felt to be cruel, unhelpful, inhuman; and so, instead of waiting to see how the symptoms develop, the doctor, to relieve his own conscience, resorts to routine, wholesale reassurance or supportive therapy. We often ask in the seminar the unpleasant question, "Reassurance or support—for whom?" In most cases it is the doctor who needs—and gets—reassurance and support. Whether patients benefit from it is another matter.

Let me reiterate what I said in Chapter X, that reassurance is not in itself necessarily wrong. It may even be a powerful drug which, if correctly prescribed, can be highly beneficial. The trouble with it is that it is prescribed wholesale, without proper diagnosis. Describing the same process from the opposite angle, reassurance is much too often administered for the benefit of the doctor, who cannot bear the burden of either not knowing enough or of being unable to help. More often than is admitted, the same is true of the various specialist examinations asked for, and of many of the drugs prescribed.

On the whole there is a good deal of truth in the paradoxical statement that "reassurance" and *placebos* have a much better effect in physical conditions, especially in the case of fairly normal, not very neurotic people afflicted with some organic illness; but their effectiveness decreases rapidly the more that personality problems become the important factor. Although this is a fairly well substantiated experience, doctors have to go on giving "simple supportive treatment," "advice" and, above all, "reassurance," proving to their own satisfaction that they are good doctors and that only the illness—or the patient—is to blame if things do not improve.

We all know the extreme case of this urge to help, the *furor therapeuticus*, against the dangers of which every experienced medical teacher should and does warn his students. On the other hand, little has been written about the compulsive need of certain patients to have a "bad," useless, therapeutically impotent doctor. This is because few practitioners can tolerate this rôle, and still fewer can adapt themselves to it with their eyes open. The overwhelming majority of us, driven by our apostolic zeal, have to

do everything possible to impress our patients—and ourselves—
that we are good, helpful, doctors. These two opposing tendencies
—the doctor's need to be helpful and the patient's need to prove
that his doctor is useless—usually lead to strain. Our next case
history, Case 26, reported by Dr. G., shows this strain, and
the somewhat unorthodox methods chosen by the doctor to
relieve it.

CASE 26

Mr. Z.* is a man of 58 and has been on Dr. G.'s list since May 1939;
but his medical history goes back to 1925, i.e. for thirty years, sixteen
of which were with his present doctor. During all this time he has
never ceased complaining. He has had pains in his rectum which "made
him faint," numbness in his left leg, bad headaches "only relieved by
military march on the wireless." He feels terrible when waiting for
trains and buses, and becomes giddy when standing about. He knows
"he will never get rid of the giddiness until he is in his box." His
indigestion is "shocking," and to prove it some of the interviews with
his doctor are punctuated by belches. In addition, he suffers from
shortness of breath, "nerves," and always feels blown up, has pains in
every part of the body, and so on.

Of course he has been seen during the thirty years by innumerable
specialists; in fact his notes require a special case. The diagnosis has
varied from neurosis, through nervous debility and hypochondriasis,
to neurasthenia. Apart from these rather irrelevant and unhelpful tags,
the specialists' reports contain only negative findings such as no
carcinoma in rectum, barium meal and cholecystography negative,
chest clear, and so on. I have to add that the psychiatrist's report is in
exactly the same vein .

In spite of all this, the patient has been able to maintain a good
enough relation to his wife; and, although they have no children and
intercourse occurs but rarely, his wife describes him as a "good
husband." Moreover, in the past twenty-five years he has only been
away from work for two to three weeks, though he had been in a
responsible and at times strenuous job as an examiner in a large factory.

Mr. Z. must have come to the conclusion a good many years ago
that doctors can do nothing for him, as no medicine has ever made
any difference to his complaints. Still, during all this time he has come
almost every Friday evening for a bottle of medicine. Every time he
says, "Nobody can do me any good." The doctor has learnt to accept
this criticism and to go on prescribing a new medicine if it is asked for.

* This report was published in *The Lancet* (1955), April 2, pp. 683–8.

Sometimes he has even taken down the pharmacopœia and said, "I have given you everything in this book, and nothing has done you any good. Will you choose now what you would like?" Mark you, this was never said in irritation or annoyance, but in a friendly and, although defeated, still sincerely sympathetic tone. Mr. Z., incidentally, seems to like these scenes; perhaps he accepts them as a sign of confidence in him!

Dr. G. summed up the situation as follows—

Over the years I have established a relationship with the patient in which I accept that nothing does him any good, and commiserate with him; we metaphorically slap each other on the back, more or less cheerfully, when he attends for his weekly bottle of medicine, which we both agree will not do him any good. He has no resentment towards me, and he does not regard me as incompetent because I cannot cure him. In fact, I am a good fellow; not like some of those other doctors. He has some pride in his toughness in resisting the bad effects of my medicines and tablets, and especially in his ability to carry on in spite of the considerable cross he has to bear "unlike some of the weak-kneed younger men of today." He is no worry to me. He senses when I want him to go, and disappears quickly. If I am busy, he comes in, and is prepared to leave without much discussion, telling me happily that, "there is a mob in the waiting-room." He is on my side, in fact.

Dr. G. could have ended his report equally truthfully, "I am on his side, in fact have been for many years."

It is obvious that the patient has been offering his doctor illness after illness. Faithful to his training, and to his apostolic function, Dr. G. patiently examined every offer, and then asked the counsel of his more learned brethren, but had to reject every offer as unacceptable. During this "unorganized" period, the patient gradually withdrew into his "you doctors are no good but I can take it because I am tough" attitude. If we accept the year 1925 as the beginning of the "unorganized" period—very likely it started earlier—the patient was then twenty-eight. As the history shows, Mr. Z. has developed and "organized" a fairly severe illness during the years, and some people may think it improbable that any medical treatment could have had much effect on him. It must be stated, however, that he was never given the opportunity "to start." It is legitimate to ask what Mr. Z.'s fate would have been if, instead of sending him to specialist after specialist and prescribing him bottles and bottles of medicine, early in his history some doctor had sat down with him for a "long interview" in the right way and at a right moment. Who knows?

Anyhow, Mr. Z. settled down and created and "organized" an impressive illness involving his whole life. Although the superficial symptoms varied and changed, the b..sic structure of the illness remained the same, and became firmer and firmer with the years. One aspect of his illness was to play hell with his practitioner, to rub in time and time again that he was "no good" and "absolutely useless." The possibility cannot be altogether excluded that this was partly a revenge for Dr. G.'s rejection of the patient's "offers." It is not mentioned in the report, but we can well imagine that there were a number of not very pleasant periods for Dr. G. He asked for help from his specialist colleagues, but received only negative advice; that is, he was told what *not* to do, but no help whatever was given him on how to help his patient and, in particular, no advice on "how to start." I wonder how many of us, whether general practitioners, specialists, or even psychiatrists, would have remained, under this irritating fire, as calm and imperturbable, as friendly and sympathetic, as Dr. G. How many of us would have thought of taking down the pharmacopoeia from its shelf and in all sincerity offering it to the patient so that he might choose a medicine he thought might help?

It was this atmosphere of unshakable, friendly sympathy that enabled Mr. Z. to make his peace with his "bad" and "useless" doctor and to accept his companionship through all the troubled years of illness, pain, and suffering. He was obviously badly in need of company, and without his doctor he would not have been able to keep going and maintain a tolerable, or perhaps even a not completely unhappy, private life.

To sum up. In this case all the organic illnesses proposed by the patient were rejected one by one, but the doctor accepted the pain and the suffering and honestly tried to relieve them. This counter-proposition of his was in turn rejected by the patient, who—perhaps prompted also by his resentment—wanted his doctor to be bad and impotent. The doctor accepted this last proposition, i.e. that he could not relieve the suffering and pain, and also agreed to remain friendly and sympathetic. On these terms a working compromise was established, and patient and doctor settled down to a form of illness acceptable to both.*

Now suppose that this patient had been on the list of a doctor who, because of his personality, must be a good and helpful man, whose apostolic function compels him to try everything in his power to cure his patients without exception—or mercy. . . .

Let us now return to the main topic of this chapter, the doctor's apostolic function. Every doctor willy-nilly creates a unique atmosphere by his individual ways of "practising" medicine and then tries to convert his patients to accept it. To demonstrate the unique atmosphere characteristic of every doctor—the most important phenomenon on the apostolic function—it was decided to identify by a letter of the alphabet each practitioner who took part in our seminars. In this way, while preserving anonymity, the individuality of each is easily recognizable. I should like to add that no criticism is implied in any of this drawing attention to individualities; on the contrary, it indicates the greater potentialities inherent in medical "responses." It is extremely doubtful whether any doctor is capable of achieving a degree of elasticity sufficient to include all the helpful variants reported in this book, and others besides. But there is no harm in setting one's aims high.

Now let us review these individual atmospheres. In this book, cases of fifteen doctors are quoted. Twelve belong to the "old guard" of fourteen who were my companions in the first full-scale project, one (Case 6) dropped out, and two (Cases 17 and 27) belong to a more recent group. In what follows I propose to use only those who are represented by more than one case. There are six of them. I wish to apologize to the other nine for leaving them out, and to the six because my description will almost certainly strike them as a kind of caricature. The picture, though not complete, will be recognizable to their colleagues, while the victim will certainly feel indignant about nice things about him being omitted, not nice things being exaggerated, thus unfairly distorting the result.

Let us start with Dr. S. As shown by his cases (15, 25 and 28) he is a benevolent authoritarian; kind, good-humoured and patient, and willing to put up with a good deal of awkward behaviour so long as the patient accepts him as a "wise old bird"

---

* See, however, the follow-up of this case in the Appendix.

who knows best and does his best. But when the patient defies his avuncular authority, shows lack of respect, or even rejects his help, Dr. S. can be hard and difficult to reconcile. For the same reason he is very cautious not to go out of his depth. Until that point he gives good service, beyond it he simply stops.

Compare him with Dr. R., perhaps the most marked representative in the group of the irresistible urge to be a good doctor. He is conscientious, circumspect, willing to go well out of his way to discover the psychological roots of his patient's behaviour. He is generous with his time, but his patients have to recognize him as a good doctor and sooner or later have to show their recognition by responding to his treatment; in fact, it is very difficult for him to accept failure. Three of his cases reported here, Cases 4, 10 and 23, all show these features. In addition, he is deeply convinced, and we had several opportunities of witnessing him converting his patients to the "psychosomatic belief." (One example is printed in Chapter XIV, Case 23.) In his apostolic zeal he can be intrepid, even impetuous.

Quite different is the atmosphere created by Dr. G. He is cautious and expects to be respected, somewhat like Dr. S. Similarly, he dislikes going out of his depth; on the other hand, once the patient has been started off, Dr. G. can follow him— though somewhat reluctantly—to rather surprising depths. But as soon as possible he returns to safety, and then it is difficult to take him for a second ride. He has had enough, and the patient is invariably converted to being content, and making do, with what he has got. Remarkably, Dr. G. is able to achieve so much in one "long interview" that his patients apparently are able to accept this policy and benefit by it. His cases 16, 19 and 26 illustrate all these points.

Dr. C. is our senior member, with a sheer inexhaustible patience. We were more than once amazed at the tolerance and equanimity with which he put up with patients of the most exceptional awkwardness and difficulty, whom all the rest of us would long since have given up, got rid of, or firmly restrained, while he carried on unperturbed, shrugging his shoulders at our short patience and hasty opinions—often to the successful conclusion of a difficult treatment. Neither of the two cases which are quoted here (Cases 12 and 20) shows the full extent of his patience, but both show enough of it to make an impression.

His patience enabled him to accumulate a rare collection of impossible cases—among them a woman who has been pregnant since 1947; several paranoias rejected by mental hospitals; a woman of fifty, for several years a chronic invalid with rheumatic backaches, unsuccessfully treated by several hospitals, who has been working since Dr. G. "treated" her back; about fifty Pakistanis who cannot speak English but come to complain about their sexual difficulties, and so on. May I add that on more than one occasion he has warmly thanked me for having saved him from the boredom of routine medical practice, but, once added, "Sometimes, after a very long day, I wish you hadn't."

Then there is the versatile Dr. M. (Cases 1 and 21), who was able to carry out with one and the same patient a fairly deep-going psychotherapy, enabling her to accept womanhood and pregnancy, and then—without any jolt—switch over to mid-wifery, looking after her during the pregnancy, delivering the baby, and ending up as the trusted doctor of the whole family.

And lastly Dr. H., whom we followed in Chapter XV from crisis to crisis, weathering all storms and eventually achieving a very remarkable cure.

All these six atmospheres are unique, each of them utterly different from any of the others. Moreover, what can be said about these six doctors could be said about every doctor. What is equally remarkable is the patient's adaptability, or, to use our newly-coined term, convertibility. The doctor, it is true, cannot help but be himself, and, however elastic in his "practice," must act as his apostolic zeal prompts him; as a rule it is the patient who is converted, and then can make use of the doctor's services.

In the seminars we often played the game of asking what would have happened if patient X. had gone to another doctor. It is an instructive and amusing game; imagine, for instance, Miss F.'s fate (Case 12) if she had been on the list of the intrepid Dr. R. or the versatile Dr. M. instead of on that of the patient and long-suffering Dr. C. What would have happened to Peter (Case 19) under Dr. S. or Dr. H.?

Implicit in this parlour game, however, is a serious problem, namely, which atmosphere, which apostolic belief, would give the patient the best chances for recovery? Would Peter have fared better without the "Smith" and under the benevolent, avuncular guidance of Dr. S., or with a fairly deep psychotherapy under Dr. H., possibly involving several upheavals? Which of these doctors would have given him the best chance? Or, would Miss F. have been converted successfully to Dr. R.'s psycho-somatic belief, ending up in marriage, as happened in Cases 10 and 23? Would Dr. M. have been able to make her accept the feminine rôle as he did in Case 21? Or would she have run away from either of these doctors?

These are cardinal problems, not only of general practitioner psychotherapy but of all psychotherapy, and they are far from being solved. They are, in many ways, unsolved problems for the psychiatrist too. Most of what he knows about these processes is contained in the psychoanalytic literature on the theory and practice of "interpretation." It must, however, be stressed that, in spite of the many papers written on this subject, our knowledge is very much in its infancy. Then there is the much smaller litera-ture on "acting out" by patients, and how the therapist should deal with it. But all this refers only to events in the strictly controlled psychoanalytic situation. The extent to which these findings will prove to be applicable in general practice remains to be seen. In Chapter XIII, I discussed some significant facts which cannot fail to make us psychoanalysts cautious in extending the rules of psy-choanalytic technique in their present form to psychotherapy in the doctor's surgery. We know too little to be dogmatic.

The seminar found the consequences of this unsatisfactory but undeniable state of affairs difficult to accept. Time and again general practitioners asked the psychiatrist to teach them what was right and what was wrong. Only with reluctance did they come to accept the fact that we do not know enough to be able to lay down hard and fast rules, to state categorically that this approach was definitely wrong, that technique questionable, this attitude certainly helpful, that interpretation timely and correct. The psychiatrist, however pressed, could point out problems and possibilities, but only seldom could he give positive advice.

His chief way out was to emphasize again and again that we were members of a research team, exploring and trying to map out hitherto unexplored regions of medicine. This leads us back to our point of departure, the recognition of the need for a pharmacology of the most frequently prescribed drug, the doctor. The study of the "apostolic function" is perhaps the most direct way of studying the chief—the therapeutic—effect of this drug.

CHAPTER XVIII

The Doctor and His Patient

IN the two previous chapters I discussed at some length the doctor's apostolic function, which compels him to convert his patients to his own standards and beliefs. From another aspect the process of conversion may be described as education or training. I have mentioned several times that in the last hundred years or so we doctors have successfully trained our patients, in fact the whole population of the western world, to expect a routine clinical examination and to accept it without much embarrassment or apprehension. I have also pointed out that doctors have not trained their patients to expect a frank discussion of their personal problems as a necessary part of the examination. This lack of training, however, does not seem to be an insurmountable obstacle. To repeat what was said in a previous chapter, several doctors reported that, as the rumour of their psychological interest had time to spread in the neighbourhood i.e. a year or so after they had started to give "long interviews," patients on other doctor's lists came to them for psychological examination.

Some more or less spectacular examples of this sort of education were discussed in Chapter XVI, such as the problem of night calls, of changing from one doctor to another, etc. Another, more important field of this education is the training of the patient to adopt the right attitude towards his illness. By right attitude I mean one that creates good possibilities for therapy.

It is difficult to describe in detail what this process of education should aim at and what methods it should use, because it has so many different aspects. In general, one would like to say that patients should be educated to mature responsibility towards their illness; but it is necessary to add a rider; with certain outlets for dependent childishness. As so often in medical practice, here too the problem is that of proportion; how much maturity should be demanded, and how much childlike dependence on the doctor should be tolerated? Or, in other words, how much pain suffering, discomfort, limitation and restriction, fear and guilt, should the patient bear unaided, and at what point should the doctor start supporting him? In general, the greater the maturity of the patient, the better will be the results of a purely "objective treatment" and the less will be the patient's need of "subjective sympathetic therapy," and vice versa. Here we find another important field of medical practice unconditionally surrendered to the doctor's common sense, i.e. his apostolic function. This is the more regrettable as by his approach he prepares the ground for the future. One might almost say that the general practitioner, in fact, starts the treatment while the patient is well, and that the actual treatment prescribed when illness occurs is only a continuation of a treatment already in progress. Incidentally, this is not necessarily the case with us specialists.

Of course, the process of education is most intense during an illness, either of the patient himself or of one of his close relatives, neighbours or friends. In the initial stage of an acute illness, when the patient is still under the impact of the first shock, that is, his illness is still "unorganized," the doctor is usually a support, allowing the patient to become dependent on him. When the first shock has passed, and the illness, instead of disappearing, becomes "organized," takes up a chronic form, if at all possible the general practitioner will try to enlist the patient's collaboration in working out an acceptable compromise between his accustomed ways of life and the demands of the illness. In other words, the aim should be to make the patient the umpire in this compromise, but it is rather seldom that this can be fully achieved. Few people have the degree of mental and emotional maturity necessary for such a difficult task. The two well-known extremes are the over-exacting patient, who cannot allow himself any relaxation, and the over-demanding and over-anxious patient, who cannot have enough. Here obviously great variations are needed, according to the patient's mental and in particular emotional maturity. Every illness, however slight, always means acquiescing in the renunciation of part of one's accustomed freedom and pleasures. Incidentally, it often happens that young people are able more easily to accept these bitter facts than older ones.

In educating the patient the doctor is greatly helped by what may be called the patient's pride in his illness. This is especially noticeable if it is a rare illness, or if the patient succeeds in coping with it to a commendable degree. This attitude is in no way peculiar to illness. Every form of growing up or maturing is greatly helped by the individual's pride in his achievements.

One must not forget, however, that the doctor is faced with great technical difficulties in this field. We have not had time to study this question in detail in our research, so all I can do is to make some brief and disjointed observations on the matter. One of the problems is *how much regression*, i.e. *returning from adult to more primitive, childish behaviour, should be permitted to the patient, and when*. In some cases the doctor may be compelled to advise his patient—or to push him gently or even forcibly—out of his maturity into some regressive, dependent attitude. There are some people who have to assume and carry more responsibility than is good for them, especially when they are ill. The opposite problem is *how much maturity should be demanded from any individual, how fast, and at what point*. As is well known, some people simply cannot bear any increase of their responsibility or apprehensions, and if it is thrust upon them they have to shed it by becoming dependent on some authority.

A well-known way of helping patients suffering from some irreversible, chronic illness which has to be accepted with all its consequences is to arrange for them to meet somebody who has achieved a good adaptation to the same problem. For some people it is easier to imitate than to devise a method for themselves.

The doctor must be on his guard, however, because *any privation imposed on the individual by his illness may be felt as coming from the doctor*. For instance, many patients feel that if only the doctor were kinder or more sympathetic, he would allow them more drinks, later hours, more interesting food, more smoking, etc. It is easy to observe the gradual emergence of this resentment, but it is much more difficult to cope with it or to prevent it. This resentful fantasy often leads to feelings of anger and hatred against the doctor for his lack of understanding, unsympathetic prescriptions and strict dietetic regulations; leading to irritation, and often—as a reaction to it—to fears and anxieties that the doctor might retaliate in kind. On the other hand, for some people, especially those suffering from unconscious guilt or those of masochistic tendencies, any strict diet or mode of life is readily acceptable, because suffering means some relief from their guilt.

We know much too little about these problems. On the other hand, for the study of the problem of maturity—or, in psychological terms, of the strength of the ego—general practice is a most promising field. People's behaviour when falling ill or when first realizing that they are ill, and their ways and methods of coping with the consequences of chronic illness, could provide as rich material as have observations of maturing children. Some intriguing problems belonging to this sphere are: What are the factors that determine the development of a childish-dependent, or a mature-independent attitude towards the illness? Are these attitudes inherent in the illness, in the patient's individuality, or are they brought about—or perhaps only reinforced—by the interplay between the patient's "offers" and the doctor's "responses?" We have come back again to the pharmacology of the drug "doctor," this time to one of its most important side-effects. And again, I have to ask for more research by general practitioners, because it is they who first see the patient when he falls ill, and it is they who can continuously observe the development of his ways of coping with the illness.

Every doctor will, I think, agree that *the patient's attitude towards his illness* is of paramount importance for any therapy, and that it is the doctor's task to "educate" the patient to become co-operative. I wish to illustrate some of the difficulties encountered in this field by a case history. The case chosen, though somewhat complicated, is not unusual. The complications were caused by the interaction of several factors, some of them already discussed: the child as the presenting symptom (Chapter III); the intervention of a consultant, leading to all the complications described in Chapters VII–IX; and the consequences of giving or not giving a name to the illness (Chapter VI). Then there was present a not admitted disagreement between consultant and general practitioner about the aims and methods of training—in this case the patient's parents; and lastly the factor to be discussed in the next chapter, the patient's—here the parents'—need for the illness to be taken seriously. The general practitioner, though right in all other points, failed to notice this need; thus his diagnosis of the whole situation remained incomplete—not "deep" enough; his treatment of the case and his training aims and methods, though objectively correct, became unacceptable to the parents and they had to change their doctor.

In one of our recent seminars a general practitioner reported Case 27 as follows—

CASE 27

A twelve-year-old girl was very ill with high temperature of unknown origin. I had no idea what was the matter with her. The parents were very, very nervous and worried people, and so the moment I guessed this I said, "Why not call someone in?" and they said, "That's just what we felt." So I said, "Shall I call somebody?" and they said, "Yes," but then the grandmother rang up and said she had a relative, a child specialist. The relative came and said, "This is paratyphoid," but in my opinion it was not.

Anyway, the next day came, and the mother said, "The child has paratyphoid, what should we do?" and, though I said, "I don't know whether this is so sure," knowing that he was a specialist, I did not dare to say I did not believe it, so I said that we must wait for the bacteriological examination and that we would leave things to the specialist. So we did. The stools were negative. The parents rang up in the meanwhile twice daily for stool reports, it was really dreadful for everybody. The specialist was called again and said, "There is no doubt this is paratyphoid."

He was an extremely nice specialist, and even came to see me. We had coffee and drinks together. I learnt from him—he stayed about an hour—his life history. He is certainly very clever, and he talked a lot. He knows everybody, he lectures and he has appointments. I explained to him there were many problems involved, e.g. that I was a National Health Service practitioner, who had to pay two calls a day and answer telephone calls during the night because a specialist said it was paratyphoid. I proposed the child should go into hospital, partly to get her off my hands, and also in order not to bear the responsibility, because I really did not know what the illness was. He said he had so much experience of paratyphoid, and he was always there if needed.

The next day I had half an hour with the mother, because she refused that the child should go into hospital. She said the child would be unhappy to go into hospital and could not get things there. I told her that *she* would be very unhappy without the child. By the way, the child is a twelve-year-old, very intelligent girl. I tried to persuade the mother to accept the view that she was approaching the situation egotistically, and that it would be best for everybody, and especially for the child, however hard it might be for her. She insisted on seeing the specialist again, and he told her the child need not go into hospital. This was on Saturday, and on the same night the father came to fetch me and I had to go there. On Sunday he came again; I was not at home, but he got from my wife the name of the doctor on duty. The doctor said the child must go to hospital, and they rang up the specialist again. The specialist said on the telephone to ring up the G.P. On Monday morning I got the blood report. It was not paratyphoid, but glandular fever. So everybody was wrong. The girl was still at home, but I got a telephone call that I need not go there any more because they realized that another doctor would be better for the whole family; and I also have come to the same conclusion.

Now, there were a number of people involved. First, the personality of the consultant. He talked much, he is a very nice, very clever man, and the diagnosis paratyphoid was certainly one of many which should be considered—but he stated his opinion emphatically and to the parents. I discussed this problem when he was with me, and he insisted it was the best thing to tell the parents the serious diagnosis. I disagreed with this. I thought of telling them it was a chill, but he refused. Now, he is a good children's specialist, and he impressed me very much, because he knows a lot better than I. I tried to insist on a less serious diagnosis, or on sending the girl to hospital. He disagreed with me, and told the parents exactly the opposite of what I had told them, and the parents lost confidence in me. Really it is not an easy problem to solve.

There are many interesting problems in this case history which were eagerly taken up by the seminar. First, was it wise to accept an unknown specialist, proposed by the family, especially as he was a relative? An unknown specialist always means hazards for the general practitioner, as no working relationship has yet been established between them. If any disagreement arises, usually the specialist's greater reputation carries the day, which in the long run may not always be a gain for the patient. This danger is doubtless increased when the specialist has ties of kinship or friendship with the family.

It was only after further questioning that we found out that at the specialist's first visit the two doctors duly examined the girl together, withdrew for discussion, but could not agree on the diagnosis. The specialist insisted that it was paratyphoid, while the general practitioner remained unconvinced, and did not want to commit himself. In the end the specialist's opinion prevailed and was communicated to the family without mentioning that the general practitioner did not agree with it; in this way the thinly disguised disagreement between the two doctors and the concomitant underground strife were started off.

Interestingly enough, the point about which the two doctors openly disagreed was whether the girl should or should not go to hospital. This was partly due to the difference in their professional relationship with the family; one was a specialist, called in only occasionally and paid for each of his visits, the other a panel doctor who had day and night to be at the service of over-anxious and rather inconsiderate parents whose demands went far beyond what was "objectively" reasonable. The problem is what to do with such people, how to "educate" them to a "reasonable" attitude. I shall come back to this, but first I wish to mention one more topic of the discussion.

We turned to the question of how it happened that the specialist visited the patient twice without the general practitioner. Should a doctor put up with this? Had the specialist behaved correctly? Further details were disclosed, and we learnt that the first such visit had taken place on the doctor's half-day off. The family had had another attack of anxiety, bombarded both the doctor's house and the specialist with telephone calls, but the specialist had correctly refused to visit the child alone. In the end the doctor's wife had telephoned him and asked him as a favour to go and reassure the family; it was only then that the specialist agreed to go.

This is a good example of how difficult it is for two doctors with different apostolic beliefs to understand each other. It is true that the issue in this case was complicated by subsidiary factors, above all their difference in status, and their disagreement about the diagnosis. The latter, however, was a minor problem in this case, although scientific, objective medicine would certainly put the chief emphasis on it. So did our doctor, who was really hurt that, in spite of the undeniable fact that his diagnosis had been correct, he was made the scapegoat and punished at the end.

This case is also exceptional in that both general practitioner and specialist were not only absolutely correct and superficially co-operative, but also tried to be really friendly, to the extent of sitting down, having a long talk and getting to know each other —a rather uncommon event. Yet, in spite of all this good will they simply did not arrive at a mutual understanding.

One of the reasons for this confusion of tongues was the difference in their apostolic beliefs about how much anxiety a patient—or her parents—should be expected to bear unaided; the other, however, was that they stopped at a superficial level of diagnosis. It is true that they disagreed on this level, but the difference between paratyphoid, glandular fever, or high temperature of unknown origin, provided the febrile condition does not last longer than, say, a week, is not terribly important in general practice, though admittedly important for scientific medicine. I am prepared to be taken seriously to task by scientifically-minded doctors, and I readily agree that in some cases the differential diagnosis may be essential for the right treatment, but perhaps I might be permitted to ask irreverently: In what percentage of the cases treated in general practice? And further, is its importance so great that it is permissible to stop at that level and totally neglect the "deeper" diagnosis? This was exactly what our general practitioner did in this case, and though his doubts about the superficial diagnosis of paratyphoid proved to be justified, his eventual punishment was perhaps not so unfair, because of his failure to aim at a "deeper," more comprehensive, diagnosis.

The seminar came to the obvious conclusion that there exist people who must be allowed to become anxious if anything goes wrong, and that their anxiety must be accepted and properly treated by the doctor. They have to be frightened, and if the doctor sets about reassuring them they have to run from pillar to post till they find a reason to be frightened. These people have to have a serious illness, a chill will not do for them. In this way the specialist was right—though his superficial diagnosis was wrong—and the general practitioner, in spite of his correct superficial diagnosis, was unhelpful. His failure was the greater as he had known the family well for years.

Thus, the doctor's first task is to arrive at a better, more comprehensive, diagnosis. The next question is what to do next. If he can find out why the patient—or the patient's parents—have to be frightened, he should obviously aim at diagnosing the cause and at treating it. Unfortunately, in fairly serious cases such as that just reported this is but seldom within the general practitioner's possibilities. But, if he cannot do this, he must still give the patient a rational symptomatic treatment. In a case of headaches, for instance, in which no cause can be found, the patient has to be given something—aspirin, codeine, and so on—or he will not be able to carry on, either with life in general or with his doctor. That brings us back to our subject, the education of the patient to a sensible attitude towards his—or his child's—illness. When should we give palliatives, how much, and for how long? When should we stop or reduce them and ask the patient, in his own interest, to accept a certain amount of suffering or anxiety as inevitable? As already stated, we do not know enough about these eminently psychological problems and must ask for further research.

In this case history we discussed the needs of over-anxious people. This, however, is only one special case. All patients "offer" us their various needs, and we doctors must "respond" to them in one way or another. By far the commonest answer is to *give* the patient something. Perhaps the doctor's most frustrating experience is being unable to give anything "rational." This giving, however, has another aspect. With it, especially if we are convinced that what we are giving is "good" for the patient, we push the blame on to him. Henceforward it will be his fault if he does not get better.

In the seminars we often had cause to wonder whether a prescription had really been given for the patient's or the doctor's benefit. It is important for any mutually satisfactory relationship that both should be able to feel that something "good" has been done, otherwise the conclusion is inevitable that the doctor is in some way the cause of the suffering by failing to cure or relieve it. Some patients slide irresistibly into this hostile conclusion, most of them because of their personality, and some perhaps justifiably. What is more interesting and more important for our subject is that there are a number of doctors who feel the same, i.e. that they have failed the patient. The majority of these are recruited from young general practitioners. Junior hospital staff have ample opportunities for diluting their responsibility, and—except perhaps during a surgical intervention—it is rare for one doctor alone to be responsible for a patient in hospital. But the general practitioner is nearly always alone with his patient, and has no institutional means of diluting his heavy responsibility. No wonder, then, that he has to try everything to convince himself that he has really given his patient something of value.

I must mention again that our knowledge of the dynamic factors active in the doctor–patient relationship is uncertain and scanty, and that we do not even know whether we are aware of all the important factors. Here at any rate is a sample of them. In the first place, the patient is nearly always frightened, though to a varying degree, and he is in the dark. He comes to the doctor, who knows. Then the patient is afraid about the future, and expects comfort. Often he is suffering, and hopes for relief. Patients have to face the fact that they are ill, i.e. temporarily or perhaps permanently incapacitated. Some are really grateful when the doctor, so to speak, allows them to be ill; others deeply resent it. The doctor has often to be the umpire in a complicated reality situation, such as when a patient is overdriving himself to cope with his responsibilities and his family expects this from him, or when a seriously ill patient is not properly looked after, or a patient with a non-incapacitating chronic condition demands inordinate attention and care from his relatives, and so on, *ad infinitum.*

As will be seen from this enumeration, there are many factors in every doctor–patient relationship which push the patient into a dependent-childish relationship to his doctor. This is inevitable, and the only question is how much dependence is desirable. The obvious answer is that it will depend on the nature of the illness, the patient's personality, and—we propose to add—the doctor's individual apostolic beliefs. This beautiful and true sentence, however, is only a cloak for our ignorance. The real question is how much dependence constitutes a good starting-point for a successful therapy and when does it turn into an obstacle. At the beginning of the chapter we discussed the necessity of educating the patient to a reasonably mature attitude towards his—or his child's—illness. How do childish dependence and a reasonably mature attitude fare together, how much of each must be taken in order to obtain a good therapeutic mixture? For the time being we can only point to these important problems, but cannot offer any well-founded answers. The only thing we know for certain is that common sense, i.e. apostolic belief, is an unreliable and untrustworthy guide.

To quote two common instances in which the doctor has to solve this problem of finding the right proportions: How often should a chronic invalid be visited, and how much time should be spent with him on each occasion? When should daily, or even twice-daily, visits be discontinued in an improving acute illness?

Apart from the complicated question of fees, what is the right "practice" that creates a good basis in the patient as well as in his environment for the treatment of any future illness? As the last case history shows, the answer to these questions is far from self-evident or a matter of simple common sense.

The lack of properly validated techniques in this highly important field is the more regrettable as the doctor's relationship with his patients—if we disregard the "nomads" (see Chapter XIX)—is lasting and intimate. Whatever he does cannot fail to influence his patient, and these influences will add up in the long run. In this respect it does not make much difference whether the patient pays fees, i.e. whether he feels in some way that the doctor is his personal servant, or whether some anonymous institution appoints the doctor, lending him a reflected halo of authority with all the ambivalence fostered by it.

The important thing is that the education is not one-sided only. Both patient and doctor grow together into a better knowledge of each other. This mutual influencing is not a simple process, developing either in an entirely good or entirely bad direction. Both doctor and patient alike must learn to bear some frustration. The doctor is not automatically available when he is wanted, he does not like to be called out during the night or on Sundays, and even if he comes, he cannot cure everything immediately; some pain and some anxiety must remain unrelieved, at any rate for some time. In the same way, the patient is often not appreciative of the great service that the doctor renders him, does not show gratitude, is inconsiderate, makes unreasonable demands, is disrespectful, etc., etc. On the other hand, there are joint memories of such things as a correct diagnosis and timely action which averted a major danger, of the many little acts of help readily given and gratefully accepted in many a petty trouble, of some serious shock which the doctor helped to bear, and so on.

It is on this basis of mutual satisfaction and mutual frustration that a unique relationship establishes itself between a general practitioner and those of his patients who stay with him. It is very difficult to describe this relationship in psychological terms. It is not love, or mutual respect, or mutual identification, or friendship, though elements of all these enter into it. We termed it—for want of a better term—a "mutual investment company." By this we mean that the general practitioner gradually acquires a very valuable capital invested in his patient, and, *vice versa*, the patient acquires a very valuable capital bestowed in his general practitioner.

In his long years of acquaintance with his patient the general practitioner gradually learns a vast amount of important details. He knows the patient's background, several members—often several generations—of his family, the type of people who are his friends, the shop, office or factory where he works, the street and the neighbourhood where he lives, etc. He knows what his friends or neighbours say or gossip about him, what his work record is, how he got to know his wife, and what kind of children he has. But these are only the minor capital assets. The real assets are—as we have just seen—the common experiences in health and especially in sickness, how often and with what sort of complaints the patient comes for medical advice, how he behaves when something unexpected happens, when a member of his family falls seriously ill or dies, or when he has a minor or major illness. In the same way the patient learns how much and what kind of help he can expect from his doctor. Obviously it is of paramount importance that these capital assets, the result of persistent hard work on both sides to gain the other's confidence and to convert him to one's beliefs, should not be wasted, that is to say, that they should be used in such a way as to yield an adequate return to both patient and doctor.

Here again I have to repeat my refrain. This is a most important field, which medical science has neglected. One of the reasons for the neglect of the problem is that the research workers—our hospital specialists—have hardly any contact with it. It is the general practitioner's domain, in fact it is his daily work. It is only he who can find out which methods can be used with profit and which methods are to be avoided when "educating" his patients, when building up and managing the assets of the mutual investment company.

The consultant, in contrast to the general practitioner, is no party to this mutual investment company; he has to start from scratch, unless the general practitioner is able to prepare both his patient and his consultant for the interview. In other words, the general practitioner should be able to mobilize and lend part of the capital invested in him by his patient to be used during the specialist's examinations. That this does not happen as often as it should is the fault of general practitioners and specialists alike. The oft-quoted request, " ? chest, please see and advise," is just as helpful in this respect as some of the letters by specialists quoted in this book. On the other hand, the consultant has advantages of other kinds; he is an outsider, a stranger, his approach is fresh, his views not biased by previous experiences with the patients The illness for him is not so much a human as a scientific problem. Similarly, to the patient the consultant is an unknown V.I.P., a blank sheet, a higher authority to whom he can look up; whereas his doctor is an old acquaintance, whom he knows only too well, with all his habits, human weaknesses, even his personal problems and shortcomings.

A further aspect of the difference between the casual consultant–patient relationship and the mutual investment company is its duration. Consultants (including those in the psychiatric departments of hospitals) usually see a patient a few times only, and hardly ever follow up the results of their examinations or therapeutic efforts. As we all know from the literature, a reliable and thorough follow-up is such a rare event that its results are usually published. The general practitioner is in an entirely different position because, whether he likes it or not, he has to follow up his cases; the majority of his patients come back to him—either grateful or grumbling—again and again. Somehow general practitioners seem to be reluctant to talk about their follow-up experiences, though in fact they could be the real judges. They content themselves with complaining about inefficient consultants, but only rarely do they pluck up courage and spare the time necessary to put their experiences constructively in writing.

CHAPTER XIX

The Patient and His Illness

THE preceding chapters—in fact, nearly the whole book—
have been taken up by discussion of the doctor–patient
relationship. This certainly cannot be altogether right. An
illness starts before the doctor appears on the scene, in some cases
considerably before. I remember well one of my clinical teachers
repeating a pet phrase to us students, "How much easier would
the doctor's task be if only cancer, syphilis and being dirty caused
pain!" Unfortunately there are other illnesses which do not cause
enough pain, discomfort or fear, and permit the patient to stay
away for much too long. Conversely, this means that there must
be a relationship between the patient and his illness, irrespective
of any doctor.

This is undeniably true, and it must be added that it is a highly
important relationship, which well merits proper examination.
There are many reasons why I have treated it so meanly in this
book. One of them is my training and practice. Being a psycho-
analyst, nearly all my experience stems from what I have learnt
in the psychoanalytic situation. Nearly all psychoanalytic discoveries have come from this source, which is characterized by a
peculiar, lopsided, two-person relationship. One partner in this
relationship is in the position of a superior, in so far as he has
more knowledge, better and deeper understanding, can and does
explain—i.e. interpret—the events that happen between the
partners. In return, highly charged emotions are transferred to
him which he has to tolerate. The other partner in this peculiar
relationship is comparatively weak, has come for help because
he cannot understand his problems by himself, because, in other
words, certain things are inexplicable to him. This creates rather
high tensions in him; one way of relieving the strain is to transfer
his emotions to the stronger partner, his analyst.

It is easy to see why we analysts cannot help explaining any doctor–patient relationship in the light of our own experience with patients in the analytic situation. It is important to bear in mind that this is tantamount to explaining it in terms of the relationship between a child and the adult. But it also means that we have a much scantier knowledge about any one-person situation; a situation in which there is no partner to whom emotions can be transferred, in which a man is essentially on his own. Situations of this kind are probably as important as the two-person situations extensively studied by analysts. A good example of this one-person situation is, for instance, artistic creation. All the psychoanalytic explanations proposed try to turn it into a kind of two-person relationship, though it is obvious that no second person is actually present, that the artist in fact creates his work of art by and out of himself. The rather pedestrian and obvious analytic explanation is to consider the work of art as a kind of child born by the creator artist. This conception is strongly supported by the imagery of the languages known to me, all of which use words borrowed from child-bearing to describe the act of creation. To quote a few: the artist conceives an idea, is pregnant with it, has labour pains, gives birth to a work of art, some of his ideas miscarry or are stillborn, etc. All this shows that this explanation, though essentially true, is rather shallow, does not do justice to the richness of the real experience.

Roughly the same is true of our theoretical conceptions about illness. We know that for some reason or other during the initial, "unorganized" period of their illnesses—which may last from a few minutes to several years—people gradually withdraw from their environment and first create and then grow the illness on their own, *out of themselves*. This period, which, according to our experience, is of paramount importance for the future fate of the illness, and of the patient, is only poorly understood. Our psycho-analytic methods do not provide us with an adequate enough technique to follow in detail the patient in his work and struggle with the growing illness. During this time, in the same way as during the artistic creation, no second person is yet present, and certainly no external partner to whom emotions can be transferred and thereby made accessible to our analytic methods. So again, as with artistic creation, one of the psychoanalytic explanations considers the illness as a kind of child, in this case a bad, damaged child which, instead of bringing pleasure, brings pain and disaster to its creator. (This imagery may become conscious and be expressed in exactly these words by certain patients, especially women suffering from a growth.) I have to repeat what I said before. Although this explanation is very likely true, it is certainly superficial and incomplete.

If direct psychoanalytical observation does not provide satisfactory data on which to build a theory, let us turn to medical science, which during the centuries has developed certain theories about the nature of illness. Apart from their scientific value and usefulness, all of them are also determined psychologically, i.e. they express one aspect or another of man's relationship to his illness. I propose to discuss only what is the most important theory at the present day—although, if I am right, its importance is gradually waning. In its simplest form this considers the individual as essentially healthy and well integrated. His harmony is disturbed by an *external agent* which penetrates the defences of the body (or the mind). The agent may be a physical force, causing bruises, wounds, concussions, fractures, etc.; a chemical substance such as acid, poison, lethal gas, caustic fluid; or a germ causing infection; or even a mental trauma. The illness, according to this theory, is the sum-total of the original damage and the body's (or the mind's) defences mobilised against it. The psychological source of this theory is the belief—and hope—alive in all of us, that we are essentially "good" and that anything "bad" must come from outside. Thus the appropriate treatment is to get this something "bad" out of us. Innumerable techniques, from primitive magic and exorcism, through "purgatives," enemata and phlebotomy to many unnecessary surgical operations, have been based on this primitive idea.

On the whole, one or both of these two opposite ideas shape— or perhaps only colour—the patient's conception of his illness. Roughly the same is true of medical theories of illness. According to the first, the patient was healthy, whole and "good" until something in him turned "bad." According to the second, the "bad" thing had nothing to do with the patient—it came from outside and is, in the true sense of the word, a "foreign body." In both cases the "bad" thing threatens him with pains, privation, or even destruction unless he can defend himself against it or get rid of it altogether, either on his own or with his doctor's help.

Which of these two opposite conceptions is true, or at any

rate, nearer the truth? The answer is difficult. The shorter the duration of an illness—and with it the period of observation—the better does it fit in with the theory of the external agent. A bruised finger or a bad attack of 'flu can be confidently ascribed to something "bad" coming from outside. But, if a patient returns periodically with some minor injury, we cannot help thinking of accident-proneness or deliberate absenteeism; and if he "catches" too many infections, we talk of hypersensitivity, allergic condition, etc. The longer the period of observation, the more the impression grows that an illness is almost as much a characteristic quality of the patient as the shape of his head, his height, or the colour of his eyes.

This leads directly to one of the eternal problems of medicine: Which is the primary, a chronic organic illness or a certain kind of personality? Are the two of them independent of each other, interdependent, or is one the cause and the other the effect; and if so, which? Do sour people eventually get peptic ulcers, or does a peptic ulcer make people sour? Are bilious attacks, or even gallstones, produced by the bitterness of some people, or do they become bitter because of their painful attacks? Until recently it was tacitly assumed that every chronic disease developed a "neurotic superstructure." In the last forty years or so, mainly under the influence of pioneers like G. Groddeck, S. Ferenczi and S. E. Jelliffe—all three originally general practitioners—medical thought has been gradually changing. This change has produced what is now called psychosomatic medicine.

This, of course, is not the end of the matter. The next step is to ask what is the origin of a psychosomatic or any other disposition. If I am right, psychoanalysis is about to develop a new conception which may be called "basic illness" or perhaps *"basic fault" in the biological structure of the individual, involving in varying degrees both his mind and his body.* The origin of this basic fault may be traced back to a considerable discrepancy between the needs of the individual in his early formative years (or possibly months) and the care and nursing available at the relevant times. This creates a state of deficiency the consequences of which are only partly reversible. Although the individual may achieve a good, or even very good, adjustment, the vestiges of his early experiences remain, and contribute to what is called his constitution, his individuality, or his character make-up, both in the psychological and in the biological sense. The cause of this early discrepancy may be congenital—i.e. the infant's needs may be too exacting—or environmental, such as insufficient, careless, haphazard, over-anxious, over-protective, or only not-understanding care.

Should this theoretical approach prove correct, all the pathological states of later years, the "clinical illnesses," would have to be considered symptoms or exacerbations of the "basic illness," brought about by the various crises in the individual's development, both external and internal, psychological and biological.

If we accept this idea, the controversy between the external and internal origin of illness resolves itself into a complemental series. The more intensive one factor is, the less is needed of the other. The picture thus emerging is that of a conflict between the individual's possibilities and his environment. Let us suppose the "basic fault" was not too severe, thus enabling the individual to develop fairly well, i.e. to adjust himself without undue strain to a large enough variety of conditions. Should, however, the strain on him suddenly increase, or involve areas which were influenced by his "basic fault," he is faced with a problem which may be too difficult for him. From this "average" case imperceptible steps lead in one direction to the extreme case of the unviable infant and of Huntington's chorea, or in the other direction to a massive infection or to a bomb dropped by the enemy.

I readily admit that my idea is far from being new. What is original in it is the bringing together into one picture the illnesses of adulthood and the experiences in the early formative period of life and relating them to each other. A further advantage of this theory is that it may provide us with a working hypothesis for the understanding of the processes in the patient while he is alone with his illness. In any case, I wish to emphasize that the little we know about this important phase is the result of reconstruction from what we learn from the patient later, after his illness has forced him to consult us. Here again, general practitioners have a unique opportunity, inaccessible to anyone else. They may know, and often do know, the patient before he becomes overtly ill, when he is alone with his illness.

This situation changes fundamentally when the patient reaches the stage of complaining. Although his illness is usually still in the unorganized state, he now needs—and finds—a partner, in one respect a superior partner, from whom he may expect help and on whom he may transfer some of his emotions. Here we analysts are at home and can use our methods with confidence, and—as I hope I have succeeded in showing—our ideas may be of some use to the general practitioner in his arduous task. The relation is by no means one-sided however. It is true that the general practitioner can learn a good deal from us about the all-important interaction between the patient's propositions and the doctor's responses prompted by his apostolic function. But it is equally true that we analysts can also learn a good deal from the experiences of general practitioners. For obvious reasons, this can only be mentioned but not discussed in this book.

So let us return to our main topic. We found that, when the patient is faced with a problem too difficult for him to cope with, partly or chiefly because of his "basic fault," his organization partially breaks down, and after some time, which may last from a few minutes to several years, he consults his doctor—*complaining of some illness*. This is a puzzling fact; in the doctor–patient relationship it occurs but seldom that patients come with a problem. In other words, patients consult their doctors only when, so to speak, they have converted the struggle with their problem into an illness. I am certain that a number of doctors will be startled by this formulation. What is wrong with this situation? they will rightly ask. The doctor's job is treating ill-nesses; of course, people come to them with illnesses. So far so good, but preventive medicine is also the doctor's task. Perhaps it would be desirable to change our apostolic function, and train our patients to consult us with their problems before the illness starts; the prospects of successful therapy might be much better in such an early phase. Then there is the possibility of an immense gain in our knowledge if we could find out what sort of people have problems but cope with them without illness, and what sort of people resort to illness. Very likely time will be another important factor. Medicine knows, for example, that cancer rarely starts before the age of forty, whereas a peptic ulcer hardly ever starts after forty. It is not impossible that these and similar empirical facts may have psychological roots, which would certainly be much more easily accessible to detailed study in the early period before the illness proper starts.

With the starting of the illness a number of secondary processes are also set in motion. One may say that the illness creates a new life-situation to which the patient must adapt himself. This readjustment drains off a good deal of his energies, much beyond what is needed by the physiological defensive processes, and the new situation may be considerably different from the immediately preceding one. This readjustment is a complicated, multi-dimensional process, and so I have to restrict myself to enumerating some of its most important aspects only.

One of the most primitive and powerful trends in the human mind is what, in technical terms, is called narcissism. This means, from our angle, that we feel ourselves whole, inviolate, imperishable, important, capable and, above all, lovable. Life and reality are not at all in harmony with this feeling; during our development and during our mature life our narcissism gets hurt time and again. It is a severe shock to realize, no matter whether suddenly or gradually, that because of illness our body (or our mind) is, for the moment, not capable, and perhaps will never again be fully capable of reassuring us that our hopes are still possible of fulfilment in some unspecified future.

Past experiences, especially during our childhood and adolescence, have taught us certain ways of dealing with such shocks. Our parents and teachers had a profound influence on this learning process and its results. Coping with an illness may be confidently compared with this process of maturing, and the doctor's rôle with that of our parents and teachers; just as the beliefs and convictions of our parents and teachers greatly helped or greatly hindered our development towards maturity, so does the doctor and his apostolic function affect us during illness.

For some people, falling ill is a severe blow, for others a welcome relief. There are people who, because of their serious "basic fault," find life too difficult, who can obtain but little gratification, whose mental or biological economy is precarious and unstable. Even minor ailments are too much for them, life is too strenuous, too frustrating and depressing, illness offers them an acceptable opportunity to withdraw and "look after themselves." No matter whether illness is a severe shock or a welcome justification for withdrawal, it is always a form of life. This is especially true of illnesses of some duration, allowing time to the patient to adjust himself to them. This adjustment is not identical with what we called "organization," but they are parallel pheno-mena, influencing each other all the time. In the present connec-tion we are concerned only with the illness as a form of life. This is a vast subject, and although we have ample empirical data about it, and a number of truly eminent physicians have tried to sum up their medical experiences of a lifetime in this field, a systematic survey is still lacking. My very modest attempt will fall far below the standard of what is needed. I shall base my discussion on the psychoanalytic theory of primary and secondary gains. Although convenient for a first orientation, this theory does not claim either to be unequivocal or to be more than a crude first attempt.

No form of life can be maintained without some gratification. Conversely, this means that if one aims at changing any form of life, one must use either compelling force or offer more acceptable gratifications in place of those to be made impossible by the change. This is rather platitudinous, but it is worth stressing that it is fully valid for the patient's relationship with his illness and also for any therapy purporting to change it. To quote a con-vincing example of many; the prevalence of "brutal" physical methods in psychiatric therapy over time-consuming psycho-therapeutic methods. The various shock treatments, and above all leucotomy, brutally force the patient to give up some of his symptoms—his forms of life—and content himself with others, less objectionable to his fellow-men. Anyone who has had opportunity to see leucotomized patients knows how painfully true this is.

So let us first of all examine illness as a source of direct grati-fication. To avoid misunderstanding, I must emphasize that, in any illness, pain, limitation, apprehension, and so on are always present. All the gratifications are only partial, additional to, or almost completely overshadowed by suffering. But it is impossible not to notice the high emotional importance of eating in prac-tically all gastric and some metabolic diseases, of the digestive functions in intestinal disorders, particularly in chronic constipa-tion, etc. An often quoted puzzling example is the frequent faecal dreams of acromegalics which are definitely ambivalently toned, partly highly disgusting and frightening, but at the same time "interesting." Psychoanalysis can offer some help in this field through *the theory of erotogenic zones of the body*. Unfortunately all this amounts only to a beginning. The reason is probably that the material observed by psychoanalysts has been highly selected, i.e. consists of patients suffering chiefly from psychological illnesses, with only a sprinkling of organic cases. The general practitioner, with his much wider range of patients, will perhaps provide us with further data to extend and deepen our psychoanalytic theories.

The second sub-group of direct gratifications consists of the opportunities offered by the illness for *withdrawal from all sorts of unsatisfactory or frustrating, demanding or over-exacting relationships with people*. Examples for it are legion—the frigid woman whose dysmenorrhoea is a welcome dispensation from marital duties; the urethritis of not securely potent men; the many eating difficulties and food-fads of over-pressed children, which enable them to escape from the clutches of their much too powerful parents, usually their mothers, by an apparent weakness; the asthma attacks which inevitably overcome the patient when visiting the home of his or her parents or spouse. The most impressive instance is the considerable narrowing of the personality during a serious illness; not only may interest in other people be gradually given up, but the patient's relationship to reality may become uncertain and tenuous. This sub-group is well known and sufficiently substantiated by observation. Unfortunately the whole field is treated mostly on the level of interesting anecdotes, and a systematic survey is badly needed.

Somewhere between the last sub-group and the next, that is between withdrawal and regression, there comes what psychoanalysis calls *introversion*. It is more than withdrawal, inasmuch as the individual's interest is not only withdrawn from his environment, but is simultaneously firmly anchored in himself. Mental processes and sensations, ideas and emotions attain an importance very seldom experienced otherwise. This phenomenon is wellknown but its finer details are hardly understood, probably because in the early stages the patient is usually alone, and has no partner yet on whom he can transfer his emotions. Thus, nearly everything we know about the events of the unorganized phase of this period stems either from a reconstruction from what the patient tells us later, when he comes to us for help, or from our subjective impressions and preconceived theoretical ideas. More knowledge about the processes in the formative phases of introversion is badly needed. If we understood them better, we could perhaps prevent the development of serious hypochondriasis, the greatest problem belonging to this sub-group.

The fourth sub-group of direct gratifications from illness can be called *regressions*. This means more than withdrawal or introversion, because it entails in addition the emergence of infantile forms in the patient's behaviour. Though its frequent occurrence is undeniable, much less is known about regression than about the foregoing forms of gratification. The connection between illness and withdrawal is fairly obvious in many cases, but the function of regression is far from clear. It may be a consequence of the severity of the illness, an extreme case of which is delirium in high fever. It may be abandoning as hopeless, as too exacting, the task of coping with life and pain in a mature way, as for instance the adoption of foetal position in a great number of painful conditions, or the willingness or even the demand of certain patients to be washed and fed well beyond the stage when this is objectively necessary, or the institution or custom of providing a nurse to hold the hand of a patient under local anaesthesia. Regression may also be an attempt at self-healing, as high temperature may possibly be in certain infections; by regressing to a more primitive level the patient may be seeking an opportunity to make a start in a new direction, avoiding that blocked by his illness.

As I said, apart from its existence, little is known about the *significance and function of regression*. This is disturbing, because the doctor's responses to the patient's "offer" to regress are of great importance for the future. We do not even know whether regression should be prevented or encouraged and, if so, in which illnesses, at what stages, or in which kind of individuals. The obvious danger is that the patient may get too well settled either in a regressed or in an over-pressed "mature" state, too well "organized" to be accessible to a real therapy. Again I have to plead for more research.

The second great group of gratifications enabling the patient to acquiesce in or accept illness as a form of life is that of *secondary gains*. Illness, as every other quality of man, can be used to obtain something useful to, or valued by, the individual. The best known example is compensation neurosis, but this is only one of its kind. To an outsider secondary gains may seem of little value, even rather silly, but they are important to the patient and must be recognized as such by his environment as well as by his doctor.

Many examples of this can be quoted; wearing an armband as a sign of having just been inoculated or vaccinated, arriving in a taxi at the hospital or at the consultant's rooms, meeting other patients—some of them obviously very ill indeed—in the hushed or buzzing atmosphere of a waiting-room; in general, being made a fuss of, being treated as a V.I.P. All this is pretty easy to notice, but in some patients it is not so easy to cope with. There are, however, more complicated forms, and the more complicated they become the more difficult it is to separate them from the forms discussed above, i.e. from direct gratifications. Withdrawal and regression in particular are most difficult to classify unequivocally.

Before going further, we must briefly discuss two important fields in the patient's relationship to his illness: *fears and pain*. Both offer great opportunities for the doctor's therapeutic skill, but both, particularly ways of dealing with fear, unfortunately belong to the domain of "common sense" therapy. We mentioned earlier in this chapter that some people experience illness as something in them turned "bad" and attacking them from the inside. This may create severe anxieties, which in some progressive illnesses, such as certain cancers, some infections or some degenerative conditions, may have biological justification. Then there are the fears and frustrations of chronically ill people who have to give up some of their accustomed pleasures, partly because of the illness itself—with impaired vision for instance, certain occupations, all ball games and fighting sports such as boxing or fencing, become impossible—or because of the diet necessary for an effective treatment. Before insulin the frustrations of diabetics were almost proverbial; nowadays the most conspicuous groups are perhaps chain-smoker ulcer patients and some sufferers from ulcerative colitis who can tolerate only a bland diet. And there is the ultimate problem, the patient's fears of death. General practitioners—and nurses—who have close contact with people approaching death have an inexhaustible supply of puzzling stories about fears, heroism, humiliation and supreme dignity in the face of death. Expert, firmly founded advice about what to do, how to help in this distressing situation would be most valuable, but unfortunately our only recourse is again to common sense.

Roughly the same is true of the patient's attitude to pain. In the first place, all doctors will agree that patients can more easily tolerate diagnosed pain than undiagnosed pain—and perhaps the same is true of their doctors. Social attitudes to pain vary widely. In certain societies it is impossible for a man to weep, in others weeping by men is tolerated. Women, as usual, are given greater freedom, but I have the impression that in this country women cry and scream much less during childbirth than in my native country, Hungary. There is no doubt which custom is better for the midwives and the doctors, but it is much less certain which is better for the women. This is yet another great problem awaiting research. Is it easier to bear unrelieved pain with a "stiff upper lip" or by breaking down and crying? Medicine until recently considered pain only from the physiological angle, resulting in the building up of perhaps the best-studied chapter of pharmacology, that on analgesics and anaesthetics, and in the creation of a new speciality. Recent years have brought us the various systems of painless childbirth, first with the help of drugs, and more recently with the help of allaying the woman's anxiety and ensuring her co-operation. This shows that in the field of relieving pain a vast opportunity still awaits the psychologically-minded doctor.

I think this is a good place to mention *the patient's subjective description of his pains* and other sensations originating in his body. It is surprising how incomparably more varied and richer one's conception of one's body becomes during illness. This is an immense psychological field which has hardly been touched by science. Why is it that people report their pains or sensations, as stabbing, lancinating, lightning, burning, pressing, constricting, gripping, stifling, throbbing, blinding, etc., or use phrases like "as if a stone were inside me," "as if a part of my body were dead," or "as heavy as lead," "a dead weight in my middle," "a red-hot poker," "as if I were made of cotton wool," "I feel woolly," or "frozen," and so on? We know that certain characteristic phrases are often used by people suffering from certain illnesses, but we know very little about which part of any of these phrases is determined by physiological processes and which by the patient's fantasies about processes possibly happening inside him. This could be a fascinating study for a psychologically-minded general practitioner who knew his patients fairly well during, before and after their illnesses.

*   *   *

To conclude this chapter I propose to mention a curious group of patients whom we called the "fat envelope" group. "Fat envelope" is a purely descriptive term referring to the copiousness of the accumulated notes about the patient. This may be due to—

(1) The patient's puzzling illness, which has necessitated a number of specialist examinations.

(2) His over-frequent visits to the surgery.

(3) His annoying habit of frequently changing his doctor.

The three factors are not obviously interlinked, but it is rare for one only to be responsible for the bulging envelope, and often all three are present. What does this mean?

When this problem cropped up in our seminars we went on to discuss the "natural" rate of change that takes place in a doctor's clientèle. Since the establishment of the National Health Service this can be easily followed. To our great surprise, we found that from eight to ten per cent of the patients on a doctor's list change their doctor in any one year. This is certainly true of practices in or near London; in rural areas the figures are somewhat lower, but just as constant. Only a small minority of these patients make the change openly by giving notice. Some change their addresses and use this as a pretext, even if they only move to another house in the same street. Most of them simply consult another doctor, and this initiates the change. Another surprising fact that emerged was that this figure is apparently practically independent of the doctor's personality, apostolic beliefs, skill, interest in psychotherapy, etc., etc. The first question we asked ourselves was why these patients changed their doctors. We had to abandon the inquiry, because when a doctor loses a patient he has to surrender his records to the local Executive Council and so no trace of the patient remains except in the doctor's memory; as these cases must be considered failures, this source could not be accepted as reliable. Other approaches were possible, such as having an immediate discussion on every patient who changes his doctor, or looking up samples of new patients taken over from another doctor. Unfortunately all of these proved rather cumbersome, and, as no doctor likes to discuss only his failures, the seminar, in spite of good intentions, always found a more urgent problem to deal with.

Nevertheless, research into the real causes of these changes would be a fascinating task. A number of these people belong to the "fat envelope" class, the problem patients in any practice, the nomads who wander from general practitioner to general practitioner, never settling down with anybody for any length of time.

A special case of this nomadism is when the change-over happens within a partnership, without any formality. For some time I thought we had found a promising way of studying this interesting group. Soon, however, we came up against difficulties. It was surprising to discover that, though the partners notice the change-overs and remark upon them, they never discuss the causes and take no apparent interest in them. The usual situation is that only one doctor in a partnership is psychologically minded; the other or others tolerate this, either with grumbles or with good humour. But this toleration was severely taxed when the doctor attending our seminars wanted to discuss with his partner why a patient had left his partner for him, or *vice versa*. So we decided— at any rate for the time being—to leave things alone. Nevertheless we collected some extremely interesting case histories, three of which, Cases 1, 5 and 9, appear in previous chapters, or in Appendix III, and illustrate some of my points.

The little we learned about the causes of nomadism can be summed up in the phrase: "Self-selection of patients according to the doctor's apostolic beliefs." If patient and doctor do not "click," and the doctor cannot convert the patient to adopt his apostolic beliefs, the only way open to the patient is to find another doctor. The self-selection and the apostolic function are counterparts of each other, it is they that build up the special and highly individual atmosphere of every practice, resulting in the mutual investment company. From this angle joint practices are valuable institutions to patients. If they cannot accept the methods of one partner they can drift to the other, who, however well adapted to his partner, still has his individual apostolic beliefs. In some cases—Case 1 is one of them—the patient used the two doctors according to her needs at the time, up to a point to everybody's satisfaction. Again, these cases could form the basis of valuable research into the kind of therapy needed by patients at different periods of their illnesses.

Perhaps the same processes are at work in the other class of "fat envelope" patients, who have to go from specialist to specialist. It is possible that in the specialist–patient relationship we shall find the apostolic function and the self-selection of patients at work in the same way as in the surgeries of general practitioners. As our research seminars have not yet been extended to consultants, I have no first-hand knowledge of the events in my colleagues' practices. For my own practice what I said above is certainly true.

The third group of "fat envelope" cases, those who come for help much too often but remain with the same doctor—Case 26 is a striking example—is a warning not to be rash in our inferences. The establishment of a working mutual investment company does not prevent a patient from becoming a problem patient. As mentioned, the three groups largely overlap, so again we can only ask for more research.

I may add that, in addition to the cases just mentioned, i.e. Cases 1, 5, 9 and 26, our Cases 2, 4, 6, 11, 12, 16, 17, 19, 21, 22 and 24 belong to the "fat envelope" class. Any research which will help the doctor to cope better with the problems inherent in this group will contribute considerably to lightening his burden. That several of them, such as Cases 16, 19, 21, 22 and 24, can be counted as real successes, inasmuch as for the time being the fatness of their envelopes ceased to increase, shows that we are going in the right direction.

CHAPTER XX

General-Practitioner Psychotherapy

A S WE have just seen, there are various stages in the history of an illness. The beginning of it all, according to my ideas, is the "basic fault"—as yet more a theory than a fact. Then comes the problem caused by a conflict between the demands of the environment and the patient's inherent possibilities which may have become more or less severely restricted under the influence of the basic fault. Some people cope with their problems by solving them, others bear the strain caused by them, while still others respond by falling ill. These last try first to struggle with the illness on their own; later, when they realize that this does not help, they consult a doctor. At this stage the illness is not yet "organized;" as we saw in Part I, there are usually several "offers" from which the doctor has to choose one to treat. His aim must obviously be to choose an illness which offers the best prospects for therapy; I mean not only a palliative help for a superficial symptom, or even for a superficial clinical illness, but a therapy which offers the best possible chances for the patient's future life.

Many cases reported in this book could be used to illustrate these points. Let us take, for instance, Miss S., Case 23. The basic fault in her case can be surmised only from its consequences. These were: a very tense relationship between a domineering and over-demanding mother and a rebellious, "managing," but guilt-laden daughter; a yearning for an understanding father who, in turn, had to be idealized; considerable difficulty in becoming, and accepting the responsibilities of, an adult woman. The basic fault in her was probably caused by the discrepancy between her mother's inadequate but overwhelmingly domineering care and her own need to be understood and in particular to be permitted to run her own life, to be herself. All this was reinforced and complicated by her parents' broken marriage, leading to an idealization of the absent father and to a hypercritical, though dependent attitude towards her mother. Her conflicts were then exacerbated by her growing sexual wishes and needs. She tried to solve her problem by becoming ill with rheumatic pains and dyspepsia. Her illness, among other things, would have prevented her from making any decision about her marriage—it would not have been sensible, perhaps even totally impossible, to think of marriage and financial hardship if she might at any moment develop a peptic ulcer. Thus, her problem would have remained unsolved, and she was in danger of developing into a sour, dyspeptic woman. For about three years the previous doctor helped Miss S. by his "agreement" to "organize" her illness on these lines. Dr. R., by his approach, first "disorganized" the dyspepsia and rheumatism, and then made Miss S. change her offer of a physical illness back into a psychological problem, and, instead of "organizing" something around it, helped Miss S. to solve her most acute problems. It remains to be seen whether this amount of help will have been sufficient for her. Without examining the extent of the basic fault, any prediction is mere guess-work.

Another sphere where these ideas may be helpful is diagnosis. In Chapter VI we discussed the various levels of diagnosis purely on the basis of direct observations in the doctor's practice. The ideas quoted above allow us to give a more definite meaning to this term. In Peter's case (Case 19), for instance, the diagnosis "headaches," "hysteria," "? migraine," "agoraphobia," were all correct and, in so far as they described an important feature of the whole picture, helpful. But they did not allow us to predict, for instance, that he would have some difficulty in acquiescing in the rôle of a father, that when this new problem turned up he would hesitate, so to speak, between health and a recurrence of his headaches and phobias, and would need some help from his doctor. They did not explain why he had had to marry a very nice and understanding but somewhat frigid woman who needed manual masturbation for her satisfaction; nor why he accepted the rôle of maid-of-all-work at home, and so on. All this, and many more features of his character as well as of his illness, become more intelligible if we take into consideration his appalling early history. Then we can feel with him in his love-deficiency condition and understand why he had to do everything and anything to get affection, why he is apprehensive of a coming rival and, on the other hand, why a too rapid disappearance of his worries was, so to speak, indigestible to him.

This is what we try to describe as an adequate level of diagnosis, and it is about as far as this that a general practitioner can and should go. Because of the many limitations imposed upon him by his practice, I think it will be only seldom that he will be able to penetrate further towards examining the nature and extent of the basic fault.

Peter's and Miss S.'s cases are comparatively simple. Peter's illness at the time of the "Smith" was not yet organized, the various primary and secondary gains not yet worked out, and still less ingrained in his personality; and thus the doctor's task was not too complicated. Miss S.'s illness was just about to be "organized," the primary gain not very great, and the secondary gains hardly existent; on the other hand, the prospects of becoming a mature and independent woman were very attractive. In her case, too, the doctor's task was not very difficult. Roughly the same can be said about Miss M. (Case 10), Mrs. Q. (Case 21), and perhaps also Mr. V. (Case 22).

On the other hand, in the case of the company director (Case 6), Miss F. (Case 12), or Professor E. (Case 8), the illness has become "organized," that is, it has become so much part and parcel of the patient's personality that it proved impossible to drive a wedge between it and the person. To describe this difference one can say that there are *some people who have an illness and others who are ill.* Some people experience their illness as something alien to them, or something imposed upon them, and welcome any offer or attempt to rid them of it; while others experience it as part of their life with which they have grown together. The prospects of therapy are obviously poorer in the latter group. In Professor E.'s case, for instance, Dr. Z. agreed with his patient; both accepted the illness, and in consequence the patient's life was adapted to it—as the follow-up report shows, apparently successfully. Our intervention in the case of the company director was futile and led only to our losing a doctor. Miss F. remained unchanged and, thanks to Dr. C.'s patience, we did not lose him. But it must be stressed that we did not succeed in any of these three cases in separating the patient from his illness and winning him over to our side as our ally against it.

Although in many of our other cases this winning over the patient to our side proved anything but easy—Case 21 (Mrs. Q.) and Case 24 (Mr. P.) are good examples—somehow the task never looked so difficult as in those three. Was this difference due to some still undefined quality of the illness, to the peculiar structure of the personality, to the nature of the "basic fault"—or to our poor technique? A pertinent question, but most difficult to answer. In Professor E.'s case, I mentioned that Dr. Z. was not an enthusiastic psychotherapist; it is possible, though far from certain, that another doctor might have converted the patient to seeking psychotherapeutic help. Whether it would have been to his benefit we do not know. But it is certain that in his case Dr. Z.'s technique must be questioned. Our doubts are on much firmer ground in regard to the treatment of the company director, Case 6. In our view, the doctor made mistakes in this case, though he did nothing contrary to accepted medical principles. But, even if we accept his technical shortcomings as proved, it does not mean that another doctor with a better technique would have been able to get the patient out of his "organized" state. Miss F.'s case, Case 12, is a useful warning against over-confidence. There we had a well-trained, very patient general practitioner and a skilled psychiatrist co-operating wholeheartedly, but the patient was not to be helped. Something similar might have happened in Case 1, Mrs. C. In spite of the promising initial success the patient was not able to make use of Dr. M.'s offer of help and for some considerable time drifted to his partner, who did not want to disturb the "organized" state of the illness by psychological investigations.

This brings us to one of the most important problems of psychotherapy in general practice: "what to treat?" This question is fairly easily answered in the acute phase or in the late stages of an illness. In the acute phase the symptoms are so overwhelming, in the late stages so ingrained—e.g. in Case 3—that we have no choice. Occasionally even in these two situations the doctor may have some freedom of choice in his point of therapeutic attack; but the problem of "what to treat" is really important in the initial, "unorganized" phases of an illness.

Our Case 28, reported by Dr. S., well illustrates this problem—

CASE 28*

The patient was a well-dressed and well-spoken, but very unhappy-looking, married woman of thirty-eight, complaining of aches and pains between the shoulder-blades. She had been on the doctor's list for many years but he had seen her only twice before, when she had come complaining about some insect bites. A physical examination revealed nothing except an almost certainly insignificant nodule in her thyroid gland. As the husband was not on the doctor's list, Dr. S. half casually asked her if she lived with her husband, to which she answered, "Yes," and continued that they had no children, although they had been married for fourteen years, and now they did not bother about it any more. The doctor then asked if she was happy with her husband otherwise, to which she replied, "Unfortunately not;" they had had nothing to do with each other for the past five years, and "his affections went elsewhere." All this was said quite dispassionately and calmly. Dr. S. then asked if her affections had gone elsewhere too. She became rather hesitant, but finally said, "No." Here the doctor stopped, and gave the patient some aspirin preparation—enough for about a week—telling her to come back if she did not feel better. He entered on her card a provisional noncommittal diagnosis of "? fibrositis." He thought that by his questions and human approach he had possibly opened the door, and that the patient would come back to him in a few days and then be able to talk more freely and openly about her real troubles.

This case history could have been quoted equally well in Chapter XI on "How to start" or Chapter XII on "When to stop," as both these problems had to be solved by the doctor—and on the spur of the moment. Leaving these two problems aside, I propose to discuss here only the doctor's choice of "what to treat."

When this patient was examined, the doctor found four possible illnesses—two physical and two psychological. There was the nodule in her thyroid gland, which could have served as a pointer. The doctor, however, dismissed it as irrelevant, probably correctly. There were then the rheumatic pains in the back. The doctor searched carefully for confirmatory physical signs and, although he found none, he still prescribed some medicine for the pains. That is, he took notice of them, but his whole behaviour was meant to impress the patient not to take them seriously. Then there was the depression, which the doctor noticed correctly but assumed to be a reaction to the unhappy marriage—a kind of secondary symptom. And lastly there was the marriage itself.

* This report was published in *The Lancet* (1955), April 2, pp. 683-8.

So at least four illnesses were "proposed by the patient": a slight hypertrophy of the thyroid gland, muscular rheumatism, depression, and chronic sexual frustration causing unhappiness.

Had she four different diseases, independent of one another? Or was one the consequence or the symptom of the others? If so, which was the real cause? Further, if it was impracticable to cure the deepest cause, where was the best prospect for any real therapy?

For instance, was she a genuine depressive, whose constant dark mood and repressed ambivalent hostility the husband could not stand, with the result that in time "his affections went elsewhere?" Or was she a fairly average woman who had unfortunately married a basically unfaithful husband? If so, her unhappiness might be the expression of her insoluble ambivalent love, which possibly had led to a reactive depression. Again, we could regard her vague pains as a kind of conversion symptom, expressing her inability either to bear in forgiving love all the strains or to free herself aggressively from them. Or did both the slight nodule in the thyroid and the vague muscular pains point to some endocrine disturbance, of which both the depression and the sexual unhappiness were possibly secondary symptoms? We might continue indefinitely this kind of speculation about the possible causes and dynamisms of her state.

We must bear in mind, however, that this speculation is not merely a useless pastime, because it is exactly in this way that the doctor comes to decide *what to treat, when and how.* The end-result of this half-conscious, half-unconscious reconstruction of the patient's dynamic pathology is the basis of the doctor's response to the patient's propositions.

What was the result, in this case, of the doctor's choice?

Nothing was heard of the woman for more than six weeks. Then out of the blue, the doctor of the factory where the woman works rang up Dr. S. He reported that the woman had complained to him of her strained family life and had asked for help. The factory doctor suggested bromide medication and asked our practitioner to let her have it under the National Health Service. Our doctor, quite rightly, told his colleague that more than bromides were needed to help this patient; that he was always available if she wanted to see him; and that he had no objection to trying bromides in the first place. In spite of his accommodating attitude the patient did not reappear.

Was this a failure, as the doctor himself called it, or a partial success? I think both. The patient was frightened away by his somewhat forceful method and did not return even after he offered her, so to speak, a golden bridge; in this sense the treatment must be considered a failure. On the other hand, when she consulted the factory doctor she did not complain of aches and pains, but of her strained marital relations. By the doctor's therapy the illness had been changed back into a problem, perhaps offering better prospects for a real aetiological therapy.

That is the second point that I wished to illustrate by this case history. As we saw in Part I of this book, one danger is that doctors, conditioned by their training, prefer diagnosing and treating physical illnesses to considering even the possibility of a psychological illness. The opposite danger, however, is that *the doctor may be tempted to brush aside all physical symptoms and make a bee-line for what he thinks is the psychological root of the trouble.* This kind of diagnostic or therapeutic method means that the doctor tries to take away the symptom from the patient, and at the same time to force him to face up consciously to the painful problem which possibly is causing it. In other words, the patient is forced to change his limited symptoms back into the severe mental suffering which he tried to avoid by a flight into a more bearable physical suffering.

We must realize that *the patient's "functional" illness is not the problem, and* a fortiori *not a psychological problem either.* A "functional" illness means that the patient has had a problem which he tried to solve with an illness. The illness enabled him to complain, whereas he was unable to complain about his original problem. The reasons for this inability may be manifold. It may be that complaining about the original problem would have been too shameful, too embarrassing, too unpleasant, too frightening, or too painful, etc. This may perhaps explain why a patient so seldom comes to the doctor openly with a problem. As a rule he comes with a complaint, and the doctor's task is to find the original problem of which the patient cannot complain and in place of which he created an illness. So, although ultimately we are concerned with the original problem, our first concern is with the illness.

Some doctors forget this, and think that their immediate task is to uncover the original conflict. This kind of psychological *tour de force*, which is really a violation of a person's private life, is attempted nowadays much more commonly than ever before. Psychoanalysis in particular has put into the hands of professional people—doctors, psychologists, social workers—methods previously undreamt of. Many of these people have become sensitive to hitherto neglected minute details, and can arrive at certain conclusions with increasing accuracy. We call this procedure psychological or psychiatric interview technique, and we seem to have inherited from our medical ancestors a not very praiseworthy indifference to it. If our diagnostic conclusions are fairly accurate, we do not appear to care greatly how much suffering is caused to the patient by our diagnostic methods. Obviously a specialist, or a psychological tester, can indulge more freely than a general practitioner in this *belle indifférence des diagnosticiens*. The patient is not his, but was referred to him only for examination; and when the examination is over is referred back. Unfortunately the general practitioner is the last line; the patient is his and he has to see him through. I wonder how many specialists trouble to find out what patients say to their family doctors about their methods and behaviour.

The real risks, however, are even more considerable. Psychoanalysis has taught us, not only to observe and interpret minute details correctly, but also to use our skill and knowledge with some assurance, even daring. We psychoanalysts can do so because, first, we have the patient's transference mostly as our ally, and secondly we remain for long periods in most intimate psychological contact with him. Should anything untoward threaten, we are at hand to notice it and to intervene in an emergency. A number of people have acquired considerable diagnostic skill and knowledge by the assiduous study of psychoanalytic literature, but they should bear in mind that in a short psychiatric, psychological, or social interview the conditions are entirely different; and I think this difference ought to be respected by both non-analysts and analysts.

Having said all that, I wish to recall the general practitioner's special position which we discussed in Chapter XIII. We saw that, if he remains true to his vocation and calling as a family doctor, he will have a much wider range of possible relationships with his patient than is available in any of the other branches of medicine. There are two important differences that I wish to stress here.

One is that he never need be in a hurry. This does not mean a free licence for procrastination, but it means that he need never be pressed for time; if the patient's resistances are too great, there is no need for him to accept battle there and then; the patient will come back in a couple of days, in a week, or in a month, and the psychotherapeutic work can be picked up where it was dropped. The other point is the great variety of possible relationships that are always at a general practitioner's command. If his open psychotherapeutic approach is blocked, he can continue by prescribing some "sensible" medicine such as a hypnotic, a vitamin, a cough mixture, something against headaches, or to improve the appetite or regulate the bowels; if this fails, he can send the patient for some "sensible" examination, such as various X-rays, E.C.G., etc., and if things seem pretty hopeless he can switch over and treat another member of the family, such as wife (husband), child, mother-in-law, or even drop in on his patient unannounced when visiting somebody in the same street.

All this means that he can take considered risks which are well beyond the possibilities of any other doctor. The one thing, however, that he must never forget is that *he is a family doctor and not an amateur psychiatrist*. I wish I could define more exactly what we mean by this most important distinction. We have made several attempts at clarifying the fundamental difference, unfortunately all of them unsuccessful. The only fact that could be established with certainty was that the boundary varies with the doctor's personality. What is general practice for one is amateur psychiatry for another. Some of these differences were discussed and illustrated in Chapters XII, XVI and XVII, to which I have to refer the reader.

For the beginner and even for the advanced practitioner the best advice is: *if in doubt, do not hurry, but listen*. True, there are serious dangers in not keeping pace with the patient, in being always behind him, so that he has not only to find his way out of his problems, but drag his doctor along behind him. These dangers are, however, comparatively small in comparison with those which result from an unjustified violation of a patient's privacy or from prematurely confronting him with a problem which he is not yet ready to face. It is equally dangerous to hurry a patient, not to allow him sufficient time to work out his own solution of the problem and to overcome his resistances to it, especially those caused by shame, embarrassment and, above all, by guilt feelings. All this needs tact, patience, and time.

In the book I have quoted cases both of doctors who like to go slow and of those who like taking risks. In fairness I must add that some of our worst failures have not been mentioned. On the one hand the aim of this book is to demonstrate what can and should be done by general practitioners and not to exhibit mistakes. On the other hand, our research was a venture into unknown territory, and mistakes are the price that has to be paid for such work of exploration. Taking these limitations into account, the cases reported in this book give a fair picture of the great variety in the techniques used by different doctors and of the advantages and drawbacks inherent in each. Again I have to admit our lack of sufficient knowledge about "what to treat, when and how" and ask for facilities for more research.

* * *

I propose now to discuss a few interesting special problems of psychotherapy in general practice. One is caused by a fact, not always taken seriously enough, that *every illness is also the "vehicle" of a plea for love and attention*. One of the commonest conflicts of man is caused by the discrepancy between his need of affection and the amount and quality of affection that his environment is able and willing to grant him. Some people fall ill to secure the attention and concern they need, and the illness is a claim to, a justification of, and simultaneously the expiation for, the extra amount of affection demanded. These interconnections are often transparent enough, but it is pointless to force the patient prematurely to recognize and then renounce them. His need of love, concern, sympathy and, above all, to be taken seriously must be accepted and to some extent gratified in the treatment before he can be expected to experiment with methods other than his illness of obtaining the affection and care for which he is craving.

Another technical problem closely related to the previous one, is *when and how the doctor should get the patient out of his fantasies*. We have mentioned on several occasions that every illness gives rise to fantasies about what its essence may be, how it started, what caused it, whether or not it will heal completely, and what its outcome may be, and so on. As we all know, these fantasies not infrequently represent serious obstacles to therapy. On the other hand, they are paths along which the patient may withdraw from reality in order to "nurse" or to "look after" himself. In other words, if the real problems in their original, crude form are too difficult, some people may resort to transforming them into fantastic forms which, among other things, have the great advantage that they can be complained of. When the doctor confronts these people with his finding that nothing is physically wrong, it is tantamount to a demand to give up the carefully constructed fantasies and to face up to bitter reality and its conflicts. This ends, often enough, in a wrangle between doctor and patient; the one emphasizing that the fantasies have no foundation in reality, the other incapable of accepting external reality as the ultimate judge and clinging desperately to his fantasies.

This dynamic picture offers us one more reason why "reassurance" is so often futile. In accepting reassurance the patient implicitly agrees that his fantasies were meaningless, unfounded and untrue. If this insight were as simple as the primitive procedure of reassurance presupposes, most patients would have arrived at it without outside help. Roughly the same is true about *placebos*. Prescribing a harmless, ineffective drug is tantamount to saying to the patient: this harmless drug will be stronger than your fantasies. Experience shows that this is easier to promise than to fulfil. Still, *placebos* are, as a rule, rather more effective than reassurance alone. This is almost certainly due to the difference between responding to the patient's complaint with something tangible as compared with mere words. Naturally, the former is nearer to taking the illness seriously.

Lastly, a third problem, which could equally well have been dealt with in the chapters on the apostolic function. I have mentioned that the patient develops an illness in order to be able to complain, since he was not able to complain about his original problem or conflict, but I wish to add that in this form the statement is unduly one-sided. *Complaining is a social phenomenon* par excellence. Although the patient's individuality is an important factor in deciding whether or not complaining about a particular thing is possible or admissible, the partner, i.e. the person complained to, is nearly as important. The third factor in this relation is the social atmosphere, which varies with the sex, age, social class both of the patient and of his doctor and, above all, with the times. If I am right, nowadays it is not so infrequent for women to complain to their doctor that they cannot get satisfaction in their sexual life. Thirty years ago a complaint of this kind was exceedingly rare, and in Edwardian or Victorian times it must have been unheard of. Perhaps doctors guessed it in some of their patients, and perhaps they even discussed it in hushed voices among themselves, but it would have been well-nigh impossible either for a well-brought up woman or for her doctor to have discussed it in a matter-of-fact objective way.

Things have changed considerably, chiefly because of the apostolic function of doctors and other professional and semi-professional people. By the change the doctor's task has become somewhat easier—he need not guess or prevaricate, but can speak frankly—but with it his responsibility has also become heavier; now he has to treat complaints which in the past were not his concern. Perhaps it is fair to add that his therapeutic potential has also increased; he has opportunity to treat illnesses in their early stages, before they develop secondary symptoms and become deeply ingrained in the patient's personality. I think this development cannot be checked, and general practitioners in particular must be prepared for more and more of their patients to come to them with straightforward psychological problems.

* * *

Before ending this chapter I propose to discuss in some detail the end-results of general-practitioner psychotherapy. In psycho-analysis the ideal case is the patient who, after an intensive period of therapeutic work is able to terminate his relationship with his analyst for good; he has solved the majority of his past problems, has learnt how to cope with his present and future problems, his dependence on his analyst has served its purpose and can now be renounced; and so, after the work has been completed, neither patient nor analyst feels the need or the urge to see each other. Not all patients finish their analysis in this way, but it remains the ideal.

Should we assume that psychotherapy by general practitioners should aim at the same end-result? I think this would be unjusti-fied, unrealistic, and, above all, would defeat its own end. *The essence of general practitioner–patient relationship is its continuity, and any treatment, particularly a successful one, should represent a further and considerable increase in the joint capital of the "mutual investment company"* as described in Chapter XVIII. A permanent severing of relations between patient and doctor after a successful therapy is tantamount to winding up the mutual investment company with the loss of nearly all its capital and a considerable impoverishment of both partners. Nevertheless, this does occur; examples are Mrs. D. (Case 7), Mrs. N. (Case 20), and Mr. P. (Case 24); perhaps even Miss M. (Case 10) should be included. I wish to point out that the disappearance of a patient has no correlation either with the success or the depth of the treatment. Mr. P. (Case 24) and Miss M. (Case 10) were helped considerably, one may even say fundamentally, and the other two—Mrs. D. (Case 7) and Mrs. N. (Case 20)—may confidently be counted as successes. In all four cases, as their history shows, therapy went fairly deep and enabled the patients to discuss with their doctors experiences which had been kept secret from everybody else.

Some of these patients simply disappear; if they are on the National Health list a printed form comes from the local committee asking the doctor to surrender his notes; if they are private patients, not even that occurs. It would be interesting to find out the true reasons why they changed their doctors, whether it was external circumstances, or resentment and embarrassment at the doctor's having found out too much about their private lives, or anxiety raised by the doctor's not entirely adequate handling of the case, and so on. The answer would be valuable, because these patients—especially those leaving without explanation—represent a serious loss to the doctor's practice. To mention one kind of loss, the doctor may not even know for certain whether his therapy was, or was not, of any use, as in the case of Mrs. D. (Case 7) or Mrs. N. (Case 20). It happens but seldom that the patient comes and takes leave of the doctor, as did Mrs. B. (Case 15), Miss M. (Case 19), and Miss X. (Case 23).

Another possible outcome is of the kind described by Dr. M. in his postscript to Mrs. Q.'s case (Case 21). The patient–doctor relationship continues unbroken; it even develops into a form more mature, more satisfactory to both patient and doctor. The doctor becomes a trusted friend, in the truest sense of the word, often to the patient's whole family. In some cases the relationship retains some sexually-coloured emotional elements, but I do not think that this amounts to more than what in any case is fairly common in doctor–patient relationships, except that in patients with a psychotherapeutic past these elements remain conscious and thus under control. Several of our cases belong to this group: Mr. K. (Case 11), Mr. J. (Case 14), Mrs. O. (Case 16), Peter (Case 19), Mrs. Q. (Case 21), Mr. V. (Case 22), and many more not reported in this book.

In my opinion these are the true general-practitioner cases. They demand a high degree of elasticity from the doctor, but they are the most gratifying—for both parties. The doctor feels that he has done a good job, and he has his reward in being able to watch the results. The patient knows that he has in his doctor's safe custody the remnants of his past problems, and that, if any new trouble should arise, he can ask for help, and doctor and patient will be able to continue their psychotherapeutic work where they dropped it. This is the most profitable way to run the "mutual investment company." We have a few impressive cases illustrating this particular outcome. Apart from Peter (Case 19)—Miss M. (Case 10), Mr. K. (Case 11), Mrs. Q. (Case 21) and Mr. V. (Case 22) are instructive examples, especially if the follow-up reports are taken into consideration. The difference in atmosphere between this group and the other two is indeed striking.

In the third group the patient remains dependent on the doctor, apparently settles down to staying with him for ever, but there is no real change for the better. Miss F. (Case 12) and Mr. Z. (Case 26) are impressive examples of this type. I must add that these two are far from being the only instances reported at our seminars.

An interesting sub-group of this type, mentioned several times, consists of patients who remain but wander from one partner to the other within a joint practice. Somehow one has the impression that something did not "click" between these patients and their doctors and, if one could only understand it, these people certainly could be helped. As already mentioned this group would be a fascinating subject for research, provided one could get good, frank reports from all the partners concerned. Unfortunately this is anything but easy. Mrs. C. (Case 1), Mrs. A. (Case 2), Mr. U. (Case 5) and Miss K. (Case 9) belong to this group.

Once again I must conclude by admitting our comparative ignorance of the processes that determine these most important events. We cannot predict with any certainty which patient will terminate his treatment in which way, whether or not the particular way of termination is desirable in his case and, above all, what kind of psychotherapeutic technique will achieve the most suitable way of termination. So I have to repeat my refrain of asking for more research.

*   *   *

To end this chapter I wish to stress that the tool in psychotherapy—the counterpart to the surgeon's knife, the physician's stethoscope or the radiologist's X-ray apparatus—is the doctor himself. That implies that he must constantly see to it that he is in good repair and in serviceable condition. Just as it is very difficult to operate with a blunt knife, to obtain sharp pictures with a faulty apparatus, to hear clearly through an unserviceable stethoscope, so the doctor will not be able to listen properly if he is in poor shape.

The other implication is that he must learn to use himself as skilfully as the surgeon uses his knife, the physician his stethoscope, the radiologist his lamps. The comparison goes even further. Just as the E.N.T. surgeon, for instance, has to learn to use his knife with his left hand as well as with his right, so must the psychotherapist learn to use himself with confidence and ease in all sorts of awkward situations. These two requirements are unconditional, and he who cannot comply with them should keep away from psychotherapy.

CHAPTER XXI

Summary and Outlook for the Future

THE more one learns of the problems of general practice, the more impressed one becomes with the immense need for psychotherapy. The present facilities for it in Great Britain —except for the wealthy few—are pathetically inadequate. The chief reason for this unsatisfactory state of affairs is that a large number of psychiatrists are either hostile to any kind of psychotherapy, or are aloof eclectics who hide their hostility behind the assertion that in "suitable" cases they advise psychotherapy and even undertake treatment themselves; or, if they are not hostile, they are interested only in physical methods, such as the various shock treatments, brain operations, and the ever increasing number of drugs.

What can be done, then, with patients in need of psychotherapy, and especially with those in need of the kind of psychotherapy discussed in this book? Our experience shows that the few psychiatrists who are not hostile to psychotherapy do not really welcome such patients, for their interest is chiefly in major psychotherapy; and the still fewer who are interested in this kind of work are greatly hampered by insufficient staff and lack of proper facilities. It is no exaggeration to say that to obtain psychotherapy for an adult under the National Health Service is nearly as difficult as winning a treble chance in a football pool.

The chief cause of this state of affairs is the lack of psychotherapeutically-trained psychiatrists. All teaching hospitals, both undergraduate and postgraduate, give a thorough training in brain anatomy and physiology and in all the pharmacological and physical methods used in psychiatry, but, so far as I know, hardly any offer systematic training in psychotherapy. In most hospitals where this is offered, it is in the form of an undefined apprenticeship of, say, six months' registrarship in the firm of a more or less psychotherapeutically-minded consultant. During this period the future psychiatrist may perhaps learn some superficial skill and a little polish, but it is highly improbable that he will achieve the "limited, though considerable, change of personality" which—as will be discussed in the Appendix on training—is the necessary basis of all psychotherapeutic skill.

As so many psychiatrists have not had proper opportunity, or have not cared to acquire psychotherapeutic skill, their attitude towards patients in need of psychotherapy—and to general practitioners who ask for it—is mainly negative. A number of negative reports by psychiatrists have been included in this book, together with some characteristic remarks they called forth from the general practitioner to whom they were addressed. If more publicity were given in the medical press both to these reports and to the doctor's reactions to them, I am sure that both would quickly vanish.

What I have just said about psychiatrists is *a fortiori* true of general practitioners who have been trained by them. I wish to put on record that in 1955, at one of the meetings of the Medical Section of the British Psychological Society, a consultant of a big London teaching hospital proudly stated that all medical students at his hospital received adequate training in the psychiatric and psychotherapeutic skills needed in general practice. This adequate training consists of a short course on the "psychobiological development of the child" during the pre-clinical year, another short course on "how to examine a patient" during the introductory clinical course, and a main course in their first clinical year, during which *the students are attached for six weeks to the psychiatric department*. Compare, with the psychiatrist's pride, the indignation of a professor of anatomy, or of an obstetrician, if anybody dared suggest that six weeks' training in anatomy or obstetrics was sufficient for future general practitioners. Moreover, we know that many general practitioners, after qualifying, will never attend a confinement, whereas all of them will have to cope with their patients' psychological problems as an inevitable part of their daily work.

This is the reason why my description of "the general practitioner" and "the psychiatrist" in this book is rather idealized and Utopian. On the other hand, as the observations reported show, it is possible to find general practitioners who are interested enough to acquire the necessary skills, and with further effort it should be possible to find psychiatrists too. Still, for the time being both are rare birds, and they have had to acquire such skill as they possess on their own, at their own cost, and mostly without help from the teaching hospitals.

But, even if we disregard these environmental, and perhaps only temporary, adverse factors, the fundamental question remains to be answered: By whom should this kind of psychotherapy be undertaken, the general practitioner or the specialist? Admittedly the scope of this field—psychotherapy in general practice—is ill-defined, and the methods and techniques to be used in it have not yet been worked out, still less properly validated and standardized. This, however, involves only a modification of the fundamental question: By whom should research in this field be conducted in order to define its scope and work out correct techniques?

The problem can be attacked from several angles. The easiest answer comes from consideration of the number of patients involved. If it is true that at least a quarter of the general practitioner's work is taken up by the psychologically ill, it is manifestly impossible to devise a psychiatric service equal to the task, unless we revolutionize both our training facilities and the whole structure of our psychiatric establishments.

Another possibility would be to create a new branch of medicine and a new breed of specialists in "minor" psychotherapy. All the arguments against the evil of further specialization of our profession can be marshalled against this proposition. There is, however, a much weightier argument. With this we arrive at the solution advocated throughout this book, namely, that the proper person for this work and for this research is the general practitioner. His position in the community admits him to a vantage point from which he can, and in fact does, keep an eye on the development of personality problems in his patients, and it is a rare exception if he is not the first to be asked for help. In this way, by his everyday work he obtains automatically all the observations which will provide the only safe basis for the new psychotherapy.

So, for part of this last chapter, let us leave the world of hard facts, such as economic limitations, ossified training methods and short-sighted professional vested interests, the unnecessarily restricted scale of the doctor's responses caused by fears and apprehensions, and all the other factors that prevent the general practitioner from achieving the "considerable, though limited, change of personality" that is required (Appendix I). Let us suppose that a basically reformed medical training—and social economy—has overcome all these difficulties and that we are about to meet the Utopian general practitioner. What will he be like? (In what follows I shall recapitulate the most important findings of our research and indicate in brackets in which chapters the particular problems were discussed at some length.)

In the first place, our Utopian general practitioner will be less impressed by the experience and skill of his hospital specialists. This involves no devaluation of the latter; on the contrary, their value will grow parallel with the recognition of their limitations. Once it is realized that the problems of hospital medicine differ to a great extent from those of general practice, and that uncritically transferring the well-proven methods of hospital medicine to general practice is a poor and impotent solution, each discipline will be able to develop freely and even benefit from the results and successes of the other (Chapter IX).

The new general practitioner will thus not apply automatically the methods worked out and validated for hospital practice. This holds true particularly for "medical history-taking," with its almost standardized sequence of questions. Though he will know the value of this kind of "relevant information," he will know also that he who asks questions will get answers—but hardly anything else (Chapter XI).

Similarly, he will be aware that complying automatically in his diagnostic work with the rules of "elimination by appropriate physical examinations" will protect him against missing a possible organic illness, but only at the price of establishing a "ranking order of illnesses and of patients attached to them" (Chapters IV and V). Another danger involved in "elimination by appropriate physical examinations" which he will try to avoid is finding some accidental and, more often than not, irrelevant physical sign and inducing and helping the patient to "organize" his illness around it (Chapter III). A number of our case histories—Cases 5, 6, 9, 10, 11, 19, 23, 26, 27 and 28—show varieties of the calamitous consequences that can follow this mechanically applied diagnostic procedure.

Our general practitioner will have learnt that the "clinical illnesses" thoroughly studied and classified by hospital medicine are only episodes, though often highly dramatic or even tragic episodes, in a long history. Although he is fully aware that it is his duty to look after his patients during these episodes—and here he frequently will need, and receive, valuable help from the specialist services—he will also know that any such episode represents only one of the several "illnesses" that a patient "offers or proposes" to his doctor (Chapters II, III and XVIII–XIX). The way the doctor "responds" to these "offers" has signal consequences for the patient's future. Much more is meant by this than the possibility of overlooking an organic process, the frightening bogy that our present training system has so successfully implanted in every doctor's mind (Chapters IV, VI and XX).

The present established method for laying the bogy, and with it the not fully admitted, but nevertheless fully felt, responsibility for one's "responses," is diluting responsibility by the "collusion of anonymity" and the "perpetuation of the teacher–pupil relationship" (Chapters VII–IX). In Utopia these ways have been given up, because specialists have long realized the advantages of relinquishing the rôle of superior, omniscient mentors, and have accepted the much more realistic and rewarding rôle of expert assistants to the general practitioner, who now remains in full charge of his patients. For short periods, when the necessary therapy or examination requires expert specialist skill, a patient may be handed over to the consultant, but only for a limited time and for a limited purpose, as happens today with a patient requiring a pathological or radiological examination.

The doctor, left in sole charge of his patient, is able to follow the developing history in all its serious and all its petty details, both during health and in illness. Hospital doctors, from junior housemen to senior consultants, can at best get fragments of this history, as much as the patient's answers to their well-proved questions reveal. The general practitioner, especially if he has some experience in managing the joint capital of the "mutual investment company" existing between his patient and himself (Chapters XVIII and XX), will need little additional information, as most of his patient's background is known to him. Thus he has no need to ask all the well-proved questions; instead he must find time for his patient and then "listen" (Chapters XI–

XII, XX and Appendix I). This, I am afraid, will perhaps remain a real difficulty, even in Utopia. However favourable the Utopian economic and medical system might be, the commodity which is always and everywhere in short supply is general practitioners' time, especially during the winter months.

Still, just as time has to be found at present for a proper routine clinical examination, however hard-pressed the doctor or the specialist is, time will have to be found in Utopia for a proper "long interview" whenever the doctor considers it necessary "to start" (Chapters XI–XII). On no account will the general practitioner be content with a superficial diagnosis as described by the hospital tags, but he will consider it his duty to arrive at a more comprehensive understanding of his patient's "offers," that is, at a "deeper" diagnosis (Chapter VI). As we are in Utopia, let us assume that psychiatrists, with the help of general practitioners, have developed a terminology which enables doctors to describe the findings of this "deeper" diagnosis, that is the various personality or psychological problems, in language as simple, concise, and generally intelligible as that in which hospital medicine describes "clinical" illnesses. In this way doctors will have no difficulty in giving a name to the psychological illnesses diagnosed in their patients (Chapter III).

I do not know what the new general practitioners will think of my proposal to differentiate the "basic fault" and the "conflict" from the "clinical illnesses" offered by the patient from which the practitioner has to choose that with the best therapeutic possibilities (Chapters XIX and III, XII, XIII, XX). Should these ideas stand up to the scrutiny of time and experience, Utopian doctors will be on the watch to prevent the patient from "organizing" his illness around an unimportant and accidental physical sign, thereby sapping in a futile and sterile manner both his own energies and those of his medical attendants. General practitioners will have learnt when it is essential to treat a "clinical illness" offered by a patient and when to disregard it and make a bee-line for the underlying "conflict." In other words, in Utopia doctors will have reliable criteria enabling them to decide "what to treat" (Chapter XX). On the one hand, their teaching hospitals will have taught them the skills required when "listening" during a "long interview" (Chapters XI–XII and Appendix I); on the other, the whole community will have been educated to expect the doctor to examine a patient both physically and psychologically (Chapters III, VI, XVIII and XX).

We have only vague ideas of what the technical solution will be of the many difficulties caused by this combination of physical and psychological examinations. Will the psychological examination, the "long interview," follow, precede, or coincide with, the physical examination? Will it be possible to establish a routine as reliable as that which we possess for the classical clinical examination? (Chapters IV, XIII and XX). Our knowledge is too scanty to permit any prediction in this field. But if we recall that two essential techniques of the classical clinical examination, percussion and auscultation, are comparatively recent innovations—percussion dates from 1761 and auscultation from 1819—perhaps it is not too ambitious to hope that during the next hundred to a hundred and fifty years our future colleagues will be able to standardize a reliable routine for the "long interview," and even for its combination with a physical examination.

Does this mean that all medical students in Utopia will have to acquire a modicum of psychodiagnostic skills to pass their finals? These skills, though not exacting, demand a certain amount of elasticity of mind and personality, as well as a certain degree of overall maturity; for the time being I do not see how facilities can be provided in an academic curriculum for all students to acquire them as well as the "limited, though considerable, change of personality" which is the unconditional basis for these skills (Appendix I). Further, I do not know whether it is desirable, or even feasible, to demand this change from every student (Appendix II). On the other hand, every doctor possessing these skills is a better doctor than he would be without them.

What I have said about psychodiagnostic skills applies even more stringently to psychotherapeutic skills. In this field, no doubt, even in Utopia there will be a selection (Appendix II); only some will feel attracted to psychotherapy, and of these only a few will be masters of their craft. This, however, is true for every branch of our profession.

If my ideas about the "basic fault," the "conflict" and the various "clinical illnesses offered" prove acceptable in the light of experience, the tasks of the general practitioner in this field may be tentatively outlined. As mentioned above, he will look after his patients during a "clinical illness" and, if necessary, call on his consultants for help and advice, as he does now, but he will also aim at preventing his patients from "organizing" their illnesses round an unimportant physical finding. If there is no danger, or as soon as the danger has abated, he will try to get to grips with the "conflict" which prompted the patient to complain (Chapters III and XVIII–XX). He certainly will have learnt not to "reassure" his patient before he has found out what the problem is (Chapter X). How far he will be able to penetrate into the patient's conflict will depend chiefly on his own personality, i.e. his apostolic function (Chapters XVI–XVII). Part II contains case histories illustrating the various techniques used and the various depths reached by general practitioner-psychotherapists who took part in our research; I expect that similar differences will exist even in Utopia.

Although there is an unmistakable line running through the "illness offered" to the "conflict" and, deeper still, in the direction of the "basic fault" (Cases 10, 19, 21–24), I do not think it will prove possible within the framework of general practice to reach the "basic fault" and still less to redress it in a seriously ill patient. This will probably remain the domain of major psychotherapy. But, having said that, I wish to point out that any psychiatrist would be proud of some of the successes reported in this book. Obviously the frontier between general practitioner and major psychotherapy cannot, and should not, be strictly defined, perhaps even in Utopia.

I have mentioned that in Utopia the specialist will not be a superior mentor, but the general practitioner's expert assistant. Conversely, this means that the general practitioner will no longer be able to disappear behind the strong and impenetrable façade of a bored, overworked, but not very responsible dispenser of drugs and writer of innumerable letters, certificates and requests for examinations; instead he will have to shoulder the privilege of undivided responsibility for people's health and well-being, and partly also for their future happiness.

What part will psychiatry play in Utopian medicine? The answer depends on one's views about the future of psychiatry, which at present is in a bisected, or perhaps only bifurcated, state. Some psychiatrists almost exclusively advocate physical treatment by drugs, shocks of various kinds, and brain operations; others advocate psychotherapy; and in spite of many finely, or not so finely, minced words the representatives of the two trends do not see eye to eye. It is a matter for conjecture whether these two trends will diverge still further, each ultimately becoming an independent speciality, or whether they will converge again at some fairly distant point. Obviously I cannot start writing a treatise on this point, so I must content myself with pointing out this uncertainty.

Fortunately, general-practitioner psychotherapy, not only in its name, but in its essence, is independent and largely uninfluenced by this controversy. The problems with which a general practitioner has to cope only very rarely call for a leucotomy. The fact that he prescribes drugs and refers his patients for shock treatment as often as he does is mainly due to convenience, to his training, but, above all, to his inability either to obtain psychotherapy for his patients or to undertake psychotherapy himself. Thus the two foremost tasks for at any rate one branch of psychiatry in Utopia will be to train general practitioners in psychotherapy and to provide psychodiagnostic and psychotherapeutic facilities for at least a fair proportion of the patients who need it.

Psychodiagnostic facilities in Utopia will probably be modelled on our emergency service (Chapters XII–XIII). After examining the patient referred to him, the consultant will not content himself with attaching to him some irrelevant diagnostic tag and advising the doctor to reassure him and give him a tonic, an antidepressant, a tranquillizer, or a sedative. Instead, he will describe where, in his opinion, the real problem lies, what methods the general practitioner might adopt to bring it to light, and how this particular patient can be helped by this particular doctor to solve his particular problem. This will not be too difficult to the consultant because he will have a sufficient knowledge of the doctor and his individual apostolic function.

The psychotherapeutic facilities will not have to be on such an enormous scale as now appears necessary. In the first place, general practitioners will themselves be able to treat a large proportion of patients in need; secondly, people will be less secretive and inhibited, they will come for help earlier, and will be able to complain about their conflicts before they develop an illness. It is almost certain that doctors will be able to cure patients in these early, "unorganized" stages, and in consequence the number of chronically neurotic patients will considerably diminish (Cases 8, 10, 11, 13, 14, 15, 16 and 19–24).

The most rewarding task for psychiatrists of the future will be to study, in co-operation with general practitioners, the fundamental pathology of the "basic fault." Some of our findings relate to the early stages of its development and thus offer a possible way of studying it; these are the "child as the presenting symptom" and the "neurotic tradition" passed on from generation to generation (Cases 2, 7, 23 and 24). If general practitioners and psychiatrists can co-operate in this field, the development of a pathology of the whole person, and with it a better theoretical grasp and a more efficient therapeutic skill in both general practice and in psychiatry, is perhaps in sight. Parallel with a better understanding, a more exact and more concise terminology will develop. Only he whose knowledge is patchy and scanty has to use long phrases to describe the little that he knows.

In the field of medical technique the new psychiatrist, in collaboration with the new general practitioner, will have to establish the criteria for the three interrelated problems of "when to start," "when to stop" and "what to treat" (Chapters XI, XII and XX). We have found in the course of our research that there are periods when patients need to be left alone, or only nursed, without anybody's expecting anything from them, and that there are other periods when they need someone to whom to complain, someone who will "listen" with a sympathetic and understanding mind. These periods may alternate quickly or each may last long, but little is known about the forces that govern them.

Closely connected with the previous problem is that concerning regression and maturity (Chapters XVII and XIX). When, and especially in which direction, should a patient be allowed to regress, that is, to become infantile and dependent on his doctor or on his environment? How long should a regressive period last and to what limits is it advisable to allow it to develop? In Utopia general practitioners and psychiatrists alike will know a good deal about these questions, and their treatment of patients will accordingly be more purposeful and effective.

In particular, both general practitioners and psychiatrists will have criteria at their disposal enabling them to decide what kind of termination is advisable in any individual case (Chapter XX).

They will also know how to see to it that a successful therapy, physical, pharmacological, or psychological, increases the joint capital of the "mutual investment company" (Chapter XVIII) and does not, if it can possibly be avoided, lead to doctor and patient parting for good. If, on the other hand, such a parting is advisable for a reliable and lasting result, they will be able to wind up the relationship while saving the mutual investment company's most important assets.

And lastly, the greatest problem of general practice, the doctor's "apostolic function" (Chapters XVI–XVIII and XX). Will the Utopians have a real pharmacopoeia of the drug "doctor," indicating in what form and what strength it should be administered, i.e. what its correct curative, maintenance, and preventive doses are? I think they will have, perhaps not a rigid code, laying down hard-and-fast rules for all doctors, all occasions and all patients, but an elastic one, allowing great latitude, but not surrendering the most important drug in our therapeutic armoury to unbridled "common sense."

*　　*　　*

The chief results of our more than five years of research are a number of problems, many of them awkward and uncomfortable. In comparison with the many problems we have raised, we have only few answers to give, and in particular we have hardly any "advice" to offer the doctor about what to do or what not to do; still less does this book offer any "reassurance." My colleagues on many occasions complained of this, both during our joint work and afterwards.

Those who do not start with the last chapter but have read the book, will know my answer. "Advice" is usually a well-intentioned shot in the dark, is nearly always futile, and that applies even more strongly to "reassurance." We have found that it is more profitable both for doctors and patients to diagnose the problem; more often than not, when that is done there will be no need either for advice or for reassurance. The real problem is likely to be unpleasant or even painful, but it will be real, and with hard work it is probable that something real can be done about it.

My diagnosis is that general practice is seriously ill, but the illness is benign and, provided the right therapy is applied, the prognosis is good. Hospital or scientific medicine, however, is not ill, but is hale and hearty, rich in achievements and successes. True, she treats her ailing sister, general practice, rather condescendingly, as a kind of poor relation. Hospital medicine charitably distributes alms and allows her poor sister to feed on the crumbs that fall from the opulent table of medical science.

Should general practitioners be "reassured" that things are not so bad and comforted by the fact that a consultant is always ready with some "advice" when a real problem or emergency arises? Is it not more profitable and realistic to demonstrate the extent to which the present symptoms are their own creation and to enable them, on the basis of the diagnosis, to take their illness seriously, i.e. instead of being "reassured," to do something real about it?

All the general practitioners who took part in our research accepted this hard fact after some remonstrance. What they resented most was that their work and their responsibility had not been made easier by their new experience and their newly won skill. This is understandable; while a patient is ailing or convalescing life must be made easier for him; as he gets better, the burdens will inevitably increase. This happened with my companions; as they learnt to see more, more exactly and more deeply, their work became more complicated, their responsibility heavier.

All of them without exception complained about this, but all of them without exception found their work incomparably more interesting and more rewarding. During all these years I have not heard one practitioner say that he would like to go back, still less that he had gone back to the old ways and techniques he used before joining our research team.

Appendixes

APPENDIX I

Training

THIS chapter is intended in the first instance for psychiatrists who may consider undertaking the training of general practitioners or students in this field of medicine—and not primarily for general practitioners. This explains why its tone is somewhat different from that of the rest of the book, psychiatric technical terms being used more freely.

On the whole, qualified doctors are much better material for training in psychotherapy than medical students.* In the first place, the training is not compulsory; it is not done for examination purposes. Doctors come voluntarily, a self-selected group, who want to acquire a particular new skill because they are interested in it. Secondly, a general practitioner has the inestimable advantage over a medical student of having been knocked about by life. He has seen successes and failures, and witnessed a considerable amount of human suffering, which it was his responsibility—at least in part—either to alleviate or to make tolerable to his patient. He has had time to test in his own practice what he was taught in his medical school and hospital, and he has thus become both less dependent on authority and less rebellious against it, that is, more humble.

Moreover, a general practitioner is, as a rule, older, more mature, than a medical student. It is questionable whether a young man or woman of twenty to twenty-three years of age, who could hardly have had any real experience of a stable sexual partnership of some duration, who possibly has never earned his living and still less been responsible for a family dependent on him, will be able to understand the subtle and complex ramifications of marital relations and the often profound conflicts between

---

* In the light of my experiences with medical students at University College Hospital, London, the statements in this and the next paragraph will have to be qualified. [Added in 1963.]

self-centred needs and obligations towards others. In this respect, too, a general practitioner in his late twenties or early thirties is more promising material.

Another promising group could be recruited from registrars (and possibly senior housemen) working together in a not too small general hospital. I have not yet experimented with such a group, but should be most interested to do so. Consultants and specialists appeared as occasional visitors in one or the other of our seminars. Although their patients' problems are the same, a specialist's technical approach to them, in fact the whole atmosphere of a consulting-room or of a hospital department, is so different from that of a general practitioner's surgery, that we had to content ourselves with recognizing this difference. It remains to be seen whether it will be possible to organize a seminar for consultants for research into the psychological problems of their practice; if so, it would certainly be most interesting.

Psychotherapeutic Skill

So let us return to general practitioners and repeat that at least a quarter, possibly much more, of their daily work is taken up with psychological cases. This being so, it is a puzzling fact that the traditional medical curriculum does not take this into consideration and therefore does not properly equip the doctor for such an important part of his work.

The realization of this shortcoming has been the cause of the ever-increasing demand by general practitioners in the past thirty years or so for some kind of training in psychotherapy. All over the world psychiatrists have tried to respond to this demand, and have arranged various "courses." But, in spite of hard work, interest and enthusiasm on both sides, the results have on the whole proved disappointing. In my opinion the reason for this relative failure is the fact that tutors and their students have taken over uncritically the forms and methods of the teaching hospitals and the traditional refresher courses; that is to say, concentrated, almost full-time courses were offered lasting a couple of weeks or so, and the mainstay of these courses were lectures and ward rounds illustrated by case histories and clinical demonstrations. It has been completely forgotten that *psychotherapy is, above all, not theoretical knowledge, but a personal skill.*

The only way to acquire a new skill is to expose oneself to the actual situation and to learn to recognize the problems in it and the methods of dealing with them. Being lectured to about problems and methods can help, but can never take the place of direct experience.

A further reason for the failure of the traditional courses is that they have not taken into consideration the fact that *the acquisition of psychotherapeutic skill does not consist only of learning something new: it inevitably also entails a limited, though considerable, change in the doctor's personality*.

Training in Psychotherapy

The only systematic course of training in psychotherapy is the psychoanalytic system (which was adopted to a certain extent by the Jungian school). It consists of three separate parts: personal analysis, theoretical courses, and practical work under supervision. In the classical form, as developed in Berlin and taken all over the world, the three parts are kept fairly separate from one another. The only exception is the Hungarian system, with its insistence that the supervision of a candidate's first case or cases should be carried out by his training analyst.

This difference has many important repercussions, and that relevant to our present topic is as follows. In the Berlin system the counter-transference of the candidate to his patient is, by tacit agreement, not dealt with in the supervision, but is left to be worked through in the personal analysis. Thus the emphasis in supervision is focused on the understanding of the peculiarities of the patient's psychodynamics, which is usually expressed in the standard question: "What does the patient try to convey to his analyst?" In the Hungarian system, the interrelation of the transference of the patient and the counter-transference of his analyst is in the focus of attention right from the start, and remains there. What is studied is the interaction of these two transferences, that is, how they influence and modify each other. It is not easy to integrate this kind of supervision into the classical system, with its clear separation of supervision from personal analysis. The examination of the transference phenomena inevitably leads to an examination of the habitual reaction patterns of the candidate, i.e. of his personal conflicts and difficulties, of his unsolved and often unconscious problems. This kind of supervision therefore always contains some elements of personal analysis, its aim being that the candidate should at least become aware of his automatic patterns and the anxieties causing them, even though they may remain unsolved for the time being.

When Enid Balint and I started our first training scheme at the Family Discussion Bureau (London) we were faced with the problem of how to train social workers, dealing with their clients' marital problems, to become aware of, and sensitive to, unconscious processes—without offering them the well-proven method of personal analysis. In fact, we had to be very careful to prevent our training scheme from becoming a therapy for the workers, at least to prevent its main objective from becoming therapeutic, because therapeutic facilities were prohibitively expensive and so had to be ruled out.

Faced with this problem, I decided to use my experience with the Hungarian system of supervision, and to work out a training in psychotherapy based chiefly on the close study by group methods of the workers' counter-transference. In order to be able to examine the latter in detail I had to create conditions in which it could be shown as freely as possible. I therefore did not tolerate the use of any paper material in the case conferences; the worker had to report freely about his or her experiences with the client, in a way reminiscent of "free association," permitting all sorts of subjective distortions, omissions, second thoughts, subsequent interpolations, etc. I used this report—as it is used in the Hungarian system of supervision—as something akin to the manifest dream text, and tried to infer from it the dynamic factors shaping it. Both the second thoughts of the reporter and the criticisms and comments of the listening group were evaluated as a kind of free association. The real proof of the correctness or incorrectness of the reconstruction of what happened between the worker and the client in the interview was the subsequent interview, in the same way as the proof of a dream interpretation is usually the subsequent dream.

The method, as we jointly developed it further for training general practitioners in psychotherapy, is based on the same ideas. In our research seminars we have no facilities for personal analysis. The whole training is carried out by discussing the reports of the individual practitioners on their patients to the group consisting of their colleagues taking part in the course. The most important material used is the doctor's counter-transference, i.e. the way in which he uses his personality, his scientific convictions, his automatic reaction patterns, etc.

Two Tasks in acquiring Psychotherapeutic Skill

Two tasks thus faced us when we launched this experiment; we had to create conditions—

(*a*) in which the doctors would from the outset be able to do psychotherapy under supervision, and

(*b*) which would enable them to view their own methods and responses to their patients from some distance, recognize traits in their particular approach to their patients which were useful and might be understood and developed, and others which were not so useful, and, when their dynamic significance was understood, needed to be modified or even abandoned.

The two tasks are very closely linked, but for the sake of clarity I shall deal with them separately.

(*a*) As soon as it is realized that a great part of the general practitioner's daily work consists of treating neurotic complaints, the first task does not seem very difficult. The only essential is *not to take the doctor out of his practice*, to encourage him to go on doing what he is doing in any case, and give him ample opportunity to discuss his day-to-day work.

So far so good, but there are many difficulties involved in this apparently simple scheme. They were discussed mainly in Part I, especially in Chapters VII–IX, when we dealt with such things as the "dilution of responsibility" by the "collusion of anonymity" and the "perpetuation of the teacher–pupil relationship."

(*b*) To start with, there is no proven, established method in general use for training in psychotherapy, that is, for helping the candidate to achieve the *"limited, though considerable, change in his personality" necessary for his new skill*. So far as I know them, the various methods adopted are based on a kind of undefined apprenticeship. The only exception is psychoanalysis (and to some extent the Jungian school) which were discussed above. To state it rather strongly, it could be said that the only systematic training in psychotherapy, that is psychoanalytic training, has turned into a therapy with exaggerated demands. I am fully aware that here I am on largely unexplored and rather uncertain ground, but I think it should be stated that for the time being we have no agreed criteria of what are the minimal and the optimal standards in the desirable personality change necessary for a psychotherapist. The analytic system works on the rather expensive principle of "the more, the safer."

As such a system and such standards were beyond the realms of possibility for our scheme, we had to devise our own methods and to define our own standards.

The Use of Group Methods

The mainstay of our scheme is the weekly case conferences, about ten to twelve in each of three annual terms. To secure intensive participation and, on the other hand, to obtain sufficiently varied material, we have found it advisable to have groups of about eight. In addition to the conferences, we offer any doctor who asks for it individual supervision of his cases, i.e. about an hour per week of "private discussion."*

I have already pointed out that we try to avoid, as far as possible, the ever-tempting "teaching-being-taught" atmosphere. Our aim is to help the doctors *to become more sensitive to what is going on, consciously or unconsciously, in the patient's mind when doctor and patient are together.* This kind of "listening" is very different from "history-taking," and we encountered considerable difficulty when trying to free doctors from the automatic use of this kind of approach. This difference was discussed to a certain extent in Chapter XI, and I have to repeat parts of what was stated there. The main difference is that history-taking is concerned almost exclusively with objective events, or with events that can easily be expressed in words; and towards such events both doctor and patient can adopt a detached, "scientifically objective" attitude. The events that we are concerned with are highly subjective and personal, often hardly conscious, or even wholly beyond conscious control; also, as often as not, there exists no unequivocal way of describing them in words. Nevertheless, these events exist, and, moreover, they profoundly influence one's attitude to life in general and still more so to falling and being ill, accepting medical help, etc.

It may safely be said that these events, happening all the time

* Subsequent experience cast some doubt on the value of "individual supervision" for our form of training. [Added in 1963.]

in everybody's mind, are only in part sensible adaptations to the ever-changing environment; to a large extent they are governed by almost automatic patterns, originating mainly in childhood but influenced by emotional experiences in later life. Our first task was to awaken in the doctors an awareness of these automatic patterns, and then to enable them to study in greater and greater detail how they influence the patient's attitude towards his illness, and on the other hand how they colour or even determine his relations to any human being, and especially to his doctor.

Another factor affecting the patient's developing relation to his doctor is the doctor's response, which is also partly governed by automatic patterns. The interplay of these two sets of patterns, whether and how they "click," to a large extent determines the efficiency of any treatment. Its influence is less important in short-lived, acute illnesses, but in chronic illnesses it is almost crucial. In order to be able to "click" better, and with more patients, the doctor must have a wide choice of responses, which means that he must become aware of his own automatic patterns and gradually acquire at least a modicum of freedom from them.

The Limited though Considerable Change of Personality

Intellectual teaching, however good, has hardly any effect on this process of liberation and general easing up. What is needed is an emotionally free and friendly atmosphere in which it is possible to face the realization that one's actual behaviour is often entirely different from what it was intended to be, and from what one has always believed it to be. The realization of the *discrepancy between one's actual behaviour and one's intentions and beliefs* is not an easy task. But, if there is good cohesion between the doctors in the group, the mistakes, blind-spots and limitations of any individual member can be brought into the open and at least partially accepted by him. The group steadily develops a better understanding of its own problems, both collectively and individually. The individual can more easily face the realization of his mistakes when he feels that the group understands them and can identify with him in them, and when he can see that he is not the only one to make them. Moreover, it takes only a short time for the group to discover that the technique of each member, including the psychiatrist group leader, is an expression of his personality, and that the same of course applies to his habitual mistakes.

Crises

Admittedly crises occur from time to time when one or other member finds it difficult to accept the full implications of some of his ways of handling his patients, or the realization of some facets of his personality that he has previously been only dimly aware of. These, however, can be borne, as they are also group events and do not solely concern the individual. It has been easy to describe this state of affairs, but it is rather difficult to explain its dynamism. So long as the mutual identifications of the members are fairly strong, any individual member can face strains, because he feels accepted and supported by the group. His mistakes and failings, although humiliating, are not felt as singling him out as a useless member of the group; on the contrary, he feels that he has helped the group to progress, using his failings as stepping-stones.* *Crises may occur when there is some tension between one or other member and the rest of the group* which the leader has not detected soon enough (I would add that neither his rôle nor his psychiatric training confers on the group leader an absolute immunity against this hazard), and, instead of re-establishing good cohesion, his criticism may help to widen the gulf.

Signs of this isolation, or tendency to isolation, and the accompanying touchiness can be regarded as equivalents of what psychoanalysts call resistances. On the one hand, they are premonitory signs that some major personal attitude of the individual is being tackled in the group situation; on the other hand, by the way in which the isolation is achieved and maintained, they show what the problem is. In the same way the reaction of the integrated group towards such an attempt at isolation reveals the other side—that is, the counter-transferences of the group to the particular personality problem. The way in which a member isolates himself, as well as the way in which the group deals with it, must be shown up. They represent very valuable

* In psychiatric terms, the depression caused by the realization of one's shortcomings must be fully accepted; identification with the common group ideal must remain, now as before, a desirable and attainable aim, but the group leader must watch very carefully when and how any member is forced or allowed to slide into a paranoid position of an individual who has been "singled out."

material for studying inter-personal relations, and their full realization is necessary for the re-establishment of a workable cohesion.

If such crises occur too often, or leave bitter resentment behind, it is a sign that the pace of training has been too exacting and that the group has been made to work under considerable strain for some time. It is an equally ominous sign, however, if no crises occur; it means that the sensitivity and grasp of the group are not developing and that the group and its leader are in real danger of degenerating into a mutual admiration society in which everything is fine and the whole group consists of nice, clever, and sensible people. It is a fact that the acquisition of psychotherapeutic skill is tantamount to the discovery of a number of hard and unpleasant facts about one's own limitations. This unpleasant strain must be faced, and the group develops as long as it can face it, and stops developing as soon as it tries to avoid it. It is the task of the group leader to create an atmosphere in which each member (including himself) will be able to bear the brunt when it is his turn to bear it.

It is a precondition of our technique that this kind of atmosphere shall be established in the group, and it is only in such an atmosphere that it is possible to achieve what we term "the courage of one's own stupidity." This means that the doctor feels free to be himself with his patient—that is, to use all his past experiences and present skills without much inhibition. At the same time he is prepared to face severe objections by the group and occasionally even searching criticism of what we call his "stupidity." Although every report and case conference is definitely a strain and an effort, the result is nearly always a widening of one's individual possibilities and a better grasp of the problems.

Importance of Timing

One of the most important factors in this kind of training is timing, which in the first instance means not being in a hurry. It is better to allow the doctor to make his mistakes, perhaps even to encourage him in them, than to try to prevent him from making them. This sounds rather foolhardy, but it is not; all our trainees have had considerable clinical experience, and this "sink or swim" policy was justified. Apart from not undermining the doctor's confidence and dignity, it had the advantage of providing ample

material for discussion, as everybody was seeing patients all the
time and was anxious to report his findings and discoveries, his
successes and difficulties.

If the timing is good enough, the doctor feels free to be himself
and has "the courage of his own stupidity." Gradually he becomes aware of the type of situation in which he is likely to lose
his sensitivity and ease of response, or, in other words, to behave
automatically. Meanwhile the reports of other doctors have
shown him what other methods might be adopted in similar
situations. The discussion of various individual methods, the
demonstration of their advantages and limitations, encourages
him to experiment. (One practitioner announced the result of
such an experiment thus: "I have done a real 'Smith' in this case
—and it worked,"* meaning he had adopted the attitude he felt
Smith usually adopted.) Every such experiment means a step
towards greater freedom and improved skill.

Attitude of the Group Leader

Perhaps the most important factor is the behaviour of the
leader of the group. It is hardly an exaggeration to say that if he
finds the right attitude he will teach more by his example than
by everything else combined. After all, the technique we advocate
is based on exactly the same sort of listening that we expect the
doctors to learn and then to practise with their patients. By
allowing everybody to be themselves, to have their say in their
own way and in their own time, by watching for proper cues—
that is, speaking only when something is *really* expected from
him and making his point in a form which, instead of prescribing
the right way, opens up possibilities for the doctors to discover
by themselves *some* right way of dealing with the patient's
problems—the leader can demonstrate in the "here and now"
situation what he wants to teach.

Obviously no-one can live up to these exacting standards.
Fortunately there is no need for perfection. The group leader may
make mistakes—in fact he often does—without causing much
harm if he can accept criticism in the same or even somewhat
sharper terms than he expects his group to accept. This must be
watched very carefully, and any hesitation by the group in
exposing the leader's mistakes must be pointed out. Obviously

* See Case 19 in Chapter XII.

this freedom cannot develop if the leader tries to hedge or to explain away his failings. It is a wholesome sign if the group can run him down, even if they have some fun at his expense, provided they can do so without rejecting him or turning hostile to him.

The Doctors' Counter-transference

I mentioned above that the most important material for our training method was the ways in which the doctor uses his personality, his convictions, his knowledge, his habitual reaction patterns, etc., all that can be summed up by the term "counter-transference."

In our setting this counter-transference has three aspects, and in our scheme we use these three in varying degrees; they are—

(1) The doctor–patient relationship.
(2) The doctor–group leader relationship.
(3) The doctor–rest of the group relationship.

We use the *doctor–group leader relationship* very sparingly, as in the group situation we try to avoid the discussion of emotions of a personal and intimate nature; that is to say, we try to avoid allowing the group to develop into an openly therapeutic venture. In order to achieve this, the group leader tries to merge as far as possible into the group. Interpreting consistently the ever-present, ever-changing transference feelings of the various participants would focus emotions still more on the leader—as happens in therapeutic groups. We all know what the conse-quences of these consistent interpretations are. The transferred emotions—except perhaps for the very last phase of the thera-peutic situation—become intensified and increasingly primitive. In our method we try to avoid this kind of development, although we are fully aware that it is impossible to do so completely. The group leader is unavoidably singled out by his place and function, and a great deal of emotion is centred on him. This fact must be recognized and accepted, but we refrain from interpreting it in detail. The few occasions when we have had to interpret it have been exceptional, and we are uncertain whether or not they could have been avoided by more skilled technique, i.e. by paying closer attention to the counter-transference in other fields.

Nevertheless, the importance of this relationship cannot be minimized. The group leader represents the standards aimed at by the training scheme. Whenever a patient is interviewed by a practitioner, in his mind the group leader is always present. Thus the interview, depending on the practitioner's actual emotional attitude, is conducted in order to show off to the leader, or to prove that he was wrong, or to demonstrate that the practitioner has learnt his lesson and that he can get on well without him, or that his opinion was most valuable and penetrating, and so on. Of course the same emotional attitudes colour the reports presented to the group. Although we are fully aware of these implications, we make hardly any allusions to them and, as stated, the group leader tries to merge into the rest of the group. I think that by using as the main field the doctor's counter-transference to his patient we enable the practitioner to acquire a modicum of the required "considerable though limited" change of personality without the necessity of a long personal analysis. Perhaps what we use most often is *the contrasting of the doctor's individual methods with those of his colleagues in the group*. With some simplification, this can be described as using the brother horde instead of the primal father. To achieve this the group leader must do two things. First, he must liberate the rest of the group sufficiently to allow them to express their criticisms in a constructive-aggressive form. Both aspects are equally important; sheer aggressiveness, i.e. destructive hatred, is as useless as highly mitigated, sugar-coated constructiveness. It must be stated, however, that even if one bears in mind that the creation of this atmosphere is one of the main tasks of the group, achieving it is no easy task.

In order to enable it to develop it is essential for the group leader to hold back, to refrain from making his own comments and criticisms until everyone else has had ample time and more to do so. To be able to make a true comment on an involved doctor–patient relationship it is necessary for the listener to allow himself, in his fantasy, to become involved in the situation and then to listen to his potential reactions to his involvement. Because of the ubiquitous resistances this happens rather slowly, and so both the group and its leader must learn to be patient. Even after the participants have learned to listen pretty freely to their internal involvements, experience shows that one usually becomes aware of one's own responses in only a piecemeal fashion, and thus time and patience are of the first importance.

This is especially difficult when *the group for some reason is hesitant or is obviously pulling its punches to spare the reporting doctor.* When this occurs the correct technique is to interpret the hesitation or the excessive kindliness of the rest of the group, and not to criticize the reporting doctor. As I have said, this requires a good deal of self-control on the leader's part, especially as it is so tempting to be helpful, understanding, and, above all, constructive. If one gave way to this temptation *one would teach excellent theory, but only at the expense of the training.* The result would most likely be that the promising doctors would gradually grow bored and drop out, and the hopeless ones would admire and idealize the leader, introject his teachings—and stay with him for ever as his faithful and loyal pupils.

It is much more difficult to deal with the opposite situation, when after a report *the group is either hypercritical or blatantly indifferent and unco-operative.* This is usually a symptom only of one of the members having been "singled out," as we call it. There are many possible causes of this strained situation; I shall enumerate a few, but I am fully aware that I shall not deal exhaustively with the problem. The most frequent is that the "singled-out" member is out of step with the group in his development, especially in regard to the stage reached by his emotional understanding of the doctor–patient relationship. He may be either well ahead of, or far behind, the rest; the fact is that either causes great irritation and can be tolerated only with difficulty by the rest of the group. There are various methods of dealing with this situation, all amounting to a kind of interpretation. The leader can demonstrate how the group behaves by his own behaviour, which of course should be as far as possible imperturbable, and certainly not irritated. If this is not enough, he can contrast the reporting doctor's work with that of the rest of the group and show in which ways they differ, and what the significance of the difference is. This is usually enough, because it helps both the reporter and the rest of the group to become conscious of their different rates of development and to see the causes of the irritation. In the whole course of the scheme we have not found it necessary to interpret this situation in so many words.

The most difficult problem of all arises if the cause of a member's being "singled out" is his insecurity. Usually this is covered up by reaction formations. In his reports a doctor may overstate his initial successes, and omit to report further developments until a crisis occurs. Then he may report on his apparent failure with bitterness, putting the blame on the course. Another symptom may be a doctor's more or less complete withdrawal, his hardly ever reporting cases and restricting his participation to acid comments showing his bitter disappointment in psychotherapy, or limiting himself to sterile, automatic repetition of one and the same comment. In such a case the doctor is well defended by reaction formations; he feels that his bitterness is justified by his experiences, and he thus plays into the hands of the unconscious resistances of the rest of the group. For the time being our method of dealing with this situation is to play for time in the hope that the development of the rest of the group will in due course draw the "singled-out" doctor out of his withdrawal. This policy is not too good, not too bad; we have had a modicum of success with it, but we expect that in the case of really insecure doctors this playing for time might not be enough. We are rather uncertain what to do, because a proper interpretation of the whole situation would go beyond the limits we set ourselves, that is to say it would lead in the direction of therapy and outside the borders of training.

The Doctor's Counter-transference to his Patient

With the foregoing I have been able to show some of the most frequent problems arising when dealing with two of the three transferences mentioned above, namely, the transference of the doctor to the group leader on the one hand, and to the rest of the group on the other. The main part, however, of the everyday work of the group conferences is concerned with the doctor's counter-transference to his patients.

Examples of how this counter-transference is dealt with in concrete cases have been given already. Chapter XV is a good instance, as are Cases 5, 6, 15, 17, 19, 23 and 28.

I hope these reports show that it is the group conferences that provide the motive power for the "considerable, though limited, change of personality" on which, in our mind, any training in psychotherapy must be based. What happens at our conferences is that the doctor becomes aware of—and to some extent even understands—his involvement and personal resistances in his relations with his patient and with the rest of the group. In this respect I wish to emphasize again the importance of timing, that is that the psychiatrist-leader must go with the practitioners, helping them to become aware of the stage their understanding has reached—but he must not be too far ahead of them. Being ahead of them theoretically does not matter much one way or the other. *Being ahead of them emotionally and showing this too early creates a superior-inferior atmosphere in which teaching begins and training suffers.*

If possible, the aim should be to create an atmosphere in which anyone can speak unhurriedly, while the others listen with a free, floating mind, in which some silence is tolerated and time is allowed to everyone to find out what he really means or what he really wants to say. Unexpected things can be said and examined at times without any drama, while at other times they are allowed to cause mirth, surprise, embarrassment, or even pain. But, whatever the group's reaction, the emotions emerging both in the reporter and in his audience must be accepted and evaluated as expressions of unconscious processes activated by the report. Once the doctor is free enough to watch, to experience and finally to listen in the group conferences instead of being anxious about understanding the psychodynamics of his patients, he can start to listen in his practice to transference and counter-transference phenomena between his patient and himself.

A most important point is that the group conferences—and for that matter the supervision sessions—offer possibilities to observe at one and the same time how doctors behave when they are themselves in authority and when they are with someone in authority. In fact, these are only two facets of the same relationship and, if understood, will inevitably make sense together. We have found that if the doctor can be helped to see them when they are particularly alive in his relationship with his patient, he may get a new outlook on his work.

If a discussion of these and other transference and counter-transference relationships is left out altogether, the patient who is being discussed may become increasingly involved with the doctor, very often in rather a bewildering way, and more often than not the doctor does not know what has caused this. What is likely to have happened is that the patient has become involved, not only with his doctor, but with the doctor-training-scheme unit, and all the ambivalence that goes with it. This difficulty, although probably the most important, is not of course the only one the patient comes across when his doctor is a member of the course. All the difficulties, only too well known, caused by the doctor's partial and patchy understanding of the case are there too, multiplied by the doctor's problem of how, when, and what part of his understanding he should convey to the patient.

Comparison with other Training Schemes for Psychotherapy

It will be seen from the two previous sections that the interpretations of the doctor's transferences and counter-transferences were deliberately and definitely limited. A rough idea of what we have in mind may be arrived at by bearing in mind the fundamental difference between training and therapy. This difference corresponds approximately to that between working with the public overt transference and working with the private hidden transference of any individual doctor. The first may be obvious to the whole group; moreover, it is their concern, since they have to adapt themselves to it at each conference, e.g. by supporting it, criticizing it, being impressed by it, rejecting it, etc. But the doctor's private counter-transference is known only to himself, perhaps not even consciously. Moreover, to change this latter counter-transference would necessitate a deeper study of the doctor's personality, amounting to a kind of therapy. I am aware that by all this I have not said much about these self-imposed limitations of our interpretations, and furthermore that by this simplified description I have deliberately disregarded a number of dynamic complications. Lastly, whether or not these limitations can be adhered to in the long run, or how necessary or desirable it is to adhere to them, is another matter, and only further experience can decide.

It may be interesting at this stage, by way of comparison, to look at the ways in which these transference relationships are used in analytic training and—in a more superficial way—in the two training schemes developed by Enid Balint and myself; that for social workers at the Family Discussion Bureau, and that for general practitioners at the Tavistock Clinic. In all three schemes there is a three-tiered structure which it is perhaps simplest to describe in the case of the Family Discussion Bureau scheme. In this the chief object on which our attention was focused was the worker–client relationship, the close study of which at our group conferences enabled the worker to understand the primary problem which brought the client to ask for help. This was a strained relation leading to or threatening a breakdown between the client and his sexual partner. The three tiers of the structure are therefore: the client–worker relationship, the client's relationship to his partner, and the worker's relationship to the group and its leader. The focus of attention is on the client–worker relationship as reported to the group conferences.

In psychoanalytic training interest is focused on the "hre eand now" relationship between the candidate and his analyst, and this relationship is understood in terms of the candidate's past relations with his parents. The analysis goes back to unresolved emotional relationships of infancy, childhood and youth, and it is these relationships which are both transferred and analysed. For quite a long while there is only this two-tiered structure—the primary problems in the candidate's childhood and his present problems in the analytic situation. Only when he has progressed a fair way in his understanding of these two is he permitted to start treating a patient. He then, so to speak, inserts a third tier—i.e., his relationship with his patient—between his primary problems and his relationship with his analyst. Consequently there is a reasonable tendency to understand and describe this third and new relationship in terms of the two which haʌe already been studied.

The same three-tiered structure exists in our work with general practitioners, but with significant differences. The chief interest is concentrated on the doctor–patient relationship; secondly, there is the patient's relationship to his illness; and thirdly, the doctor's relationship to the group and its leader (and the supervisor). The main concern of our scheme is the simultaneous study of these three relationships. In spite of this similarity in the work with practitioners our interpretations have hitherto been more limited and less detailed than in either of the other two training schemes mentioned. I cannot yet give a satisfactory explanation of this. It is possible that our scheme is still too young for us to be able to say whether this limitation is only temporary, i.e. whether we shall have to go deeper and into greater detail as the course develops.

On the other hand, there is another important factor which is peculiar to this field of work. At the Family Discussion Bureau, which is the nearest parallel to our work with doctors, the primary problem is the relationship between the sexual partners, which can be understood as a relationship with an outside object. It is to be expected that in a relationship with another outside object—the worker—the same fears, defensive mechanisms, apprehensions, desires, will be at work. The primary problem facing the doctor is of an entirely different nature. In the patient's relationship to his illness there is no obvious external object. Its most important aspects are physical pain, impaired physical functions, possibly visible changes in the body, new and frightening sensations, etc. Psychoanalysis knows a good deal about anxieties and neurotic inhibitions. It also knows something—not very much—about mental pain, but hardly anything about the nature of the problems which face the doctor.

The primary problems at the Family Discussion Bureau scheme were essentially libidinal relations to objects of love and hate. In our present scheme we have to study the relationship of the suffering patient to his illness, of which we know very little. So it will be a fitting conclusion if I repeat for the last time my refrain that we need more research, and research which can probably be undertaken only by general practitioners.

APPENDIX II

*Selection**

GENERAL PRACTITIONERS

SELECTING the right people for the job is obviously a most
desirable aim. Unfortunately we are only beginning to form
an idea what the job is, and it will take some considerable
time before we can formulate it even approximately. When the
training scheme started, our ideas about psychotherapy by general
practitioners were so vague that I decided that the only honest
policy was not to select, but to rely on self-selection by the
doctors; that is, we advertised "Introductory Courses on Psychological Problems in General Practice" in the medical press and
accepted every practitioner who applied.

I knew that this meant taking risks, but the advantages were
perhaps equal to the drawbacks. By accepting everybody we
were able to form an opinion about what sort of doctors were
interested in psychotherapy, what their needs were, and what
sort of "treatment" they demanded. It was obviously impossible
that the "treatment" given, that is, our training scheme, should
suit everyone, and a number of doctors dropped out. At the
beginning of the course our "casualty rate" was high, about
60 per cent in my first groups and about 35 per cent in recent
ones.

As was to be expected, in nearly every group there were a few
seriously neurotic doctors who in reality sought therapeutic help
under the disguise of training. Fortunately, most of them soon
"selected themselves out" when they realized that our training
scheme did not offer them what they needed. The one or two
who did not or could not leave were either advised to seek
therapy or were asked to discontinue attendance—a most unpleasant task for the leader.

* A book dealing with this topic by E. and M. Balint, R. H. Gosling and
P. Hildebrand is in preparation.

Another group of early leavers was made up of "superior" doctors. These were well-established, experienced practitioners with a good reputation both among their patients and among their colleagues, and with very strong "apostolic zeal." From the outset they preached their own well-proven methods while being practically incapable of listening to, and still less of seriously considering, any methods other than their own. This inevitably brought them into competition with the psychiatrist-leader, representing the aims of the seminar, and this resulted in a rather strained and awkward atmosphere. After some unsuccessful attempts at converting the rest of the group to their "faith," these doctors dropped out, almost certainly dissatisfied and hypercritical.

A third group of early leavers was made up of "one-term" doctors. They attended regularly, took an active part in the discussions, seemed to benefit a great deal from the conferences, and soon began to experiment with the new ways the seminars opened up for them. In fact we thought highly of them, but after the end of one term, or at most two, or rarely three, they never returned. Either they were lost to us completely and no more was heard of them; or they followed the further development of their former group with friendly interest but from a safe distance; or, lastly, some of them became critical of our aims. The most frequently reported criticism was that our kind of work was nothing but a time-wasting unnecessary fuss.

The fourth group of leavers were very conscientious, sensitive practitioners to whom their practice and their patients meant a great deal; they were apparently more than willing to learn. The first impression was that they were certainly a most promising group. Moreover, they remained with us two or three terms and left us reluctantly, struggling with a conflict. All of them were what may be called with some exaggeration obsessionally conscientious characters. What they repeatedly asked for and apparently needed was reliable rules, efficient, time-saving methods, intellectual problems which could be discussed and solved with detachment and objectivity and, above all, no personal psychological involvement. To them our rather casual, adventitious and deliberately unpremeditated ways made no sense. Possibly they did not recognize the need for the "considerable, though limited, change of personality" which was the chief aim of our training scheme. The obverse of the coin, however, shows the shortcomings of our scheme. The tempo of progress and the atmosphere of the discussions were allowed to develop to suit the majority of the group and, I readily admit, the personality of the leader; this does not mean that the scheme was rigid and inconsiderate, but that it paid less attention to the needs of minority groups.

These are, however, only first impressions. The training technique described in the previous chapter is still in its experimental stages—that is, it is crude. We were fully aware of this, and we decided to accept the risks involved. Our first consideration has been to develop a technique that is workable for a reasonable proportion of the doctors interested, in order to test out whether such a training technique is possible at all. The results of the two pilot projects—the Family Discussion Bureau scheme for social workers and the Tavistock Clinic scheme for general practitioners—are highly encouraging, though not yet final. As soon as our technique is fairly securely settled, our next concern will be to examine our "casualties"—that is, the reasons why a number of our entrants left us. It is true that psychotherapy, like surgery for instance, is not within everybody's reach; nevertheless, our "casualty rate" is considerable. Conversely, this implies that our training technique is, for the time being, inelastic and too exacting for a number of practitioners.

There is, however, an important difference between training for psychotherapy and training for any other of the many specialities in medicine. Any advance in therapy demands a new skill from the doctor, even if it amounts only to learning the correct ways of prescribing a new drug. In other words, mastering a new therapy involves a change. But, while the changes required by new techniques in other branches of medicine do not make much impact on the doctor's personality, the technique of psychotherapy involves the personality fairly deeply. From this angle the action of some doctors in dropping out was perhaps a sensible defence against an unauthorized violation of their private mental life, and must therefore be treated with respect. The diametrically opposite danger is that the group training may degenerate into therapy pure and simple. We are fully aware of this danger, which in fact is present in every form of psychiatric training, but we have hitherto succeeded in avoiding it.

Before going further, I wish to illustrate what I have just said by our figures, which, however, do not amount to more than a rough approximation. They are too small to be reliable; by some administrative mishap the records of two groups were lost; and the greatest shortcoming is that the groups of leavers are not unequivocally defined. In a number of cases it was purely subjective judgment or lack of reliable information that decided whether a leaver was classified as neurotic, obsessionally conscientious, "one-term" doctor, and so forth.

We have proper records of six groups, that is of sixty-one entrants. To show the limited reliability of the figures, they were subdivided into two, one column analysing the earlier groups Nos. 2–5 and the other the recent groups 7 and 8. (The records of groups Nos. 1 and 6 were lost.)

ANALYSIS OF ATTENDANCES

Entrants	Groups 2–5		Groups 7–8		Total	
	Number	Approx. per cent	Number	Approx. per cent	Number	Approx. per cent
Regular attendants	14	39	16	64	30	50
Seriously neurotic	4	11	2	8	6	10
"Superiors"	2	6	2	8	4	7
Obsessionally conscientious	8	22	3	12	11	18
"One-term" doctors	8	22	2	8	10	16
TOTAL	36		25		61	

I am rather uncertain in which direction our scheme should develop. The two possibilities open to us are—

(*a*) Selection.
(*b*) Extending the scope and elasticity of the training.

After more than five years of experiment, and after watching the fate of eight groups, that is, of about seventy-five doctors,

I have decided to interview henceforward all applicants before accepting them for the seminars. It is probable that in this way most of the seriously neurotic and the "superior" doctors can be dissuaded. According to our figures, these two groups amount to about 15 per cent of the applicants.

The real problems are, however, provided by the other two groups: the "obsessionally conscientious" and the "one-term" doctors, each of them, as just mentioned, represent about 20 per cent of the applicants, the two together about 30–40 per cent. Moreover, most of them appear to be worth-while candidates for training in this field, and, as mentioned, the decision to leave us cost most of them conflict, bitterness and disappointment, i.e. unnecessary strain. In retrospect, I think that in an initial interview about half the "obsessionally conscientious" and about one-third of the "one-termers," i.e. about 20 per cent, could have been picked out as bad risks. I shall return presently to the problem caused by the remaining 15 per cent.

The other possibility is to make our training and research scheme more elastic. Here I am very uncertain what to recommend. It would not be too difficult to devise methods which would enable a greater proportion of our applicants to remain longer. But would it not be a waste of time for the others and for the psychiatrists? And, still more important, would this perhaps unprofitable prolongation not be unfair to the potential leavers? Perhaps the "limited, though considerable, change" might be a danger to a cautiously balanced-out personality, who is better left undisturbed with his own solutions and with his individual apostolic function. On the other hand, the "limited, though considerable, change of personality" might be exactly what these people need, and might provide the solution of some of their personality problems as well as of some of their individual difficulties in their practices. I do not expect that the inevitable limitations of an initial interview will allow me—or even a more experienced interviewer—to reach reliable decisions on this most important point. But I hope that it will be possible to dissuade some of the least promising candidates from starting the course and to reduce our "casualty rate" to about 25–30 per cent.

In view of the casualty rate in other training systems, from the training of medical students to psychoanalytic training—to quote two extremes—our initial figure of 60 per cent failures was definitely high. Our present figure of 35 per cent is acceptable, and if it can be brought down to 25–30 per cent it may be called creditable.

PSYCHIATRISTS

In the foregoing I have tried to give some idea of the kind of problems encountered in selecting general practitioners for training in psychotherapy. I hope it will be clear that in exactly the same way not every psychiatrist, not even every psycho-analytically trained psychiatrist, is suitable to undertake this task: the two disciplines mentioned are perhaps necessary prerequisites, but are certainly not a sufficient basis for it by themselves. Apart from knowing a good deal about psychotherapy and medicine, about unconscious urges, needs and emotions, their ways of emergence and about how and when to interpret them, the psychiatrist must also be trained in group therapy in particular and group management in general. In addition, and above all, he has to realize that his specialist skill is limited by the conditions of his setting, and that a different setting, such as the doctor's surgery, requires different methods. This difference was discussed on several occasions in this book, particularly in Chapter XIII, and Chapters XVI to XVIII.

A wholesale transfer of psychiatric or, for that matter, psycho-analytic methods into general-practitioner psychotherapy creates over-exacting, unrealistic and unnecessary limitations, and is thus unhelpful. Another undesirable consequence of this approach is that by it the impression is evoked in the general practitioner that psychotherapy is a higher, worthier, more profound occupation. Should this happen, he might lose interest in his practice and apply for training at one of the psychotherapeutic schools and, if accepted, be lost to general practice, or, if rejected, might become a frustrated and discontented practitioner. A still greater danger is that he might, on his own initiative, turn into an amateur, not properly trained, psychotherapist. In either case a potentially good practitioner will have been lost to the profession.

The aim of the trainer-psychiatrist should—as emphasized many times in the book—be to enable the practitioner to become a better doctor, with a deeper understanding of his patient's problems and with a greater skill to help them. Once this is realized, the psychiatrist will not be tempted to "teach" his own skill in a diluted, inferior form; instead he will join forces with the practitioners for the purpose of finding out what part and how much of psychotherapeutic or psychoanalytic knowledge and skill can be applied with profit in the doctor's surgery. This, as I can testify from experience, is a really fascinating task in comparison with that of being a knowledgeable, or even omniscient teacher.

On the other hand, it demands a great amount of elasticity and freedom from preconceived ideas. At nearly every case conference one comes up against a problem necessitating a searching re-examination of one's accustomed techniques or even of theoretical ideas which one has always believed to be firmly based. Some psychiatrists may find this constant revision too difficult or too exacting. Unfortunately, there are various ways of avoiding this onerous task, all of them highly plausible and tempting, both to psychiatrists and practitioners.

One is to teach well-founded psychodynamics, and establish thereby a teacher–pupil relationship in which the psychiatrist can excel and the practitioners can acquire rewarding knowledge— at the expense of developing their skill.

Another way is to allow the case conferences to develop in the direction of therapy. This, too, is gratifying to both parties. The psychiatrist becomes a good, helpful doctor who really gives something valuable; the practitioners, especially in the initial stages, benefit greatly, and, to quote Gilbert, "all is right, as right can be." This is the more dangerous as any reasonably good therapy is as a rule accompanied by an improved standard of work; this improvement can then be taken as proof of the correctness of the training technique. My long experience in psychoanalytic training made me wary of this possibility, with the result that I have no first-hand experience of the ultimate consequences of its systematic application. I expect, as mentioned in the previous chapter, that the transferences of the participants to the psychiatrist, and with it the whole atmosphere of the conferences, would become more and more primitive and highly charged with emotion. Once this situation had developed, in my opinion, most of the time would have to be spent on therapy and only a small part could be spared for training. Whenever I succumbed to the temptation to turn into a "good doctor," all the alarming signs appeared at once; an ambivalent—eager and frightened—demand for more therapy by the doctor concerned, a curiously hushed and keen expectation of some revealing experience in the rest of the group, and a very strong urge in me to give freely. I stopped myself as soon as I realized what was happening.

The third way out is to become a superior mentor who knows what is good and wholesome for the practitioner to undertake and where he ought to stop. This safety-first policy is highly acceptable to everyone. The psychiatrist does not expect the practitioners to "sink or swim," he keeps them in safe depths, and is constantly on the look-out to warn them of any danger of deep personal involvement. The practitioners feel safe—and dependent. It is not they who make decisions, but the benign and knowledgeable psychiatrist, who can be trusted. Obviously this training method is utterly different from the spirit of our research, but it must be admitted that it might be a way out for some of our failures. Some of the "obsessionals" and "one-term" doctors in particular might find this method more congenial to their way of feeling and thinking, and thus more acceptable.

As is evident from the foregoing, the personality of the psychiatrist is a crucial factor in his selection. It is this that will decide whether he will undertake the training of general practitioners, what methods he will adopt, what atmosphere he will create—and what successes and failures he will have. What is true for the general practitioner is also true, of course, for the psychiatrist; that is to say, his "practice" of medicine, including his methods of training general practitioners (or his refusal to train them), is one expression of his apostolic function. And, of course, this holds true for me and *a fortiori* for this book.

Follow-up Reports

INTRODUCTION

T HE first thing that must be realized is that the 28 patients reported in this book are not a representative sample. They are not representative of the Metropolitan population, or of the practices of the doctors who took part in the research, or even of the cases that were discussed in our seminars. As mentioned several times in the book, the participation in our discussions was voluntary; a doctor presented a case when he had some reason for doing so; for instance: if it was a difficult case which worried him, if he wanted to prove a point and the case was a good illustration of it, if he wanted to show us how successful he was, etc., etc. When I decided to write up the research, I went through the records of our past discussions, and picked out of them these twenty-eight cases to illustrate the various problems of medical practice that our research had brought to light.

There is, however, yet another feature which is common to all twenty-eight cases, in fact to all the cases discussed in our seminars, and that is that, in addition to the traditional medical diagnosis, we attempted to arrive in each of them at a "deeper" level of diagnosis. This enabled us to give in each case, in addition to the traditional prognosis, a wider prognosis which included the patient's future relationship with his doctor and a prediction whether rational therapy would or would not be successful in this particular case.

A systematic follow-up was not part of our original plan. This idea developed gradually as we became more and more impressed by how closely the events with and around the patients followed our predictions. By the time the idea became specific and concrete enough, the draft of the book was almost finished, so it was decided to carry out a systematic follow-up, extending to

December 31st, 1955, and to include its results as Appendix III in the first edition. The occasion of a second edition enabled us to carry out a second systematic follow-up covering the time until June 30th, 1963. Since the dates when the cases were originally reported varied from 1951 to 1954, the length of the first follow-ups varied in the same way, giving a very rough average of three years.

We know, on the basis of another research, that in the London Metropolitan Area every year about 8 to 10% of the patients registered with a doctor leave the practice. We may add that in a well-established practice about the same number of patients join the doctor's list. This yearly turnover does not seem to depend—as one would expect—on the doctor's professional skill and knowledge, or personality, but chiefly on the place where his practice is situated. It is smaller in provincial towns, and still smaller in rural areas.

Taking 8 to 10% as the yearly turnover, of the twenty-eight patients reported in this book, 20 to 22 should remain on the doctors' list after three years. In fact, the actual figures were as follows:

TABLE I

At the end of Period 1 (December 31st, 1955)

Remained on the Lists	Uncertain	Left the Practice	Unknown	Total
18	2	7	1	28

The length of the second follow-up period is exact and the same for all our cases. It lasted from January 1st, 1956 till June 30th, 1963, that is for 6½ years. Taking this time as the basis of our calculations, of the eighteen cases on the lists of various doctors, 9 to 10 should remain at the end of the 6½ years' period. The actual figures were as follows:

TABLE II

At the end of Period 2 (June 30th, 1963)

Remained on the Lists	Uncertain	Left the Practice	Unknown	Total
11	1	14	2	28

The calculated and the observed figures show a satisfactory agreement which suggests that the twenty-eight cases reported behave in some respects as a representative sample of the London Metropolitan population. Of course, special emphasis must be put on the adverb "in some respects", otherwise an incorrect impression may be created.

Like the original case histories, the follow-up reports are printed here in the form in which they were either compiled in writing, or reported verbally to the seminar by the doctor in charge.

CASE 1 (Mrs. C., reported by Dr. M., pp. 11–12)

Period 1, ending December 31st, 1955

July 1954. Mrs. C. (32 years) did not come to see me for nearly two years after our last talk. During that time she saw my senior partner in the obvious desire to deal with her illness on the physical level.

Mrs. C. was seen by my partner approximately twelve times during the intervening two years. I notice also from our files that last year she was referred to a urologist, who thought her symptoms were due to nervous tension. The urologist's house surgeon referred her a few weeks later to a gynaecologist, and another two months later the urologist referred her to the psychiatrist of the same hospital. The psychiatrist reported—

8th October, 1953.

Mrs. C.

I saw this patient on the 5th October, 1953.

Complaint: Depression and crying fits for four years.

History: The patient was the eldest of five children and had a happy childhood.

The patient married in 1940, her husband being in a reserved occupation. From the beginning her husband told her he did not want to have any children. Three years after marriage she became ill with various bodily symptoms, such as fleeting pains in the chest. Her husband continued to practise coitus interruptus. The patient suffered a good deal from dyspepsia, but latterly she has had crying fits. Previous doctors have suggested that frustration of maternal feeling might be connected with her trouble.

In the last year her nervous strain got worse when a young woman came to live with her and the patient felt that her husband was paying too much attention to this woman, though there was no hint of misconduct.

The patient is very tense and over-meticulous, and there is some frequency of micturition.

One brother was enuretic till he was adult.
Diagnosis: Hysteria.
Comment: I will see the husband and see whether her marital arrange-
ments can be changed for the better.

Yours sincerely,

(Signed) Physician in Charge.

A little while ago she called us to her home; as I happened to be on call duty that day, I visited her. She was very depressed, broke down, and told me that her husband was friendly with a girl-friend of hers, and was very hostile towards her. I have seen her twice since then, when she told me more or less the same story.

She came in last night again, as the last patient (a sure diagnostic sign that she wanted to take possession of the doctor for the night), and without saying a word, started to cry very loudly and dramatically, and clutched my hand. She told me again of her husband's infatuation for her friend and, when I asked her what she intended to do about it, she became very angry, and said I did not understand her. There was nothing she could do, as her husband got angry when she talked about his affair, and he would murder her if he knew that she had talked about it to me, or if she were to tell his or her parents. She would tell the girl-friend's husband when he comes out of hospital where he is at present, and that will be her revenge.

She was very angry with me. When I asked her how she would like me to help her, she said very gruffly that she had only come to ask me for a bottle of tonic. I gave her a prescription, and left the door open for her return.

January 1956. As I reported in July 1954, I did not see very much of Mrs. C. after my original report, and after I offered her psycho-therapy. That was not what she wanted. She went to see my partner from then on, who likes to deal with physical illnesses, and, as I see from her records, she had indeed numerous physical illnesses, mainly digestive and menstrual disturbances.

Last year, however, she returned to me. She was in a deep crisis. Her husband had been unfaithful with her best girl-friend, and in such a clumsy, obvious way that I have little doubt that he wanted to be found out. She blamed the badness of man and woman for this, but also felt guilty that with her frigidity she might have caused her husband to betray her.

Our relationship was much better then than it had ever been before. Whilst in previous years I saw her as an attacking woman who wanted to seduce me and against whom I had to defend myself, my attitude now was no longer defensive. She found now that she could talk to an understanding physician, and she found it possible to talk about her hostile feelings to her husband and parents, and about her frigidity. After a while the couple came together again. I had only seen her five or six times for a quarter of an hour or so at a time.

She did not come to us for a while, then she came again to see my partner, and then me once or twice.

Her conflicts are not solved. She is still an hysteric, but apparently she can cope with it, and for the time being has no need to be ill. Perhaps I flatter myself by thinking that this might be due to my changed attitude when she found that in her relationship with me there was no need to use her usual hysterical behaviour pattern towards men.

A new problem has, however, arisen. Her husband, who is my partner's patient, has digestive troubles now, and my partner tells me that he finds it very difficult to cope with him.

This is an instructive history for many reasons. It shows that even with a correct diagnosis and with considerable therapeutic skill it is not always possible to induce a patient to give up her "organized" illness and do something about solving the original problem. It is true that this was one of our very first cases and perhaps Dr. M. was less skilled than he is now. This doubt comes out quite clearly in his sincere and frank reports.

Another interesting point is the patient's wandering between the two partners. We may even conjecture the reasons. Whenever she was able to accept the fact that she was in some psychological trouble she consulted Dr. M., and whenever this was too much for her and she wanted to get away from her pressing problems she saw his partner. This important symptom—changing from one doctor to another—of her total illness was unfortunately used only to arrive at a better diagnosis, but not for therapeutic purposes.

And lastly, this is another instructive illustration of the "collusion of anonymity" and the "dilution of responsibility." Like Miss F. (Case 12), Mrs. C. manipulated her doctors in such a way that no-one was able to be fully responsible for her. As is inevitable in such cases, a large number of consultants were also involved. Apart from those mentioned in the original report, their number was increased by a urologist, a gynaecologist and a psychiatrist. And, as in most cases of this kind, the psychiatrist's report was hardly of any use to the general practitioner.

Period 2, ending June 30th, 1963

Mrs. C. changed several years ago from our practice to that of a woman doctor, and I have not seen or heard from her since.

However, her husband stayed in our practice and is now one of my partner's patients. If you are interested, my partner would be willing to give a report on him.

As the partner's report was somewhat lengthy, I am giving here only the gist of it:

Mr. C. is a seriously ill man. He has been out of work since March 1959. The immediate cause of his incapacity was a heart attack suggesting infarction, but which was diagnosed in hospital as hysterical. For several years prior to his attack, that is since *c.* 1955, he had complained of various cardiac symptoms, all of which were diagnosed as functional.

An unsuccessful psychotherapeutic attempt by the general practitioner revealed highly intense aggressive feelings in Mr. C. amounting to murderous impulses against his wife, which—according to the doctor—were largely justified by his wife's behaviour. A psychiatrist was then consulted; he agreed with the doctor's assessment, and referred Mr. C. to a rehabilitation centre, where he spent some time, but did not benefit from this either.

In 1961 Mr. C. asked to be taken back by his old firm; he started work again, but experienced such intense aggressive feelings towards his foreman that he had to give up his attempt. Since then he has not tried again.

The doctor concludes his report:

Mrs. C. visited me on one occasion to complain violently about her husband's continued ill-health and my failure to cure him. She is certainly able to arouse violent aggression in me! I pointed out to her that she had done this and perhaps did this with her husband, to which her reply was: "You doctors are all the same"—and perhaps we are.

Thus Mrs. C.'s—and her husband's—treatment must be accepted as a failure. True, it was one of our very first cases and all of us, the general practitioner and the psychiatrist alike, did not have much experience at that time in the field of psychotherapy by general practitioners. On the other hand, it must be stated also that a number of treatments which were started at about the same time prospered favourably. So there must be specific reasons in Mrs. C.'s case that caused the failure.

The most common cause of any failed psychotherapy is failure of understanding the patient's real problems. This is definitely true in her case. Although there is some indication that Dr. M. diagnosed that Mr. C. was a neurotic man, the severity of his neurosis was not recognized by him. This became apparent only after Mrs. C. left the practice, that is much too late.

In consequence, her behaviour was only partly understood. Time and again she was described as a hysterical flirtatious woman with insincere and superficial emotions—in the same way as her husband was described by Dr. M.'s partner as a desperate man driven to extremes by his wife's impossible behaviour. There is a good deal of truth in these complementary descriptions of husband and wife. One may even add a few coincidences to reinforce them: the husband's cardiac complaints started round about 1955 at about the same time as his wife gave up hope with Dr. M. and started her wandering among the members of the partnership, becoming more and more dissatisfied and angry. Similarly, his heart attack must have happened at about the same time, or soon after Mrs. C. left the practice and changed over to a woman doctor, which perhaps meant giving up any hope of being understood by a man.

Of course it is easy to be wise after the event. What could have been done earlier? I am afraid the only thing I can do is to give the standard answer which is: not to blame the absent partner, but try to concentrate on the problems presented by the patient in the surgery, that is, the one who has come to the doctor complaining. If Dr. M. had been able to understand Mrs. C.'s flirtatious approach to him as a desperate attempt at demonstrating the way she treated her husband and her need, therefore, to be helped to understand why she had to do so, then perhaps the outcome would have been different. By the way, *mutatis mutandis*, the same holds true about his partner's treatment of Mr. C. I say, perhaps, because in this case both Mr. and Mrs. C. had been very ill for quite some time, and it is somewhat uncertain whether a general practitioner, or for that matter anyone else, could have helped them to readjust themselves to one another, so that their mutual relationship should become tolerable.

It has to be admitted that our original diagnosis and our favourable prognosis based on it were definitely wrong.

CASE 2 (Mrs. A., reported by Dr. E., pp. 12–13)

Period 1, ending December 31st, 1955

January 26th, 1956. She has had very little contact recently with me, but has concentrated on my partners, particularly the newest one, who is soft with her. Throughout 1953 she had dyspepsia, and had barium meals and enema, all negative. Consultations, including visits, for the boy averaged one a month. From autumn 1953 till the middle of 1954 she complained of her son's phimosis and balanitis. She used to come and say, "Do you think he is in need of circumcision?" I said "No." Finally she went to my partners, and they referred her to a surgeon. The surgeon reported, "He has not got a marked degree of phimosis but would benefit by circumcision." He was circumcised in April 1954, and while the wound healed the mother was terribly anxious. The wound went septic. In May, patient's mother bought her a flat and they moved into much better conditions. In June she became pregnant. Patient's mother thought she was not strong enough to take the pregnancy and that it should be terminated, but she carried on. She had a lot of trouble, toxemia, all sorts of things. Finally she had episiotomy for foetal distress. Baby was born. She had to stop breast feeding. She then started with menorrhagia and has continued ever since. She has had two admissions for D. & C. Two months before the baby was born the boy had a mild attack of pneumonia and was in hospital for a week or so. The patient said, "He has been too dependent on me. Now I have got baby, I shall have to save my energy for the baby; he will have to look after himself." Since the baby has come the older boy is getting on much better; much less is heard of him and about him. The baby is the worry now, the burden has been taken off the older boy and put on the baby. Baby went to hospital at two months with diarrhoea, and at nine months the baby passed a plastic toy.

This case is a text-book illustration of what we termed "the child as the presenting symptom" and the "neurotic tradition." The boy's illnesses were in an exact parallel to the mother's state. Whenever she was under some strain the boy became ill, and whenever the strain on the mother decreased, the boy improved. It is to be expected that now, after the birth of a new baby, the relationship between the older boy and the mother will be less close and he will have some possibility of developing. Unfortunately the mother is concentrating now on the baby and it is an ominous sign that she had to go to hospital twice in her first year. Obviously the neurotic tradition has already started.

Period 2, ending June 30th, 1963

The mother's anxieties continued to affect the new baby as before, leaving the older boy somewhat immune. For a year or two she continued desperately running from one doctor to the other in the partnership, without any sort of control being possible. Finally she left the partnership with N. After three months she asked to be allowed to return. We accepted her once more but again the same sequence of events occurred and after a period of one year she once more left with N. No further follow-up available.

Rather a disappointing follow-up. The little we hear about the two children does not allow us to form a reliable picture of their development. The mother's neurosis is fairly well described. Her main symptoms: anxiety, restlessness, desperate clinging and equally desperate disappointment, are clear enough, but they are diagnosed only as a nuisance and not as an illness. In consequence, it is very likely that she did not receive specific treatment. On the other hand, it must be admitted that, with the severity of her symptoms and with her limited intelligence it would have been a difficult task for anyone to treat her properly. The original doubtful prognosis proved to be correct.

CASE 3 (Reported by Dr. P., p. 13)

Period 1, ending December 31st, 1955

Left the district. Dropped in once for a friendly chat, unfortunately Dr. P. happened to be out.

Period 2, ending June 30th, 1963

No further contact with the doctor, which was to be expected.

CASE 4 (Reported by Dr. R., pp. 14–17)

Period 1, ending December 31st, 1955

I saw her again on July 20th, 1954. She told me that while she had been at her parents' home on holiday she had had no trouble, but one week after returning to London there had been a recurrence of her rectal bleeding and pain. On examination there was a small fissure-in-ano. She was no better with simple treatment by August 9th, 1954, so I referred her to a surgeon (as a private patient at her request). The surgeon subsequently reported that the fissure should be excised.

On September 20th, 1954, she returned complaining of having had frequent periods in the past two months; there were fourteen days between the periods, and they were very heavy. I was unable to examine her at that time, as she was losing, and I suggested that she came to see me when it stopped. She then asked me whether I would be able to continue looking after her if she moved to another part of London, as she was about to do so.

After a discussion, in which I explained I could not look after her under the National Health Service if she lived so far away from me, she said she would come to see me as a private patient.

To this date I have not seen or heard from her again!

It appears that in this case doctor and patient could somehow never understand each other. In spite of all Dr. R.'s efforts, there was always some tension and friction between them. Perhaps the patient's request that her doctor should continue with her treatment in spite of her moving to another part of London was the last attempt to get the attention and perhaps also the affection that she needed. The doctor's professionally correct answer was possibly interpreted by her as a rejection, and so she had to leave him, once again disappointed and let down.

Period 2, ending June 30th, 1963

No further contact, as predicted.

CASE 5 (Mr. U., reported by Dr. E., pp. 21–22)

Period 1, ending December 31st, 1955

He has carefully avoided me, though he has seen a fair amount of my partners in turn. In May 1954 he was referred to W. Hospital for his pains. They saw him, and eventually asked him to see their psychiatrist. He no longer went to the hospital or saw that partner and for some months even stopped coming to the surgery, but carried on at work. In December 1954 he saw partner No. 3, who referred him to M. Hospital for examination. They investigated him again, but nothing startling came of it. Four months later he returned to partner No. 2, who sent him back to W. Hospital, department of physical medicine. Though the consultant did not think there was much wrong, they gave him treatment. He appears now to have resigned himself to his symptoms, and carries on as best he can. He does not come himself, only sends for a bottle of Mist.Pot.Brom.Valerian. Once in error I gave him Mist.Pot.Brom. without the valerian and this was sent back, he said it smelt different. I have not seen him for eighteen months, but I saw him once at home when I visited his child; he just said "Hello" very politely, made no comment. His wife had anxiety symptoms in the summer of 1955. Their eldest son, now twelve, is very timid and passive, rather feminine. When I tried to discuss the subject with mother I did not get very far.

The follow-up vindicates our worst forebodings. In spite of Dr. E.'s and everybody else's efforts to prevent it, the situation developed almost exactly as we predicted. Mr. U. left his previously trusted friend and has become a "nomad," wandering from one partner to the other in the joint practice and from consultant to consultant in various hospitals. The model patient as we saw him before the accident has changed into a withdrawn and suspicious man who is forced to mistrust the doctors who try to help him.

I think it is fair to say that, if the seminar had not thrown light on this case, it would have disappeared among the many other "fat envelopes" in the practice. Although we could not prevent the outcome, I think we achieved something by bringing this problem to the fore.

Period 2, ending June 30th, 1963

The younger boy with nephritis continued with very severe bouts of illness throughout the years. On one occasion, in late puberty, he had an attack of what was diagnosed as encephalitis. His schooling suffered considerably, and he was thought to be backward because of some brain damage subsequent to the encephalitis. At adolescence his physical health improved remarkably, and exacerbations of the nephritis seemed to disappear but he became a rather solitary, withdrawn, and eccentric young man. I made a considerable effort at this time with him and the family to try to avoid any deterioration of his condition, as I was afraid of a schizoid breakdown. I saw him weekly for several months and established a certain, if not warm relationship with him. I had various psychological tests carried out to show he had not sustained cerebral damage. He became less aloof, more friendly and more sociable, not only with me, but generally in his life. Then he left school and found a job in the Civil Service at clerical level; he maintained this improvement and when last seen was behaving like a reasonably normal young man.

Little contact was made with the older brother who remained when seen extremely passive and rather feminine. The mother had frequent gynaecological complaints (menorrhagia etc.), leading finally to hysterectomy. It was about the time when the younger boy improved that the father gradually became more friendly and regained his trust in me. He stayed with me, ceased to consult the other partners and no longer asked me to send him to hospital. He had become reconciled to his lot, apart from developing gastric symptoms. Barium meal proved negative and he was able to discuss the matter reasonably with me.

At this time the family were unfortunate enough to find that an espresso bar had been installed just beneath their flat, with continual noise throughout the day and continuing into the night. This external enemy seemed to unite the family and act as a cohesive force. All their dissatisfactions were focused onto the espresso bar and the noise. Recently they have moved away and have had to change their doctor.

This is a puzzling follow-up. If the seminar had still been working at the time of the events described in it, we would have spent quite some time in discussing the possible explanations, asking Dr. E. to have another look at the various members of the family U., and then trying to review the explanations in the light of his new observations. Instead all I can do is to give here some of the explanations that came to my mind.

Unquestionably the strain borne by this family remained largely unchanged during the follow-up period. It cannot be decided, however, whether the strain was caused only by the serious illness of the younger boy or, to a considerable extent, by the father's emotional crisis. In any case, the two seem to have diminished at about the same time. It is safe to assume that Dr. E.'s sincere interest in the boy and his successful help in restoring his self-confidence played a considerable part in this improvement. The boy got over a difficult period causing some disquieting symptoms, and found himself a satisfactory job in the clerical grade of the Civil Service and—at about the same time—Mr. U. got over his disappointment and again accepted Dr. E. as his trusted friend. Equally, we do not know whether the mother's gynaecological troubles were a contributory factor, or a consequence of these critical states. And, lastly, the most important question whether Mr. U. was in fact able to re-establish his old friendship with Dr. E., in which case the espresso bar was an unfortunate accident, or, in spite of some spurious efforts, he remained the same disappointed man, in which case the espresso bar might have been a welcome excuse.

However, even if we accept the most favourable explanation, Mr. U. had to go through a crisis of confidence lasting several years, because of the misunderstanding between himself and his doctor, exactly as was predicted in Chapter III.

CASE 6 ("Company Director", pp. 26–31)

No report about further developments.

CASE 7 (Mrs. D., reported by Dr. G., pp. 32–33)

Period 1, ending December 31st, 1955

Mrs. D. moved from my district and I have not seen her for some time.

As far as I can remember (the old notes have been forwarded to the Executive Council) she saw me occasionally, we had little chats—no further interpretations. Relationship was good. Michael apparently had no further attacks of asthma, at least I was never called to treat him.

We do not know for certain whether the cessation of the asthmatic attacks was connected with the "long interview," but it is a fact that it happened *post hoc.*

Period 2, ending June 30th, 1963

No further contact with patient.

CASE 8 (Professor E., reported by Dr. Z., pp. 55–56)

Period 1, ending December 31st, 1955

He is much better, and in full work. I said to him that, if he was finding certain things too much strain, he must plan his life at his department in such a way that he was not subject to interruptions. He did something which he never had the courage to do before—he locked his door for a large part of the time he was there, and was able to organize the administration in a much better way. We do not bother about hypertension now.

Apparently Dr. Z. assessed the situation correctly in 1954, and his decision about not going further was a sensible one—at any rate for the time being. It will be most interesting to follow this case, say, for the next ten or fifteen years.

Period 2, ending June 30th, 1963

The patient has held his own very well in the nine years which have elapsed since my original report.

He kept well for several years, seeing me at infrequent intervals for minor ailments, such as: a sebaceous cyst, wax in ears, eye test, occasional headaches, but always reported that he was keeping very fit. A very occasional blood pressure check showed it to be well down $\frac{130-155}{95-105}$.

Towards the end of 1959 he felt as if he were stiffening up all over, especially his legs in the morning or after sitting and listening to a lecture; he also had rigidity of neck muscles and shoulder girdle of long standing. I referred him to a physiotherapy department, where he was investigated and given a course of postural exercises. This led to limited improvement.

In the spring of 1960 his headaches became worse, and he also had some nausea; the pattern suggested migraine, but this never developed to any degree of frequency.

In December 1961 he said he was getting mild migraine about once per week and was worried lest it strike him when chairing a committee. In March 1962 he wrote for a repeat prescription and told me his chairmanship was being a great success.

During 1962–63 he has been seeing me more often with headaches and rise of blood pressure. From early 1962 he has been worried about his wife, who has been working under great strain. She has become a professor and has had an increasing number of departmental duties. She has also published several successful books over the years, all involving a vast amount of meticulous research. He says she is a competent administrator and is a most valuable member of all the committees on which she serves, but he has been afraid that the strain would prove too much for her.

Though she consulted me herself several times in 1962, she has managed with little help to remain in full activity.

Both the adopted children are doing well.

To summarize, one has the impression of an integrated family, with a husband and wife who have a deep affection for one another and common interests to a high degree. There is no doubt that Professor E. has the greatest admiration and love, in the broadest sense, for his wife and is in no way jealous of her recent somewhat greater academic achievements.

Contrary to his often voiced intention, he himself has not retired into a quieter life, but has dealt with his administrative work effectively. I do feel in this case that a better result would have been obtained by trying to re-adjust his sexual life on the lines discussed in 1954 (cf. pp. 55–60).

I have no doubt that the one interview* was of enormous help to the patient and to myself. It gave me a new light on this kindly quiet man and, on his side, he unburdened himself of material which was accepted in a matter-of-fact way, and which otherwise might have built up to a considerable tension over the years.

Report on an interview with Mrs. E.

The interview took place in 1954, a few months after Professor E.'s "long interview," during which he asked me whether I would like to talk to his wife. Unfortunately, owing to an oversight, this report was omitted from my first follow-up report.

She said that all sex life had been given up more than a year ago, after activity had been diminished over several years. She thought the cause was more the children than the war. It began to break down years ago when they had no adequate help and everyone was ill together. Soon afterwards her husband had his operation. Gradually he became less potent and there was a period when they were both unhappy because intercourse was attempted but often not achieved. During the years that she was trying to conceive, it was much better. For the first years of marriage, she was using a contraceptive.

She became pregnant a few times but miscarried at 3 months, and was eventually advised that she should avoid conception.

This is a most interesting follow-up. In many respects it proves that Dr. Z. in 1954 assessed the most complex situation of this family correctly, and that the therapeutic approach adopted by him was realistic and useful. It enabled him to be of considerable assistance to these two valuable people, and helped them to continue to lead an active and fruitful life. This statement does not apply only to their academic career but also, as the good report about the development of the two children shows, to their family life.

In addition, this report should silence the critics who doubt the wisdom of what we call a "long interview" during which the doctor enables his patient to talk freely—among other things—about his sexual pleasures and problems, contentments and disappointments. As the more than nine-year follow-up shows, the long interview did not cause any disturbance in the doctor/patient relationship. On the contrary, it enabled the doctor to understand

* Dr. Z. refers here to the "long interview" in 1954 described in the original report (pages 55–56).

his patient better and, possibly, eased the tension under which the patient laboured.

This is the positive side of the picture. There are, however, some negative sides, too, which, in fairness, must also be mentioned. Although Professor E. has maintained, or even improved, his professional status and efficiency, there cannot be any question that during the last few years it was his wife who made the greater strides. Although Dr. Z. states explicitly in his report that this did not cause any disturbance in the affectionate relationship between husband and wife, I think it ought to be pointed out that it was during these years that both husband and wife presented some psychosomatic complaints to their doctor. I mean the migraineous headaches and the muscle pain of the husband, and the less impressive complaints of the wife.

If we add all this together, we come to the conclusion that the situation may well have remained fundamentally the same throughout the period of follow-up. The considerable strain that we diagnosed in 1954 is still there in both partners, as well as in their marriage. But, apparently because of their good potentialities for sublimation, they seem to be able to tolerate this strain, although under some difficulties. The question is still whether one can trust that this arrangement will stand the test of time.

What we learn from the additional information contained in the second follow-up—about Mrs. E.'s miscarriages and then the disappointing discovery that she would not be able to bear a child; the decision to adopt two children and the parallel gradual giving up of any attempt at a sexual life—fits in well with the picture that we constructed originally and reinforces our diagnostic assessment. It may also explain Mrs. E.'s admirable capacity for work, both as an administrator and a research worker, which now appear as perhaps substitute gratifications for a creative motherhood which was denied to her. Since both Professor and Mrs. E. are talented people, this kind of substitute gratification might go a long way to fill their life with contentment.

CASE 9 (Miss K., reported by Dr. D., pp. 60–62)

Period 1, ending December 31st, 1955

It was not long after my last report (August 1954) that she developed a young man. Finding that her parents opposed her marriage with him, she made herself pregnant on purpose, and then married him. She now has a baby. She ceased to have any symptoms from the time when she met the young man and became serious with him. The marriage is, as far as we know, happy, except for the fact that there is no housing, and the couple spend a good part of their time living separately for this reason. I am told that she is an over-anxious mother, but I personally never see her now, because she sees my partner.

This is an astonishing report. Either our whole assessment of the case was wrong, or a kind of miracle happened, something like an almost psychotic episode healing out without any trace. I cannot believe that this is the case, and I expect that the present improvement will prove only superficial and temporary. It will be most interesting to follow this case for the next few years.

Period 2, ending June 30th, 1963

Miss K.—as already reported—married and had a girl-child without difficulty in 1955. The marriage lasted less than one year. The husband was a small ineffectual man who left her and has failed to support her ever since. The marriage never seemed important in her medical story though the problem of supporting and bringing up the child has been important. She has leant heavily on the help of her mother who fills the gap generously, yet with resentment.

Miss K. has attended either my partner or myself at least once weekly since 1955. She has on the whole remained faithful to the two of us even though there are more doctors in the partnership. Until a year ago the need was invariably for reassurance that this or that bodily symptom was not a cancer or leukaemia. Most of the symptoms were at the mouth or anus but there were others elsewhere. We needed occasionally to seek hospital out-patient opinions when the pressure became very great but, in general, we tried hard to keep her away from consultants. Usually we would examine her symptom, say "it's all right," "it's one of your queer feelings" and she would leave, reassured for but a few days.

We referred her to a psychiatrist in 1958 (she had been unwilling before). His report was as follows:

Thank you for your letter about this girl whom I saw here yesterday afternoon. It seems to me that she has a number of different problems which are likely to continue to need separate approaches.

(1) Her hypochrondriacal preoccupation with her throat is, I suspect, a manifestation of a deeply ingrained hypochondriacal tendency which is unlikely to alter very much even if her social circumstances improve. I

conceive that at any rate for a considerable time, to give repeated reassurance that there is no grave organic disease and certainly no cancer, is going to be necessary to keep this symptom within tolerable limits. I wondered whether you might feel that the time had come for another specialized examination of the throat in order to reinforce reassurance, and if you felt this were so I will be glad to arrange it here.

(2) Her general tendency to worry about her future and the associated anxiety symptoms—the tremblings which she experienced a little while ago at night, and I take it also the epigastric discomfort—seem to be attributable to her sense of frustration. Her way of life clearly gives her very little satisfaction in that her earnings plus the allowance from her husband for the child hardly do more than keep her and the child and make no provision for the future. She sees no hope of getting a home of her own or of being able to lead anything of a social life or meet any new friends. I find it rather difficult to see how this can be altered unless she were to make some arrangements for the child either to be adopted or, at any rate, looked after for her. She seemed rather reluctant to consider anything of this kind but unless she does, her way of life seems unlikely to be capable of much modification.

The situation continued unchanged and resistance to any attempt at psychological interpretation also remained unchanged.

It was in 1962 that she was persuaded to return to the psychiatrist. His letter was as follows:

> This young woman did at last appear at Out-patients today.
> I am sorry I have been so long about seeing her again.
> Her severe and recurring hypochrondriacal preoccupations seem to have started when she was about 16—long before her unsatisfactory marriage and the money worries and social deprivation which its collapse entailed. Nevertheless I should imagine that the extreme restrictions of her present life—worse during the past two years since her husband stopped sending her money regularly—must be serving to maintain the anxiety and the hypochondriasis of which it is an expression.
> It is difficult to imagine that she could be helped by individual psychotherapy, but I believe there might be just a chance that she could respond to group therapy. I am therefore asking Dr. X. if he would see her to assess her suitability for one of his groups.

Since that time there has been some change. She has attended the group and also the hospital social club with regularity and enthusiasm. She has still needed to come to us about physical symptoms but in November 1962 I noted " 1 month without a visit."
Even more recently her symptoms have become less physical and

more psychological. She has complained of being unable to concentrate on her work and of wanting to run away from everything. She discusses openly the problems of living with a father who has not spoken to her for four years and a mother who looks after her child but with whom she constantly quarrels and who has no time for her complaints. She admits that her child is a drag on her "although she means everything to me." She wants to leave home but "how can I, when my husband gives me no money and I have J. to look after?"

The husband's solicitors have recently started legal proceedings and this has thrown her into such an anxiety that she became unable to work and has had to have certificates. We hope that she is soon going to spend a period at X rehabilitation centre.

It has taken us ten years to reach this point but this girl is beginning to look at her life. It is not an encouraging vision for her. As her doctor I feel I am now up against a more real problem and that there is at least a hope of helping. No solution is in sight.

Her daughter is now 9. She had nephritis but recovered. She was an undisciplined, aggressive child, about the age of 5 and her mother had no control of her. Nowadays we see little of her.

This second follow-up report seems to confirm my comments on the somewhat rosy report of the first period. From our present vantage point, about ten years after the marriage, which appeared to Dr. D. in 1955 as a possible solution of some of Miss K.'s most pressing conflicts, we can see that it was only a desperate but inefficient and hopeless attempt, which was bound to fail. It was not only that her husband was not a proper man who wanted to have a wife and a child, but Miss K. was not able either to sever the ambivalent ties that linked her to her mother. Her general situation has remained unchanged in all its essential features; in spite of her becoming a married woman and a mother, she remained a dependent child who could not create a life of her own in which she could forego her mother's help; similarly, in spite of the fact that she started to have an adult sexual life, she could not give up her displaced exhibitionism, she had to go on insisting that her doctors should look into her throat and anus to see that there was no cancer in either. The report does not say anything about her continuing the same ritual with her mother, so there is a possibility that she was able to give up that part of her symptomatology.

During all these years she was seen, once a week, by Dr. D. or his partner who consistently tried to get her to accept the possibility that her symptoms have psychological origins, and that a psychiatrist should therefore be consulted. These attempts were met first with a point-blank refusal, then, in 1958, with an abortive visit to a psychiatrist, and in 1962 with an apparent acceptance. A possible explanation for this change may be found in her partly successful projection. She succeeded in finding a most suitable object, her husband, to blame for everything that was unhappy and wrong in her life. It was this wicked man who left her, who did not give her enough money to bring up her child properly, and thus prevented her from taking her proper place in social life. This partial success in relieving herself of blame and the subsequent guilt feelings is a possible explanation for her recent willingness to consult a psychiatrist and to accept the group therapy offered to her.

On second thoughts this last statement ought perhaps to be qualified. Examining more closely the two psychiatric opinions contained in the second follow-up report, as well as the one in the first report in 1954, it has to be admitted that they amount only to a correct, though somewhat superficial description of her symptomatology, quite well known to her doctor, and that there is hardly any attempt in them to understand the dynamics that led to the development of her hypochrondriacal symptoms and to her pathological form of life. In consequence, instead of therapy based on proper understanding, all the help that the psychiatrist could offer to the hard pressed general practitioner was to resort to advice, reassurance and elimination by appropriate physical examination. The very limited usefulness of these methods was discussed in Chapters IV and X.

CASE 10 (Miss M., reported by Dr. R., pp. 63–65)

Period 1, ending December 31st, 1955

The case was followed up to Christmas 1955 in Chapter XIII (pp. 160–162)

Period 2, ending June 30th, 1963

Miss M. returned to me on the 8th July, 1957, simply to tell me that "I am afraid that things did not go well—my marriage broke up." She went on to tell me that "he stopped caring for me very early". I did not have to do anything more than discuss with her her present situation. She had no symptoms but was clearly depressed. I saw her again on the 11th July, 1957, when she seemed to be adapting well to her new situation which was that of living in rooms on the other side of the river and working again. I was interested to note that, although the last time I had seen her was in March, 1955, she had not changed to another doctor until the present time. I had to tell her that, as much as I regretted it, I could not keep her on my list as she was now living in a district very far from mine. I then received the usual form asking for her medical records to be sent in as she had transferred to another doctor in her new area in August, 1957.

I did suggest to her that, should she ever feel that I could be of help to her, I should be pleased to see her, but I have not seen her since July 1957.

A sad story but a most interesting follow-up.

First, I think, it ought to be pointed out that when Miss M. met with the disaster of the breakdown of her marriage, she came to her old general practitioner complaining, not of some minor physical ailment, but of her present distress. A great change, an unquestionably excellent result of her previous treatment by Dr. R., and a promising opening for another piece of therapy.

It is unfortunate that Dr. R. did not do more on this occasion than accept the facts: that her marriage had broken up and that Miss M. was now living in a district too far away from his. What he could have done was to examine with his patient the finer, that is the more important, details of the marriage breakdown. For instance, what happened to make Miss M.'s husband "stop caring for her," apparently in the same way as the Armenian did? It is quite possible that the result of this examination would have revealed faults in Miss M.'s methods of finding partners for herself, as well as faults in her methods of treating them. Another aspect of the same examination could have been centred on the doctor-patient relationship, which started so to speak on the wrong foot by Miss M. choosing rooms in an impossibly distant area of London. This could be considered as a sample of her relationship to men in general; she must create conditions which make it extremely difficult for any man—including her doctor—to keep up a mutually satisfactory contact with her.

Of course if Dr. R. had started on an examination of this kind, this would have meant a continuation of his medical responsibility for Miss M. for some considerable time—a responsibility not easily accepted by a busy practitioner for an N.H.S. patient living far outside his area. As we all know, there are various second-rate methods for dealing with this difficulty; unfortunately, each of them has the unavoidable additional disadvantage that it restricts the free and easy relationship between a general practitioner and his patient which, especially in this case, proved so valuable for the treatment.

Whatever his motives were, Dr. R. decided not to embark upon these examinations, and so we do not know the answers to our questions. As pointed out several times in this book, if a patient and his doctor have to part after a period of psychotherapy which has led to some insight and understanding, this inevitably means the winding up of what we called the "mutual investment company" with considerable losses to both of them. This is what happened in this case and as the examination was not carried out, we do not know whether this outcome could or could not have been avoided.

Dr. R. obtained from the Executive Council Miss M.'s present doctor's name and address. Through this doctor's help we were able to get hold of a few details of Miss M.'s recent medical history which—though by no means complete—shows what may happen to a patient after the "mutual investment company" has to be wound up.

Miss M. transferred to another general practitioner in the London area, with whom she stayed till the beginning of 1960. When, in July 1957, she consulted Dr. R., she was depressed and complained about her broken marriage but no psychosomatic symptoms were offered. After losing Dr. R. apparently she returned to her old habits and eventually she was referred to A. Hospital, whence her general practitioner received the following letter:

2nd December, 1959

I saw the above named patient of yours in Medical Out-patients. She complained of vague epigastric discomfort periodically for the past 6 months. She thought the recent attack was just preceding her menstrual period. When I saw her she was symptom free.

I was unable to detect any evidence of an organic lesion on clinical examination. Associated with some of her attacks there was some diarrhoea, as you mentioned in your note, but I agree with you the diagnosis may well

*be emotional diarrhoea. As you know, she was divorced during the past
week.*

*I did not consider any treatment at present indicated apart from re-
assurance, but would like to see her again in 3 weeks, in order to reassess
her case, and to determine the relationship of her pain to her period.*

(Signed) Consultant Physician.

and about six weeks later, a second letter:

19th January, 1960

*Further to my letter of 2nd December, 1959, I saw Miss M. again
yesterday in Out-patients.*

*She tells me that she has felt better for a few weeks, but her symptoms
of abdominal colic and loose motions have recurred 3 weeks ago. No obvious
organic lesion was detected clinically, and I considered her symptoms to be
due to an emotional diarrhoea. I thought this should improve following the
course of a tranquillizer such as Stelazine, 1 mg. b.d., and Mist. Kaolin,
½ oz. t.i.d., which she could take while her symptoms are present.*

I should like to see her in 2 months, re progress.

(Signed) Consultant Physician.

We who know her medical history of the past years can see that
she has now re-produced all her old symptoms. However, instead
of any attempt at understanding her actual conflicts and their
connexion with the symptoms presented by her, we witness in
her case the routine inconsistent handling that most patients of
her kind receive: in the December letter the consultant states that
he does not consider that any treatment is indicated apart from
reassurance, while in his letter in January, for the same condition—
although the patient has in the meanwhile improved—he recommends a tranquillizer and some Kaolin. Of course he does not
give any explanation for his change of policy for the simple reason
that it cannot be explained rationally.

Miss M. was then recalled from London to a country town to
help to nurse her mother who was seriously ill. The last letter is
from her present doctor:

18th July, 1963

Thank you for your note re Miss M.

*You say that she was your patient until August 1957. You will therefore
remember that her marriage broke up, following which she became rather
disturbed.*

She contracted various symptoms—abdominal pains, diarrhoea, irregular menses, etc. She was seen at A. Hospital by Dr. X.
She eventually settled down.
I have known Miss M. for the past 16 years and I would say that now she has become thoroughly adjusted. At the present she is caring for her mother who is quite ill.

A typical well-meaning, hopeful letter. Although with some doubt, let us hope that the future will prove that the doctor's assessment of Miss M.'s present state was correct.

CASE 11 (Mr. K., reported by Dr. Y. pp. 69–71)

Period 1, ending December 31st, 1955

After the original report in May 1952, Dr. Y. started psychotherapy with Mr. K. As the treatment came up against some difficulties Mr. K. was referred to our emergency service and was seen in September. Here I cannot report in detail about his complicated psychological problems and the ways he developed for coping with them. Suffice it to say that Dr. Y. was able to make use of the help given by the conference, and Mr. K.'s treatment continued. In spite of some serious setbacks in his employment, the intensity of Mr. K.'s symptoms gradually diminished. By July 1953 his condition improved so much that it was possible to discontinue regular psychotherapeutic sessions. Since then he reverted to the status of a "normal" patient and has been seen only rarely, about three or four times a year, for minor ailments. The only trace of his past is that he still occasionally takes some alkalines.

Period 2, ending June 30th, 1963

After 1953 Mr. K. only came to the surgery at three-monthly intervals, sometimes sending his wife for his Alkali cream. He was quite happy, in a masochistic way, not to be recognized as the capable person he knew himself to be, looking forward to his retirement, when he would be neither persecuted nor suppressed and making his colleagues envious of his way of enjoying life.

His physical condition, though not completely cleared up, remained under control until 1957–58, when he showed symptoms of a hiatus hernia, which was confirmed by barium meal. He was given and accepted general rules of behaviour in order to avoid discomfort. At the same time an E.C.G. was taken, as he complained of pain in left lower chest and breathing difficulties. The cardiogram showed "some, though not very convincing, evidence of myocardial degeneration". He retired about this time.

1958—He was given a truss for a right inguinal hernia.

1959—He was suffering from strain of the rotator cuff of his right shoulder, which subsided with hydrocortisone injections.

I gave up my N.H.S. practice in January 1960.

In March 1960 Mr. K. had a slight coronary attack and was sent to hospital by my successor. E.C.G. showed "left axis deviation, otherwise was within normal limits." Chest X-ray n.a.d.

He was kept in hospital for a short while and then returned home. My successor said he was "no trouble" and was scarcely seen in the surgery.

There were no more entries on his card.

For the sake of this follow-up, I visited Mr. K. and found him slightly euphoric, enjoying life—but not "tremendously" as I had suggested in a leading question. He had gained too much weight, looking rather coarse, only his slim hands still reminding me of his former appearance. He is spending his time mainly in "doing" things in the house, some carpentry, decorating, gardening, growing cacti. He does not make music any longer, reads little and has in general settled down to dull ordinary life. He has taken up making jewellery, but in a purely mechanical way, inserting stones into prepared patterns.

With regard to his previous work and the people he worked with, he is somewhat paranoid ... "they were such a mean crowd, conditions stunted you, you could not talk to anybody. . . ." In contrast to this he boasted how many friends he had made since his retirement. Everybody knows him in the neighbourhood (and of course looks up to him), he feels himself cherished and valued.

He still does not like crowds, does not go to the cinema—he has television—but he does not travel, except on his holiday.

His tummy trouble is under control. He knows what to take and when to take it. Very rarely he still experiences sudden panic, for instance when invited to dinner he suddenly gets the old butterfly feeling in his stomach, with a burning sensation and feeling of vacancy. But he reassures himself by thinking that, after all, he is among friends.

His heart attack took place after sawing down a tree in the garden. To his mind it was an accident without further consequences.

He explains the fact that he is enjoying life, but not to the full, by his nostalgia for youth and, generally, by his loss of zest. "One lives from day to day." He is not afraid of death, as he has become a spiritualist. Many years ago, when talking to his brother, he saw his mother's ghost standing between them. He took that as a favour shown to him and in his rivalry with his brother, did not draw his attention to it. Also he is now singled out to advantage (if only the fellows at work knew!). He attends séances regularly and has a "blue aura," i.e. he is considered a "healer."

Men still play a much greater rôle in his life than women. He is either equal to or better than other men—mostly better though. He dreams a great deal, but finds it impossible ever to recall a dream.

Women are scarcely mentioned. His wife, who used to be the "rocher de bronze" through all the years of his continuing illnesses, has succumbed to Menière's disease. She attends X Hospital once in three months, and though the complaint is not very bad, she gets his attention, especially since the attacks are brought on by stooping—a thing which he strictly avoids because of his hiatus hernia—"and one of us must do it!"

His daughter, now in her early thirties, a conscientious civil servant, with an hysterical episode ten years or so ago, when she had to be admitted to a mental hospital, has made many efforts at getting married, without success. She manages to attach herself to unobtainable men.

While Mr. K.'s pride is hurt as his daughter is still a spinster, he feels gratified at the same time that she stays at home, embellishing the home with her presence and income.

In his relation to me Mr. K. made it clear that he is quite independent. He does not "trouble" any doctor now. He buys his own medicine (as my successor did not continue to give him what I prescribed, and he does not like what he prescribes) and he is a "healer" after all.

On the whole he seems content with his life as it is.

The report contains a good deal of interesting detail, enabling us to follow adequately Mr. K.'s later development. His attacks of pain, doubling him up, disappeared completely; the cholecystectomy seems to have been justified. All the other pain and discomfort which plagued him so much after the operation and prompted Dr. Y. to try with psychotherapy, has been considerably reduced almost to insignificance; thus psychotherapy seems to have been equally justified. I wonder how many doctors will realize and accept the full implications of these two parallel statements for their everyday practice. In other words, how many doctors will see that the process described in this book as "elimination by appropriate physical examinations" is in many cases a most costly procedure, both for the patient and the doctor, and should not be used in a routine way automatically.

After this general statement let us examine in detail what happened to Mr. K. A man of many abilities and good promise was not able to develop into an active and efficient individual because of his many inhibitions, both in relation to men and women. Although every doctor who attended him recognized and diagnosed promptly these inhibitions, nothing was done for them; instead of it about two decades were spent in chasing various, more or less irrelevant, physical conditions which he offered in addition to his psychological symptoms. Mr. K. was already in his fifties when Dr. Y. realized the futility of this medical policy and offered him psychotherapy.

As we learn from the first follow-up report, this proved anything but easy and it is not surprising that, at this comparatively late age, Dr. Y. could help him only in a limited way. As the second follow-up report shows he has become a pompous, overbearing, narcissistic man who must always be right, who apparently has only pride and vanity but not much love for anyone else, including his wife and daughter. Moreover his gaining weight, apart from not being a good prognostic sign for his heart condition, suggests a chronic depressive state, against which he tries to defend himself by over-eating and by reassuring himself that he is enjoying life and is much better than anybody else. This suggests a precariously balanced situation, and therefore the prognosis must remain uncertain and guarded.

CASE 12 (Miss F. reported by Dr. C., pp. 76–80)

Period 1, ending December 31st, 1955

January 14th, 1956. She has not improved. Her periods are pretty regular and her babyish behaviour is unchanged. She still comes spasmodically for injections, is childishly flirtatious, she is ever so grateful to me and she thinks I am wonderful. Nobody gives injections so painlessly as I do, and she is getting on splendidly. She sent me a Christmas card, with love, and signed with her Christian name (but she did that last year too). Rashes on her face come and go as before, and she demands antihistamine ointments regularly. She does not say so, but I am pretty sure she is not taking her hormone tablets regularly as she used to. Her demands for prescriptions are less frequent.

I myself thought I was improving with her. I have not had to swallow my irritation at her out-of-hours and meal-time visits. I was managing to accept (as I thought) all the little inconveniences she inflicted on me, and was hoping that I was changing myself into the benevolent, good person she would be able to come clean to if she ever did.

I was disappointed therefore when a week ago she called and, after her injection and the usual childish babble, said she might possibly take a job in the country, in the town where her parents had recently bought a house. "I love the country you know." I didn't know what to make of it, whether it was an empty threat or a serious one. Here I had been managing her better, and she threatens to desert me. All I could think of was that she felt if she stayed longer she might have to drop her pretences, and was running away from the danger. Is that right?

The interesting aspect in this history is the overwhelming power of the repetition compulsion. As we saw it in the original report in Chapter VII, nobody is allowed to be properly in charge of the case of Miss F. Should this event threaten, she either produces another doctor and then plays one off against the other, or runs away. Apparently she is about to resort to the latter in the case of Dr. C. It is difficult to say whether this repetitive pattern could have been changed before it became firmly "organized," or even prevented from developing in the first place. Unfortunately, it seems that very little can be done now.

Period 2, ending June 30th, 1963

Miss F. left the district. No news.

The apprehensive predictions of the first follow-up period were correct. It is a pity.

CASE 13 (Reported by Dr. Y., pp. 82–83)

Period 1, ending December 31st, 1955

The patient came to see me from time to time. I tried to make her talk, and to relate her symptoms to her past life and her present worries. As far as her past life was concerned, she was so well defended that she would admit no interpretation at all.

Her present worries were—

(1) The impossible situation of constant rows with her lover's mother.

(2) The worry about her daughter, who was on the point of repeating her own pattern of life, namely, living with a man who could not get a divorce from his wife.

She felt relieved through being able to discuss her problems with me, but the headaches remained.

A few months later her lover's mother, also one of my patients, came to tell me that she and her husband were moving away, as she could not stand life in her house any longer. From then onwards my patient's headaches improved, as she was so obviously relieved of the everyday quarrel. Her daughter broke with her lover, and has since concluded an ordinary marriage.

My patient is now quite well. The everyday life problems on top of her deep-level problems proved too much for her and must have caused her symptoms. Through the solution of her present problems she fell back into her old status of well-defended balance. She has been quite well since.

Period 2, ending June 30th, 1963

After her operation for varicose veins the patient was not seen until January 1958, when she developed pneumonia after influenza. This cleared up completely. By now she seemed a much happier person. Circumstances had improved in so far as the old people had moved away, and she had the house to herself and her lover. Her daughter had dissolved the relationship to her boy-friend—(married and unobtainable, just like mother's) and had got married to an Arab who had settled in England in a good job after studying engineering.

1959 (November) complaints of constant indigestion.

1960 Barium meal and gastroscopy showed nothing but " mild gastritis." By now she had given up her job as saleswoman in a big store in the neighbourhood and had become manageress of a small shop in the City. She was feeling well, apart from occasional dyspepsia. Headaches had disappeared. She was working very hard, leaving the house at 7 and coming home at 8, though being free at weekends.

February 1962. She woke up one morning feeling very giddy with a pain in her chest. She thought this was indigestion, went to the City with great difficulty and walked through the streets "like drunk." At lunch time she was taken home. My successor—by this time I had given up N.H.S. practice—sent her to hospital. The hospital reported "E.C.G. n.a.d. Her pain is not typical of any particular cause. Heart-burn symptoms were worse on bending and lying. Ba-Meal." She was sent home, but seen again in March 1962, when the report reads: "I thought the patient's chest-pain was rather typical(!) Straightforward E.C.G. normal, but exercise test shows *definite evidence of ischaemia*. Barium meal was quite normal. She should lose a stone of weight and be put on nitrites and sedation."

When I saw her for the follow-up she seemed well and happy. She has had 2–3 more minor attacks of angina pectoris, but knows now what to do. She is not frightened when the attacks come, does not think of death, but only how to handle the situation technically. She tried not to let anybody know about it (including her present doctor) because other people get so worried. When a neighbour recently "popped off with coronary" she thought—"This will happen to me one day," but she does not brood on it. She has never been frightened of death. When she had her severe mastoid operation as a young woman, shortly after her husband's accident which turned him into a mental case, she dreamed that she had died. She saw her own funeral procession with all her relatives, a coffin covered in flowers; but she herself was outside the coffin, flying over it, though her body was inside. She felt very happy and only wished she could make the situation, as it really was, clear to the mourners. Ever since then she had no fear of dying. She looks upon this experience as a personal favour shown her by fate, singling her out for a "happy ending", as in practically all her life situations. So far all her problems have been solved in a satisfactory way; true her husband who is still alive and in a mental home has been an inmate there for almost thirty years. He still wishes badly to come home, but this is impossible, as he is confused and suicidal! She has not been to see him for years, neither has her daughter, who used to visit him regularly, though at long intervals, and saw him last three years ago. They left off visiting because it upset *him* so much. The patient feels that she has paid off her debt towards him by bringing up her two children, and working so hard that she managed to give them both a good education. Also, until the advent of the Health Service, she had to pay £3 a week for his upkeep.

She lives very happily with her man; the fact that they cannot get married—as his wife declines to divorce him—does not worry her at all. He is accepted by her children and she by his family.

The patient ignores her coronary to such an extent (or perhaps covers up her fears in that way) that she intends to give up her present job and open up a shop of her own.

Her daughter's marriage has turned out very well and she is expecting a baby. Her son is also happily married with two children.

A remarkable development, but in good agreement with the previous report.

CASE 14 (Mr. I., reported by Dr. B., pp. 86–90)

Period 1, ending December 31st, 1955

I have seen Mr. I. professionally only once since my last report in March, 1955, when he had a mild bronchitis with underlying depression, of which he was aware and about which he realized it was a matter for his analyst, whom he had not been able to see for a few weeks. He got over his depression quickly when he returned to treatment. I have met him in the street several times and his general style is greatly improved and he seems to be happy and working well.

Period 2, ending June 30th, 1963

Dr. B. gave up his practice and moved out of London. In consequence Mr. I. could not be followed up.

CASE 15 (Mrs. B., reported by Dr. S., pp. 109–115)

Period 1, ending December 31st, 1955

I have not seen Mrs. B., only her mother, who tells me that Mrs. B. and her child are getting on very well. The mother goes to see her and is allowed to stay with her, but not for the night. While she is there, the son-in-law is out. She never sees him. The mother is quite satisfied with the progress of her daughter and the child.

This is a highly interesting development. Apparently the daughter was not able—and perhaps was not willing—to break completely with her mother. Very likely the mother threw her whole weight into the scale in order to re-establish her hold on her daughter. In any case, the ambivalent mother–daughter relationship has been apparently re-established, and the son-in-law-husband is again excluded from it, as previously. No wonder, then, that the mother "is quite satisfied with the progress." The question is whether the husband will be able to stand up to the strain, especially if, as is possible, the mother–daughter relationship becomes closer and more intense with time. If Mrs. B. were still under Dr. S.'s care I should strongly advise him to try to clarify with her her rôle in this triangle, as a preventive measure against future complications. In any case, a most interesting case to watch.

Period 2, ending June 30th, 1963

From the mother I heard that my former patient, Mrs. B., developed diabetes about three years ago, but can cope better with her husband and two children. The relationship between the couple and her parents has also improved, and they are now on visiting terms. Lately Mrs. B. was supporting her mother morally, when her father stayed in hospital with haematemesis from a peptic ulcer.

Postscript

Since my last follow-up report I happened to meet Mr. B. in a big department store, on 29th August. He looked well and prosperous, seemed pleased to see me again, and told me that he is one of the senior salesmen in the department, and that he has also been successful as a writer. He publishes articles, has published two books, and a third is in the making.

He referred proudly to his two girls, aged nine and five, and to his wife as an excellent mother and housewife, who, in spite of her diabetes, which was detected two years ago, keeps it under control most intelligently.

They live outside London in a pleasant house, and manage to see his wife's parents frequently. They are anxious to invite the grandparents, offering them transport both ways in their car.

His mother-in-law would accept the invitation gladly, but father, an invalid with a peptic ulcer, is reluctant to travel.

Encouraged by my interest in the family the next day the couple presented themselves with the children in my surgery. They were on the way to supper with the parents. Mrs. B. looked healthy, self-assured, well-groomed, and was very pleased to show off her well-developed and well-mannered two girls.

They seemed to me a contented, normal family, and I could not have wished for a better success with my endeavour to help the couple in their chaotic state while struggling for adjustment in the house of the parents-in-law.

Apparently, the "common-sense" in this case made me hit the target well.

A most satisfactory development, in the same direction but definitely better than my guarded prognosis in 1955. A "peaceful co-existence"—or should it be called an armistice?—has been established between mother and husband, but no one knows, certainly not Dr. S., at what price and at whose cost. The development of a diabetic condition in a young woman of barely 30 may be interpreted as a pointer that Mrs. B. has to bear the lion's share of the burden. This, however, may be a much too pessimistic view and perhaps it would be fairer to concede Dr. S. the success of his "common sense" therapy. Or should one wait till the next follow-up?

Case 16 (Mrs. O., reported by Dr. G., pp. 122–126)

Period 1, ending December 31st, 1955

There is not a lot to add, except that Mrs. O. is now in hospital with a slight recurrence of urethral caruncle. I feel a lot of good has been done here. There has been no recurrence of her chronic complaints and she sees me but rarely. In the last six months I have seen her about twice, whereas she used to come almost every week. Last time I saw her she was in the house of another patient whom she was helping to nurse.

Our predictions seem to have been correct. The frustrating

relationship between doctor and patient has disappeared completely and the saving of the doctor's time continues, to the satisfaction of everyone concerned.

Period 2, ending June 30th, 1963

I see her reasonably often, mainly for recurrent bronchitis and more recently for post-menopausal bleeding and a recurrence of urethral caruncle, which was again removed. Relationship remains good. She comes and talks freely when she feels like it and I myself have no anxiety about her.

I would say the chief gain in this case is to the doctor. She no longer depresses me and I can keep her going without any difficulty.

I can only repeat what I said in 1955, namely that our predictions seem to have been correct..The saving of time still continues and, what is more important, the frustrating relationship between doctor and patient has completely disappeared to everybody's satisfaction. Considering that the "long interview" which fundamentally changed the situation happened in March 1954, this long follow-up amounting almost to ten years, is an important support for the recommendation that tiresome patients should not be automatically fobbed off with some more or less rational prescription or with a common sense placebo.

CASE 17 (Mr. Y., reported by Dr. K., pp. 127–131)

Period 1, ending December 31st, 1955

About a month after the first report, Dr. K. mentioned Mr. Y. again—

He came back . . . having talked him out of having the X-ray and reassured him. You said there was a lot more coming—sure enough he did come along again two to three weeks later saying roughly the same thing . . . and could he have an X-ray? as if we had had no previous conversation at all. Knowing the man, and thinking that obviously he would have to be reassured, I did not go into a lot of details that time, I said, "Say that X-ray does show the tiniest ulcer, the fact is that the treatment isn't going to be any different, is it?" But it was very curious; if you started explaining . . . "What are you worried about, are you afraid of a growth?" he would say "No, no, no." "What do you want the X-ray for?" . . . All he says is, he must have the X-ray. It's extraordinary, this feeling. He has got to have that X-ray, although he doesn't know really why he wants it. As soon

as you start cross-examining him he has got nothing behind it. And
he will not allow you to suggest that that isn't the problem really.
As he could not get this X-ray without seeing the physician whom
he saw before at the hospital about his chest, I referred Mr. Y. to him.
So I am now awaiting this report.

At this point we can see two forces at work. On the one hand
there is the patient, who cannot be reassured, who must have an
X-ray, without knowing why. Obviously he cannot express his
fears, but he feels them the more. He is definitely on the danger-
list, and must be taken seriously. On the other hand there is the
doctor, who now has better insight but still has not the skill and
the confidence necessary to convey his ideas to the patient in
mutually intelligible language. Talking at cross-purposes is painfully present, and the only way out—the only course acceptable
to both patient and doctor—is to ask the opinion of a consultant.
The consultant in question is a general physician, and it is doubtful
whether he will be able to assess Mr. Y.'s case deeply enough.

The usual, easy answer is that nothing has been or will be lost
by asking for the consultant's opinion. If the finding is positive,
the examination was necessary; if it is negative, both doctor and
patient will feel "reassured" and, if thought advisable, a psychiatrist can then be consulted. What is completely neglected, or
even repressed, is that by this procedure the patient is forced (or
helped) to "organize" his illness on physical lines and the chances
of any psychotherapeutic help are considerably diminished. It
is probable that the mere suggestion that he should consult a
psychiatrist will become unacceptable to him, as no steps have
been taken to prepare him for this possibility.

Because of this lack of preparation, it will be rather difficult
for the doctor to switch his patient's way of thinking from
physical to psychological lines. This difficulty is great enough if
the consultant's findings are negative, but if the slightest positive
sign is found it will be practically insurmountable. In the latter
event, Mr. Y. will be another illustration of the danger of finding
a "physical illness." The case history leaves no doubt that he is
struggling with his neurotic conflicts, but if he has the bad luck
to have the slightest physical sign, it will be practically impossible
to offer him help for his real trouble.

Early in 1956, Mr. Y. was mentioned again. There was some
hitch and he had not had his X-ray yet. The delay did not worry

him, he was waiting patiently. Dr. K. added to his report that he had forgotten to mention that Mr. Y. had another, elder, daughter, who was married and living on her own, not in the district.

Period 2, ending June 30th, 1963

I continue to see Mr. Y.—from three to ten times a year, mainly for renewal of prescriptions for his indigestion or for the seborrhoeic eczema on the sides of his scalp. He has had indigestion for about 22 years, and scalp irritation for 8 years. He has had no further trouble with his chest. There has been no further psychotherapy as he has never really wanted to talk about his problems. He likes to brush his problems aside with a joke. "I'm worried about my skin today, doctor, not my stomach. I can look after that. It's just a matter of being careful and avoiding fried food," and then with a broad grin "You know a wife could murder her husband by the judicious use of a frying pan." On another occasion when he was complaining of his indigestion, he said he was sorry he could not enjoy his food as it was "the most enjoyable pleasure of life," and also mentioned a row he had had with his wife over who was running the shop. I have referred him to hospital on two occasions in 1956 and 1961 for a barium meal, and on both occasions the X-ray showed no abnormality. A gall-bladder X-ray in 1961 was also negative.

Mr. Y.'s youngest daughter, the one with the Bell's palsy, got married a year or so after the original interview, is living abroad, and he occasionally goes over with his wife to visit her. Mrs. Y. had an operation in 1956 for hysterectomy for fibroids which had caused her menorrhagia for the previous 2 years. I learned that her mother had died in 1955 and that she had been disinclined for intercourse since then, and thought it might well have been that some of Mr. Y.'s symptoms at that time were related to his feeling of rejection by her.

On the whole Mr. Y. seems on balance and able to manage the ambivalent feelings he must have towards his warm-hearted wife. He continues in his shop to meet his customers with an amusing banter and a large smile. He and his wife know all their customers' affairs intimately, and indeed their customers bring them their problems because of the relief they know they will get—Mr. Y. to laugh them off and Mrs. Y. to supply sympathy or praise.

This follow-up report contains a few new details which confirm our original tentative diagnosis. We learn from it that Mrs. Y. had already in 1955, at the time of her husband's original visit to Dr. K., severe bleeding which then led to a hysterectomy a few months later; and, further, that it was at about that time, if not earlier, that she stopped having intercourse with her husband. Another important point is that his younger daughter got married a year or so after the original interview, which means possibly that she was already at that time involved with a young man; a point in support of this interpretation is that she went back to live in the country, from which she returned rather reluctantly when her parents became agitated about her Bell's palsy. All this strongly suggests that towards the end of 1955 Mr. Y. was indeed under a serious strain, feeling that all his women—his wife as well as his favourite daughter—were deserting him; it is no wonder that under this pressure he came to his doctor to find out whether he was man enough.

The original report, the discussion in the seminar, and the first follow-up well illustrate the difficult situation that developed between doctor and patient. Both of them tried their best, but all that they could achieve was talking to each other at cross purposes. Mr. Y. mentioned his real worry only half-heartedly when his doctor was occupied by writing his prescription; and the doctor, although noticing and reporting the event, could not really listen to it. In consequence the case followed the usual course of "elimination by appropriate physical examinations." The opening, offered timidly and half-heartedly by the patient, was not taken up, and this experience almost certainly reinforced his defences which were strong anyhow. Although it is quite possible that he offered a few more timid and half-hearted openings to his doctor, it is more likely that he did not. Whatever the case may be, the result is the same: an almost impenetrable brick wall defence camouflaged as a pleasant and co-operative appreciation of the doctor's work.

There will certainly be a number of people who will disagree with this description and will point out that the overall results are not so bad. The daughter got married, got away from her somewhat over-protective and over-pressing parents, and is now living at a fair distance from them, possibly happily. True, Mrs. Y. had to undergo a hysterectomy and to give up her sexual life perhaps too early, but she became a sympathetic woman, well-liked by everyone. And lastly, the real patient, Mr. Y. had no serious illness for the last ten years or so, and has been able to keep up his pleasant and cheerful character in spite of his annoying chronic indigestion. Unquestionably, his doctor has been a great help to him during these years, reassuring his patient when he thought it necessary by appropriate physical examinations. We hear of two X-rays and one gastroscopy in eight years, which is reasonable in view of the fact that Mr. Y. is in the age group when one ought to be cautious about the possibility of a growth.

All this must be conceded to our critics. The only thing I can do is to ask the perennial question—what the price of these results was. The answer is: a geographical separation of parents and daughter; a probable premature cessation of sexual pleasures for the couple, with the consequent strains that they have to endure, and perhaps more. It is possible that Mr. Y.'s ability "to laugh things off" which is mentioned several times in Dr. K.'s write-up, is a kind of clowning, hiding his bitter disappointment behind the mask of laughter. His joke about the wife who can kill her husband off with a frying pan, agrees well with this supposition. In this case his chronic indigestion might be another symptom suggesting that he had to swallow much more than he could easily digest. Mrs. Y.'s sympathy and praise bestowed upon everyone so conspicuously may be an attempt at self-justification —a kind of defence against her guilt feelings; as if she were saying it is not true that she is a hard woman—to her husband; on the contrary she is very nice and sympathetic—to everybody else. Her dyed hair and the "kick" that she got when she saw the picture in Dr. K.'s waiting room, agree well with these assumptions.

Of course all these are, as I said, assumptions; but it is equally an assumption that these two people are happy and well-adjusted. The trouble is that it is almost impossible to find out the truth because all of them, especially Mr. Y., have been well-trained to expect physical examinations from their doctors, and any attempt or suggestion of a psychological investigation will cause a surprise or meet with misunderstanding, or even icy resistance.

CASE 18 (Mrs. J., reported by Dr. P., pp. 137–139)

Period 1, ending December 31st, 1955

Dr P. has not heard anything about this patient, as was to be expected.

Period 2, ending June 30th, 1963

No contact whatsoever. The initial prediction seems to have been correct.

CASE 19 (Peter, reported by Dr. G., pp. 139–147)

Period 1, ending December 31st, 1955

March 12th, 1956, Peter's wife was in to see me last week with her baby, who had a cough. I enquired about Peter. "Since baby was born he has been a changed man. Very little in the way of headaches, no feelings of fear. Even her parents have noticed it. He idolizes the baby. He is no longer moody or quick-tempered."

The improvement has been definitely maintained. Shall we accept this as the happy ending of the story, i.e. assume that Peter has received sufficient help to overcome his "basic fault," or is it still justified to remain unconvinced? It will be most instructive to follow this family, in particular the baby's development, for the next few years.

Period 2, ending June 30th, 1963

I must be pardoned if I regard this case as a triumph. He must have known about your letter to me because he came in this morning! His wife is in hospital, having just had an appendicectomy and he has been coping with three children—normal children I may say. He would like a rest from work for a few days because he had had a rather difficult two weeks previously.

Other than that, he had had "none of his old trouble for years," an "occasional headache" and feels fully confident that his previous trouble is a "thing of the past, thanks to you, doctor."

He has a lovely family of three normal healthy children, none of them problem children.

I am trying to find flaws in all this, searching for clues of what his "feeling all right" might be a prelude to, but I cannot find anything. True it seems too good to be true, and we doctors are loathe to accept these quick cures, which seem too *pat* since "we have not resolved anything really" and "have not touched on his psychopathology to any depth," etc., etc. But if he carries on like this for another twenty years, I do not think Peter will worry much about this technical problem.

I think that Dr. G., backed by a follow-up longer than 10 years, is justified in his claim of calling his treatment a triumph. His "long interview" in March 1953, and his subsequent handling of the case, changed a seriously neurotic youngster, who had to go through an appalling childhood and adolescence, into a normal adult man with a satisfied wife and three normal children—not a mean achievement by any standards.

CASE 20 (Mrs. N., reported by Dr. C., pp. 148–150)

Period 1, ending December 31st, 1955

After a few tries I got Mrs. N. on the telephone. She is now working as a sort of clerk in the almoner's department of a hospital. Hence the difficulty of getting hold of her.

I began to wish I had not got hold of her, for she would hardly stop talking. She had been on the point of ringing me many times but had not liked to bother me, etc. Her headaches have gone, but not the sleepiness. She sometimes feels dreadful, because people notice it. She is a regular consumer of Drinamyl. If she misses it she feels as if she had been chloroformed and couldn't come round. Falls asleep on buses. Whenever she relaxes she falls asleep. She fell asleep at the dinner table yesterday. She would like to see me again to talk about it, and I gave her an appointment. And now I am wondering what to do about it. She has shifted her ground, and it looks as if she is trying to force my hand. As she is now appealing for help, I don't see how it can be refused, but I don't see how I can find time for her—though I am sorely tempted. Would a group do for her, do you think?

Apparently our uncertainty in assessing the therapeutic results in her case was over-cautious. Her headaches have disappeared, but not her "basic fault." From this angle the decision "to stop" was perhaps right. It is difficult to evaluate the nature of her sleepiness on the basis of a telephone conversation only. It could be caused by an insidiously developing narcolepsy, but might equally well be due to a deterioration of her old hysterical symptom, or even to a combination of the two. Obviously further examinations, both psychological and neurological, will be needed.

Period 2, ending June 30th, 1963

Mrs. N. had a recurrence in 1957 and came back for a few sessions. Less for headaches this time than for a number of other subjective symptoms, such as insomnia, nightmares, nervous dyspepsia, "dreadful feelings," etc. Still falling asleep in daytime. Hostility to men in general and her husband in particular came out clearly. Same pattern as before, seduction and then refusal. Complained of her husband's lack of interest in her, and yet she blocked any advance by him, i.e. went to bed an hour before he did and pretended to be asleep when he came to bed. She had some insight into this and agreed that it expressed an inner resentment. Her symptoms cleared up and she stopped coming. In the end she was not falling asleep in tubes and buses, except when coming to see me.

No more contact till two months ago, when she rang for an appointment. Free from headaches for seven years or so, that is till the last four years when they had returned. She apparently took four years to make up her mind to come back. She had been working in the office of a big hospital and one of the doctors suggested she had an examination. She was passed through all the departments and everything was negative. Then, she put it—"I went through all the drug lists and nothing did any good". Then, she went to the neurological department and nothing was found and they advised her to go to a psychiatric department but she would not go. Said—"It was bad enough talking here, I did not want to talk to them." She had relaxing exercises and by the time they finished with her she had a worse headache than before.

When she arrived she was the same stylized, well-defended, seductive, rather precious woman. Well preserved, youthful appearance. She came to me because some of her friends had said hypnotism was a very good thing and could I recommend a hypnotist to her?

I could, of course, have easily done this but I was curious and did not want to lose her, especially as I knew a follow-up would be wanted sooner or later. I hate hypnotism. I suppose we have all had a shot at it, and most of us get fed up with it. I always feel such a charlatan and have never had any lasting results. But, as I did not want to lose her and as hypnotism anyhow does not take very long, I said I would do it for a few times to see if she got any benefit from it. So, we started every session with about a quarter of an hour of hypnotism, and then came the first surprise. For a woman with hysterical symptoms I expected her to go pretty deep easily, but she did not. She got as far as a moderately light hypnosis, but no further. It took a long time for the penny to drop and for me to see that she was playing out on me her old seductive and repelling pattern. Inviting me to a sort of sublimated hypnotic-erotic relationship and at the same time holding me off.

There have been two special strains on her: her daughter had left home to share a flat with other girls; and she herself had had an affair with a Scandinavian for five months before the headaches came back. It fizzled out as he had to leave London, but it need not have fizzled out if she had not let it. Her husband found out about the affair and she confessed; but it looked as if she wanted him to find out, and I am sure she could have easily dissembled and put him off if she had wanted to. He had, in the meantime, grown jealous of other men who were paying her attention. She said it was a great shock to him; he asked her if she wanted a divorce, and she said she did not. Thereupon, the husband changed his behaviour; whereas he used to be out most evenings and she considered herself neglected, now he was at home whenever he could be and became much more demanding sexually. She complained of this just as much as she had complained of his lack of attention previously. If only he would leave me alone, etc. Would she feel the same if it was from her Scandinavian lover? Well, er, No. The Scandinavian was always immaculately dressed and the husband was always a bit careless. (Father was always a great dandy about his clothes.)

The headaches were typically during the week-ends. They wore off during the day and during the week when she was away from home working in her office. The daughter annoys her by coming to see them apparently only when she wants something, either bed linen for her flat, or something similar. She dislikes the feeling that she is being made use of.

What came out new was that her continual talk about wanting a house of her own with her own front door and a garden round it separating her from her neighbours, bore no relation to her early upbringing; it was thought that this attitude was dictated by her father's profession which compelled him to live with his family in other people's houses. In fact in all his employments he had had a house of his own and thus her longing could not originate from this source.

After eight interviews, the headaches had almost gone, and then she left to go abroad on her summer holiday with her husband. She pointed out that the headaches were always better on holiday. I thought she had gained a little insight and realized that her resentment against her slow-coach husband was partly realistic, and partly determined by her wish that nobody should come up to the childish picture of the immaculate father.

She said she would ring me up on her return from holiday, which she did. She said that her headaches had completely vanished, although the husband was with her all the time. There were the usual (for her) excessive sexual demands but that apparently did not bring on the headaches. She came to see me and the headaches had apparently gone and we left it that she would ring me if they came back. She rang me three or four days ago saying that the headaches had returned as bad as ever and made an appointment. So the case is still on.

I am rather at a loss. I feel she is bringing me around to her own opinion that it is the frustrated wish for this sort of dream-house which gives her the headaches, and yet I don't feel that this can be true. I feel a bit stuck with her and am tempted to get rid of her, say, by referring her for group therapy. I did this once seven years ago, but unfortunately the group therapy did not work and she left; this makes it rather difficult for me to suggest the same thing again. And yet, my curiosity wants me to get on with it and do it myself.

The follow-up is in good agreement both with our initial assessment and the predictions, with one exception, namely, that the idea of narcolepsy on organic basis may now be dropped. The course of treatment, taking the whole ten years, is typical of what we called "the special psychological atmosphere of general practice." Mrs. N. was able to consult her doctor whenever she wanted and, in response to this, the doctor continued with as much or as little psychotherapy as the situation warranted.

CASE 21 (Mrs. Q., reported by Dr. M., pp. 162–169)

Period 1, ending December 31st, 1955

The follow-up is included in Chapter XIII (pp. 168–169).

Period 2, ending June 30th, 1963

(*a*) Till August 1960

This case history was used again in the book by Michael and Enid Balint—*Psychotherapeutic Techniques in Medicine*, London and New York, 1961—as Case 1. Its history was followed up there, till August 1960 on pp. 12–16 and 212–213. A précis of the follow-up is reprinted here:

As the years passed Mrs. Q. became more and more independent. Parallel with this she felt that her marriage was increasingly unsatisfactory, especially so sexually. She struck up a friendship with another man, an Indian, who was kind, generous, very fond of her and treated her gently. Thus he was utterly different from her husband. After some time she decided to leave her husband and to ask for a divorce on grounds of cruelty.

First she moved with her child to her parents but remained on the doctor's list. The parents did not approve of her affair and refused to look after her child, insisting that this was Mrs. Q.'s duty. On the other hand they were willing to allow her to stay in their house. Under these circumstances she had to accept support from her Indian friend.

During this period Mrs. Q. came occasionally to tell the doctor about developments and eventually asked him to be a witness in the divorce proceedings, which he accepted. Mr. Q., however, defended the suit, promised at the hearing to mend his ways and offered reconciliation, which Mrs. Q. refused. Under these circumstances the judge did not grant a divorce, but gave the custody of the child to Mrs. Q.

Now she is living with her friend, officially as his housekeeper, facing the difficulties of her position amazingly well, and she hopes to have a child by him in due course.

She has had no illnesses in recent years. No further work has been done about her jealousy of her sister and sister-in-law, in fact the doctor thinks that she sees very little, if anything, of them.

In the doctor's opinion she certainly has become more mature, dresses neatly, and is no longer sluttish. She knows that if her husband can prove adultery her son may be taken away from her. She says that she loves him very much but feels that she should not sacrifice her life and independence completely to him. She had to make a difficult decision whether to stay with her parents, who did not treat her very well, and be sure that she could keep her child, or go and live with her friend and risk losing the child. After long consideration and without any outside help she decided on the second choice.

(*b*) Rest of the period.

Dr. M. mentions that in the meanwhile Mrs. Q. got a divorce from her husband, and then continues:

In my last report I told you about Mrs. Q.'s alliance with an Indian. The Indian's wife came to this country to join him here, and although for a while Mrs. Q. remained friendly with him, even hoped that he would send his wife back to India and marry her in the end, she gradually began to take a more realistic view of the situation, and about three years ago broke off all contact with him.

She was very unhappy for a while, but then took on a job as a saleswoman, which took her all over England. She proved to be very competent and efficient in her job, gained promotion, met another, older, man, whom she married a month ago. I have seen very little of her, except that once or twice a year she came along to tell me how she was getting on. She had during that time hardly any physical complaints. Her relationship with her parents was not too happy, though her child stayed with them. I believe she intends to take the child into her new home, but I am not certain about this.

Dr. M. then adds to his report that Mrs. Q.'s parents have been for some time on Dr. E.'s list, who reports about them as follows:

The family, consisting of Mrs. Q.'s parents and her son, moved into my district, and after some while Dr. M. persuaded them to join my list. Mrs. Q. lived with them but stayed with Dr. M.

I found the grandparents, that is the parents of Mrs. Q., two of the most unpleasant people I have ever encountered: they were smiling, slimy and insincere. I was most interested in the family set-up because of my acquaintance with Mrs. Q.'s case but, after a time, I found myself completely unsympathetic to the parents. Dr. M. and I have often discussed how difficult it is, in general practice, to take on one another's patients. I saw a fair amount of Mrs. Q. and must say that, contrary to my expectations, I found her a pleasant person, quite unlike her parents. It was hard to recognize her as the same individual as described in the psychiatric and psychological reports of 1952. She had left and divorced her husband and was contemplating making another marriage. It was interesting to watch the efforts that the parents made to play me off against Dr. M. The boy is the apple of his grandparents' eyes and very much spoilt. In spite of this, he has quite a pleasing little personality. Both parents had had very serious illnesses which they had coped with, on the whole, satisfactorily. When I last saw them, Mrs. Q. had left to take a job as a commercial traveller in the North. The boy was left with the grandparents and appeared to be getting on quite well. I believe since then the family have moved away from my district.

Apparently the improvement in Mrs. Q.'s condition is still continuing. She is getting more and more independent of her parents and, parallel with this, becoming more mature. True, she could not avoid committing a few blunders on her way to maturity but we must not forget that this happens to quite a number of people. And, if we call to mind, as Dr. E. does, the extremely poor condition in which we met her in 1952, we cannot but be impressed by the great changes that she was able to achieve. Unquestionably she still has a long way to go, so let us hope that she will find, in her new home up in the North of England, a doctor as versatile and as helpful as Dr. M.

CASE 22 (Mr. V., reported by Dr. H., pp. 174–181)

Period 1, ending December 31st, 1955

January 26th, 1956. I have seen Mr. V. three times since Christmas. By the way, his wife is pregnant. When he first came he told me that he had changed his job in October (after eighteen months at one firm where he was very happy). He had again taken the blame for something; he could not bear it, and chucked his job up. He had spent Christmas with his family, had got bad there, the change of job had depressed him so much. A week after Christmas he had phoned the manager of his old firm and asked whether they would take him back. I said, "Why didn't you come and see me all these months after you had changed your job?" He said, "I didn't want to disappoint you." He only came to see me after he had made up his mind to go back. They took him back, and told him that they knew all the time it was not his fault. He repeated the same situation we had before. I said, "You say I am your mother and you don't want to disappoint me, and you react to your manager as to your father. This fear of disappointing me is only because you make me your mother, but I am not your mother, and you could have come." He came the following week when everything was all right again; no pains, no depression. I think it was really a good result that he had the courage to go back to his old firm.

April 1956. He phoned me up last week to say that his wife has had a baby boy. He said he considers himself a very lucky man.

A most interesting follow-up. It well illustrates what we mean by the "mutual investment company." After the psychotherapy was terminated, patient and doctor did not part, but only reduced the frequency of their meetings. When further trouble occurred, the patient, after some hesitation, was able to come to his general practitioner for help, and the two could pick up the threads where they had been dropped. Very little psychotherapy was needed to reinforce the processes already at work in the patient.

Period 2, ending June 30th, 1963

(a) This case was followed up in Michael and Enid Balint's: *Psychotherapeutic Techniques in Medicine*, London and New York, 1961, as Case 2 till August, 1960 on pp. 16–22 and 214–215. Unfortunately the structure of the case is so complex that any abstracting would amount to distortion. So, for details I must refer the reader to the work just mentioned. On the whole, with some ups and downs, Mr. V. kept fairly well, had another son, and improved his business successfully. In 1960 he was so well off that he seriously looked round to buy a house for his family.

(b) Rest of the period

Dr. H. reports: Mr. V. did not buy a house but the family is living in the same Council flat in my district. All went apparently well with him until the beginning of this year. He came to me and was complaining of headaches, loss of weight and he was depressed. He told me that the partnership with his brother broke up and that he was left alone to pay off considerable debts. His business was not good during the cold winter months and he was forced to take on a job as a driver to deliver bread. He had to get up very early every morning, was working until midday and in the afternoon carried on with his decorating. At the same time his wife's father was very ill in hospital, following a cerebral haemorrhage, and he visited me shortly after his father-in-law's death. We discussed the identification with his own father and his own fears of death; I asked him to come and see me again but—as on previous occasions—he did not keep the appointment. I did not see him again as a patient, but we had employed him again to redecorate our old house last year and as there was a small repair to be done I used the opportunity to contact him a few days ago. He has given up his job as a driver and is working now on his own as a decorator. He seems to be fairly busy and satisfied. He apologized for not having come back to me but thought it was not necessary.

His wife is working as a part-time housekeeper for an old lady. She rarely comes to the surgery now. She and her mother are much better since her father, who for many years was a very ill man, died.

Mr. V.'s daughter has developed into a good-looking girl and works as a comptometer operator. The two boys go to school and are both very lively and strong.

Apparently the "mutual investment company" mentioned in my comment to the report of the previous period is still working well for both partners: patient and doctor alike. If we recall the original hospital report of 1950, and the relationship which developed under its influence between Mr. V. and the hospital doctors, and then compare this with his present situation and his present relationship to Dr. H. we cannot but be impressed by the immense difference. This difference was brought about by psychotherapy, carried out by a general practitioner.

CASE 23 (Miss S., reported by Dr. R., pp. 181–191)

Period 1, ending December 31st, 1955

January 1956. Miss S. brought her husband to introduce him to me. They were about to move from London; he got a job in a provincial town, and they came to say goodbye just before Christmas 1955. Then everything was satisfactory.

Period 2, ending June 30th, 1963

Dr. R. had no further contact with the patient.

CASE 24 (Mr. P., reported by Dr. H., pp. 194-212)

Period 1, ending December 31st, 1955

I haven't heard anything.

It is a pity, but apparently Mr. P. belongs to the group of patients who disappear after the psychotherapy has been successfully concluded. It would be interesting to know what the final results will be in some years' time.

Period 2, ending June 30th, 1963

Dr. H. has not received any news from Mr. P.

CASE 25 (Mrs. T., reported by Dr. S., pp. 219-222)

Period 1, ending December 31st, 1955

Mrs. T. during a period of a few months of the renewal of our relationship behaved meekly and gratefully for a few interventions on behalf of the children. For herself she only asked for repeats of a prescription for an antihistamine which I first gave her four years ago for an allergic nasal condition. That drug she continued taking more or less without interruption and requested it usually over the telephone.

One day, however, she came with a complaint of lower abdominal pain, which she insisted was caused by a gynaecological disease. I allowed myself to be seduced to an examination. She seemed disappointed about my negative findings and my rejection of her demand to be sent to a specialist, and went apparently straight to a colleague in the neighbourhood, new to her, who gave her a letter to a consultant. Next day she sent her cards to me, with the request to sign them for the transfer to the other doctor.

I heard a few weeks later that no organic trouble was found in hospital. Her husband, whom I once met, answered my question why his wife had again taken the cards away from me with, "You know these women."

Period 2, ending June 30th, 1963

Mrs. T. left the district about five years ago. She had no further contact with me, but I have heard from her husband's employer that she was found to have pulmonary tuberculosis.

In spite of all efforts by the doctor, no lasting relationship could be established with this woman. These efforts included all sort of medical examinations, attempts at understanding her emotional problems, tolerating her aggravating behaviour with patience, using common sense strictness to educate her to a change of her aggravating behaviour, etc., etc. None of them helped. The fault was not with the methods, each of them was sensible in itself; the trouble was that the doctor was not able to understand in this case the patient's individual problems and, in consequence, could not find a way to approach her in a meaningful manner—I mean meaningful to the patient.

CASE 26 (Mr. Z., Reported by Dr. G., pp. 232–233)

Period 1, ending December 31st, 1955

January 1956. He came early in December—seen by my locum, who left a note with a long list of his complaints. Saw me a few days later, complained bitterly of vertigo. Not so friendly. "There must be something wrong. Don't you think I ought to see a specialist and find out what it really is?"

Sent to physician—Report: "A long list of symptoms, N.A.D. organically; symptoms are functional. He is a real, old-fashioned hypochondriac." No suggestions were offered for treatment, in fact one sensed a rather affectionate use of the term "Old-fashioned hypochondriac"—like the "good old days."

He then went on the sick-list and remained on it for six weeks—couldn't get to the bus, felt so giddy. "Do you think I should give up the job and get one nearer home, which does not necessitate waiting for buses?" Then, "Everybody seems to think I'm crackers, should I see a 'nerve doctor'?"

I gave him a note to see our local psychiatrist. Report: "Chronic anxiety neurotic who has had anxiety hysterical symptoms since World War I. I do not think he could really do without his symptoms now and am afraid that no form of outpatient psychotherapy would have any effect."

I saw him twice more after that, still disgruntled, although not aggressive. He still liked me, but was not happy and proud of his disabilities at the moment.

He signed off reluctantly on January 14th, and I have not seen him since—a long spell for him!

As I said in my previous note, the worm has turned with a vengeance, and it has rather shaken me, as I really felt that I had the situation under full control, in spite of your hints to the contrary.

A further report on February 17th:

He came in. His old attitude was there—"I haven't seen you for about a month," triumphantly. Complained of pain in chest and coughs. He was friendly, non-aggressive and not especially depressed.

He admitted to feeling a little better, although still giddy. He said "You're a better psychiatrist than the one at the hospital!"

So he is back in his old form.

Apparently things have settled down, the old agreement between patient and doctor is working again. But we do not know what the crisis was about, why it happened just around Christmas, whether it is a single event of not much consequence, or a serious indication that the strain on Mr. Z. is becoming too great.

Trying to get this kind of information would obviously mean breaking the agreement, and neither the psychiatrist nor Dr. G. is keen to do so—for obvious reasons.

Being left alone with his illness was more than Mr. Z. could bear, so he had to come back to his doctor. Perhaps the short-lived rebellion, demonstrating once again that his doctor was really a "bad," impotent doctor, made the return somewhat easier. We must ask, however, how long the present peace will last.

Period 2, ending June 30th, 1963

Since the previous note on him he has had
  (1) pernicious anaemia (for which he is receiving Cytamen injections regularly) and
  (2) a mild myocardial infarction.

He is a transformed character, comes in only for his necessary tablets and Cytamen. He is apparently a normal man and does not exhibit his previously hypochondrical symptoms.

We are still pals, but with a slightly more serious atmosphere to our transactions, almost as if he now realized that what I was prescribing for him were really necessary and would do him good. In the past, the purpose of his acceptance of the medicine was to prove I was powerless to make him better. He was proof against all my magic, I was impotent. I have now become a wielder of powerful magic. In fact our negotiations are conducted on a more practical and serious level.

His organic conditions have swamped his neuroticism. In fact I feel that pernicious anaemia and myocardial infarction have paradoxically cured him, although the latter may eventually kill him.

A most intriguing development, which would be well worth a proper and searching study. Apparently Mr Z. could tolerate a "bad" doctor only as long as he was certain that his life was not threatened. It seems that as long as he could feel that his life was safe, the most important thing for him was to keep up his superiority, and it did not matter to him that he had to pay for it with considerable suffering and anxiety. The trauma of the myocardial infarction changed this situation fundamentally. As Dr. G., almost certainly correctly, points out, Mr. Z. made his doctor become a "wielder of powerful magic." And this must be so in every respect, everything that his doctor prescribes must have a good effect, otherwise he (Mr. Z.) would fall prey to intolerable anxiety.

It would be most interesting to find out how this change influenced the other areas of his everyday life, especially his relationship to his workmates and his wife.

Case 27

Period 1, ending December 31st, 1955

The doctor has not heard of the family since the break, although they have not removed themselves from his list.

Period 2, ending June 30th, 1963

The doctor had no further contact with the family, except that in due course he was informed that they had changed over to another doctor's list. Some time ago he heard from some neighbours that the family had left the district. He has not met the specialist either since the events reported.

Case 28 (Reported by Dr. S., pp. 271–272)

Period 1, ending December 31st, 1955

The patient, although still on my list, has not returned since the consultation reported.

Period 2, ending June 30th, 1963

The doctor has never seen the patient since the consultation, but knows from the patient's sister that soon after he reported his consultation with her to the seminar, the patient met a widower from Canada, married him and—according to the sister—lives happily in Canada.

SUMMARY OF PREDICTIONS

To assess the reliability of our "deeper" level of diagnosis, let us examine now how far our original assessments in the years 1952 to 1954 were confirmed by the events during the two follow-up periods. This would be a fairly simple procedure, but for the problem caused by the patients who left their doctors. There are various ways in which the event of leaving can be treated.

First, one could view it as an untoward accident with which neither the patient, nor the doctor, nor the treatment had any-. thing to do. In consequence if the doctor did not hear anything more about his former patient, the case should be classified as "no follow-up ɔvailable." This procedure would be objective and unequivocal, but would miss a number of highly important differences and might lead to some unfounded or even misleading inferences.

To show what I mean, may I quote Case 23, in which the doctor successfully rescued a young girl from the brink of a neurosis, helped her to sort out a complicated family entanglement, and enabled her to find an apparently satisfactory partner. As the husband got a job in a distant part of the British Isles, the patient came to say goodbye to her doctor, since when nothing has been heard of her. Let us compare this situation with that of Case 1, in which a woman after many years of persistent attempts still felt misunderstood by her doctor, started to wander between the partners of the practice and eventually felt compelled to change over to another doctor in the same district. Or, take Case 5, in which we predicted that a serious crisis would be the consequence of the way the doctor treated his patient. The crisis in fact lasted for many years, the mistrust created by it disappeared only gradually, but then—apparently for an external reason—the family decided to leave the district.

There cannot be any doubt that these three cases represent three utterly different dynamic situations, and should not be lumped together. If, however, one tries to find out the real meaning of the patient's leaving and classifies the case accordingly, the procedure will always have some subjective elements, and cannot avoid being somewhat equivocal.

In order to forestall either of these criticisms, I shall use both methods. As mentioned in the preamble to this appendix, at the end of Period 2, that is June 30th, 1963, out of our original 28 patients there were 11 who were still in contact with (on the lists of) their doctors.

TABLE III

Original Prediction	Total	Still in contact on *30.6.63*	Total
Favourable	10	Cases 11, 13, 16, 22	4
Guarded	9	Cases 8, 15, 17, 19, 20, 26	6
Unfavourable	9	Case 9	1
GRAND TOTAL	28		11

It is somewhat uncertain whether Case 21, for whom we made a favourable prognosis originally, has or has not left her doctor finally.

TABLE IV

Original Prediction	Total	Left in Period 1	Left in Period 2	Total
Favourable	10	Cases 7, 24	Cases 1, 23	4
Guarded	9	Case 25	Cases 10, 28	3
Unfavourable	9	Cases 3, 4, 18, 27	Cases 2, 5, 12	7
GRAND TOTAL	28			14

There are two cases about which we know nothing: one is Case 6, whose doctor abandoned the seminars in our very early stages, and about whom we could not find out anything; the other is Case 14, for which we gave a favourable prognosis, and were able to follow up till the end of Period 1. However, his doctor gave up his practice during Period 2, and left London; so we do not know what happened to this patient. These two cases must be classified as truly "unknown."

I wish to repeat that these figures are as objective as figures can be; for instance, they could have been obtained by a simple questionnaire asking the doctors to tick off whether patient X was or was not in contact with them any more. Statistically they are highly significant. Whereas about one half—10 out of 19— of the patients with favourable or guarded prognosis have kept up contact with their doctors, only one in nine of those with unfavourable prognosis has done so.

This conversely means that on the basis of our "deeper" diagnosis we were able to predict, with almost 90% probability, that certain patients will leave their doctors' list. Moreover, closer inspection of our Table IV shows that even the time of leaving may be predicted. Four cases with unfavourable prognosis left within a couple of years, two further—Cases 2 and 12—left soon after two years, and only one, Case 5, stayed considerably longer. However, as we did not pay special attention to the time of leaving in our predictions, I cannot pursue this interesting question further.

Now let us turn to the other method based on clinical judgment. This means examining each case in detail in order to assess how far the original predictions were confirmed by clinical observations. This method, of course, allows a much finer gradation but, inevitably, will contain some subjective elements.

We gave a favourable prognosis for Cases 1, 7, 11, 13, 14, 16, 21, 22, 23 and 24. Of these, by the end of the first period, Cases 7 and 24 left their doctors. True, each of them had compelling external reasons for leaving and these were frankly discussed with the doctors. Moreover, both of them paid a proper farewell visit and at that time there was no indication of any impending change in their conditions. Still, it must be stated that neither of them has got in touch with their doctors since; true, Case 7 was a simple Irish woman who could not be expected to write letters, and the history of Case 24 is such that it makes understandable the fact that the patient did not want to be reminded of his past. Although Miss S., Case 23, came with her new husband to say goodbye to her doctor before Christmas 1955, it was only in 1956 that her name was removed from the doctor's list. Since then there has been no news about her. About the same happened to Mrs. Q., Case 21, towards the end of our second follow-up period but, as far as we know, her name has not yet been removed from the doctor's list. So we labelled her as "uncertain." Truly "unknown" is only Case 14, whose doctor, as mentioned above, has given up his practice. It was only in one instance, Case 1, that our original prognosis had to be completely reversed. This was already done on the basis of the first follow-up, and subsequent events confirmed this reversed prognosis; the patient left the doctor's practice disappointed.

To sum up:

TABLE V

Favourable Prognosis

Prediction	Patient	Cases	Total
Confirmed	Still with Doctor	11, 13, 16, 22	4
	Uncertain	21	1
	Left in Period 1	7, 24	2
	Left in Period 2	23	1
Changed to Unfavourable	Left	1	1
Unknown		14	1
		GRAND TOTAL	10

A guarded prognosis was given in Cases 8, 10, 15, 17, 19, 20, 25, 26 and 28. Of these 17, 20 and 28 can be considered as having confirmed our original assessment. Case 19, Peter, has developed far better than was expected; this was foreshadowed already in the first follow-up, but the second follow-up report is so good that his prognosis ought to change from guarded to favourable. Cases 8 and 10 appeared at the end of our first follow-up period to develop better than expected; this impression, however, was not confirmed by subsequent events, so I think their original assessment should remain unchanged. Of the rest, Case 25 left towards the end of the first period, while 10 and 28 left in the first part of the second period. In all three cases it was possible to obtain more or less reliable news about the patients' conditions. This information, as well as their ways of leaving their doctors, is in my opinion good confirmatory evidence for our guarded prognosis. Moreover, in Cases 25 and 28, the leaving was predicted. Case 15 is difficult to classify, the patient left the doctor's list towards the end of our first follow-up period, but remained in touch with him both through her mother and directly. Furthermore, although she developed diabetes recently, according to the last follow-up she seems to be well adjusted. So, for the time being, her prognosis should remain unchanged.

TABLE VI

Guarded Prognosis

Prediction	Patient	Cases	Total
Changed to Favourable	Still with Doctor	19	1
Confirmed	Still with Doctor	8, 15, 17, 20, 26	5
	Left in Period 1	25	1
	Left in Period 2	10, 28	2
GRAND TOTAL			9

An unfavourable prognosis was given in Cases 2, 3, 4, 5, 6, 12, 18 and 27. Case 6 could not be followed up because the doctor in charge left the seminar; it is a real "unknown." It was predicted that Cases 3, 4, 18 and 27 will leave their doctors and will not have any contact with them in the future; all four left during Period 1, and the doctors have not heard anything about them since. Cases 2 and 12 left their doctors early in Period 2; their relationship till this point and their mode of leaving confirm our predictions. As discussed in detail in my comments on the second follow-up report, it is very difficult to assess Case 5 properly. It is possible that the patient worked himself through the predicted crisis, in which case his unfavourable prognosis should be changed to "guarded," but it is equally possible that his leaving was a further symptom of the same crisis. In this case our original assessment should stand. As there is no compelling evidence for a change, I adopted the more conservative policy and left his prognosis unchanged. In Case 9, the subsequent events, at any rate until 1962, proved that contrary to the hopeful first follow-up report our original unfavourable prognosis was nearer the truth. It is, however, possible that in the last year a definite improvement took place in the patient's condition. As this is still doubtful, I left the patient's prognosis unchanged.

TABLE VII

Unfavourable Prognosis			
Prediction	*Patient*	*Cases*	*Total*
Confirmed	Still with Doctor	9	I
	Left as predicted in Period I	3, 4, 18, 27	4
	Left in Period 2	2, 5, 12	3
Unknown		6	I
GRAND TOTAL			9

In conclusion, the reliability of our predictions assessed on the basis of clinical judgment can be summed up in a concise form in Table VIII:

TABLE VIII

At the end of Period 2 (*June 30th, 1963*)								
Column	*1*	*2*	*3*	*4*	*5*	*6*	*7*	*8*
	Confirmed				Changed			
Prediction	*Patient still with doctor*	*Un-certain if patient left*	*Patient left*		*to better: Patient stayed*	*to worse: Patient left*	*Un-known*	*Total*
			in Period 1	*in Period 2*				
Favourable	4	I	2	I	–	I	I	10
Guarded	5	–	I	2	I	–	–	9
Unfavourable	I	–	4	3	–	–	I	9
TOTAL	10	I	7	6	I	I	2	28

What do these figures tell us? Of course the findings contained in Table III reappear in Table VIII. We see that more than half—exactly 11 out of 19—patients with favourable or guarded prognosis have remained in contact with their doctors, while only 1 patient out of 9 with unfavourable prognosis has done so. However, the assessment based on clinical judgment, as was to be expected, can offer a finer gradation. Among the 12 patients who kept up some contact with their doctors, that is those in Columns 1, 2 and 5, in only one case had our prediction to be changed from "guarded" to "favourable" (Case 19, Peter). In the other 11 cases direct clinical observation confirmed our predictions. Equally, taking the 14 patients who left their doctors, that is those in Columns 3, 4 and 6, here, too, in only one had the prediction to be changed from "favourable" to "unfavourable" (Case 1, Mrs. C.). In all the other 13 cases, either the leaving was predicted or the mode of leaving was such that it confirmed our predictions. In Cases 6 and 14 we lost contact with the doctors, and so we have to classify these two as "unknown."

Or, to put the same findings in a different form, an almost ten-year-long follow-up proved that we did not make mistakes when we gave an unfavourable prognosis to a patient; but in roughly 10% of the patients with favourable or guarded prognosis, our predictions were incorrect. As it happened, in one case we gave a better and in the second a worse prognosis than was proved by the events; so it is unlikely that we were victims of a systematic error, such as a constant tendency to much too optimistic or much too pessimistic assessments.

A word about the apparently high rate of leaving in patients with favourable prognosis. Its chief cause is that this group contained two young women who were sufficiently helped by the treatment to sort themselves out, and either get married during the first follow-up period (Case 23), or get remarried during the second period (Case 21). As in both cases the husbands lived in a distant town from London, their marriage led to a severing of contact with their doctors. Apart from these two, there was only one more young girl who married among the 28 cases. She was Case 10 with a guarded prognosis. There was no such case among the patients with unfavourable prognosis.

And lastly, the problem caused by the somewhat mixed group of patients with guarded prognosis. Unquestionably some of the patients, like Case 19, and possibly Case 8, could have been grouped among the patients with favourable prognosis, while others, like Cases 25 and 28, might have been classified as unfavourable. Although justified up to a point, this classification would have still left a number of patients with truly guarded prognosis, like Cases 10, 15, 17, 20, 26, and so the gain would have been very little. Still, I wish to state that the "guarded" group is less homogeneous than the other two.

Now, let us suppose that we shall have good luck, and that a third revised edition will be required at some future date. What can one expect from a third follow-up? First, we must be prepared for the fact that some more doctors will have given up their practices, or even that some of us will no longer be here. Evidently, the same might be true about some of the patients. In consequence, what we may expect is some further interesting information about one or the other of our cases; but, since the "unknown" and the "left the doctor" must inevitably increase, the value of the collected data will diminish. This rather gloomy but realistic appreciation of our future was the reason why I added this somewhat lengthy summary to the follow-up report of the present Period 2.

I wish to repeat that our 28 cases are not a representative sample; moreover, it is quite possible that with a larger number of patients with perhaps more complex problems and certainly with less time and enthusiasm at our disposal, the results of our predictions might prove less good. Still, I think it is worth recording that in a fairly well documented research these results have been obtained. This fact might encourage other research workers to experiment with a similar approach to ours. May I add that we have the records of more than 200 patients discussed by the same group of doctors during the original research, that is in the years 1952 to 1955. It would be a most interesting project to use these write-ups as a basis for predictions and then ask the doctors to check them by following up the patients. This, however, would be a real undertaking, which would need considerable support.

An Additional Rôle for the Psychological Clinic

By John D. Sutherland

IN acquiring psychotherapeutic skill of the kind described, the learning process has two aspects. On the one hand there is the building up of knowledge and experience of psychological manifestations, and on the other there is, for a considerable period at any rate, the process of adjustment in the doctor's own personality as he encounters emotional disturbances in others which may have a special significance for himself. These two aspects are interrelated, and together they make learning slow. Indeed, it may be said that the setting of a time limit to a training period in psychotherapy is a relatively arbitrary matter because learning goes on for many years.

For practical purposes, however, a certain time limit has to be defined as "the training period;" but what happens after this period has proved to be an important issue for the Clinic. Several of the practitioners who completed the training seminars wished to maintain a continuing relationship with a consultant psychiatrist to discuss their cases or at least to have the opportunity to do so in a convenient way. The recurring situation in which the general practitioner wants advice in this kind of work is as follows—"I have tried to help Mr. or Mrs. X., with certain difficulties, in such and such a way. Things are not going right, and what is going wrong?" It is this kind of problem for which the sending of the patient to the Clinic for examination with a written report following is, as a rule, of very little help. Instead, the practitioner needs to discuss his case with the consultant, and to do so he has to know him sufficiently well to talk readily about what his own contribution to the patient–doctor relationship may have been. Correspondingly, the consultant must get to know the practitioner well enough to judge how the practitioner's contribution may have affected the patient. To get effective help, the doctor and the consultant must have a relationship that is sufficiently personal for both parties to speak freely to each other.

Providing a continuing consulting service with individual sessions is rather expensive in consultant time, and so it was arranged that one of the consultants on the staff of the Clinic would have a regular period each week at which former members of the courses could bring up their cases. This has proved to be a useful and economical arrangement. Many of the practitioners had become well known to each other during their training period, and so it was easy for them to bring up their cases in front of their colleagues at these conferences. Few of the members attended regularly each meeting and mostly they would come when they had a case they wished to discuss.

The senior members of the staff at the Tavistock Clinic have come to the conclusion that devoting a proportion of their time to such continuing "conferences" is an extremely important function for the specialist clinic in a community mental health service. There is no doubt that when the specialist can devote a proportion of his time to training and maintaining a number of general practitioners in their work with psychological problems, he can make a far more effective contribution to the provision of psychotherapy on a scale appropriate to community needs than he can by attempting to provide the treatment himself.

This kind of work with general practitioners has been considered by the consultants at the Tavistock Clinic to be so important as a contribution to the mental health services that a number of allied developments have been fostered during the last few years. Thus, as well as general-practitioner groups, requests for training from other professions whose members can play an important rôle in tackling psychological problems when the psychiatric clinic would appear to be inappropriate have also been met. These groups have been given the opportunity to acquire some psychotherapeutic skill in a similar way to the general practitioners and they have also been given continuing help with their cases through regular conferences. So far these groups have included psychiatrists who have not had any special psychotherapeutic training, family case-workers helping with marital problems, maternity and child welfare doctors and health visitors, and probation officers.

Our experience in the last few years has therefore suggested that to increase the resources of our mental health services, the specialist psychological clinic should fulfil two rôles—

(1) The treatment of the more serious and complicated psychological conditions.
(2) (a) The training of general practitioners and other professional groups.
    (b) The maintaining of a permanent consultant relationship with such groups through regular conferences.

It is impossible to define the boundaries of the kind of case that may be taken on by the general practitioner or allied professional worker as so much depends on his personality, on the skill he has acquired, and on the amount of consultant help he can draw upon. The important point, however, is that with the making available of a continuing, and therefore personal, relationship with the consultant, he can undertake a good deal of work that he might not otherwise do.

It has been our experience that when the highly specialized knowledge and skills of the consultant psychotherapist can be drawn upon by these allied groups, sound work can be done within the limits of the skills taught. The continuing relationship through the regular conferences makes it unnecessary for the practitioner or allied workers to stretch their skills beyond their resources, and the interests of all parties, the patient, the practitioner and the specialist can be safeguarded.

One further implication for the clinic providing specialist time for this purpose, is that the consultants in the clinic, or at least a self-selected group of them, should work together sufficiently, and share a sufficiently common approach to the treatment of everyday problems. Some consultants may be better at training, but there will always be the situation where training groups pass into the "maintenance" groups. The practitioner must feel that in passing from one consultant to another he is going to meet with a similar outlook and "language." From the time that our scheme was started we found it useful for a number of the consultants to attend the general practitioners' groups from time to time so that the general lines of work were familiar to all.

References to Case Material

Case Number	Clinical Details	Other References
	See pages	*See* pages
1	11–12, 325–330	19, 42, 224, 237, 265, 270, 280
2	12–13, 330–331	19, 32, 37, 266, 280, 291
3	13, 331	19, 270
4	14–17, 331–2	19, 236, 266
5	21–22, 332–5	31, 41, 42, 43, 60, 71, 265, 280, 285, 310
6	26–31, 335	42, 60, 71, 224, 269, 270, 285, 310
7	32–33, 335	279, 291
8	55–56, 335–8	68, 269, 291
9	60, 62, 338–342	65–68, 265, 280, 285
10	63–65, 342–6	3, 65–68, 160, 236, 269, 279, 280, 285, 289, 291
11	69–71, 346–9	42, 266, 279, 280, 291
12	76–80, 349–350	85, 89, 94, 108, 236, 266, 269, 270, 280, 285, 327
13	82–83, 350–2	89, 291
14	86–90, 352	94, 279, 291
15	109–115, 353–4	3, 230, 235, 279, 291, 310
16	122–126, 354–5	108, 236, 266, 279, 291
17	127–131, 355–9	3, 230, 266, 310
18	137–138, 359–360	108, 236
19	139–142, 145–147, 360–1	3, 158, 266, 279, 280, 285, 289, 291, 306, 310
20	148–156, 361–4	236, 279, 291
21	162–169, 364–6	3, 237, 266, 269, 270, 279, 280, 289, 291
22	174–181, 366–8	5, 266, 269, 280, 289, 291
23	181–191, 368	3, 224, 236, 267, 279, 285, 289, 291, 310
24	194–212, 369	3, 5, 266, 270, 279, 289, 291
25	219, 222, 369–370	235
26	232–233, 370–2	236, 280, 285
27	243–244, 372	86, 90, 285
28	271, 272, 372	235, 285, 310

References to Doctors Participating

Dr. B.   86, 352

Dr. C.   76, 148, 236, 349, 361

Dr. D.   60, 338

Dr. E.   12, 21, 48, 330, 332

Dr. G.   32, 122, 139, 232, 236, 335, 354, 360, 370

Dr. H.   174, 194, 237, 366, 369

Dr. K.   127, 355

Dr. M.   11, 45, 162, 237, 325, 364

Dr. P.   13, 136, 331, 359

Dr. R.   14, 63, 160, 236, 331, 342, 368

Dr. S.   109, 219, 235, 270, 353, 369, 372

Dr. Y.   69, 82, 346, 350

Dr. Z.   55, 335

Index

Figures in heavy type denote pages on which the topic is the principal subject matter.

Round brackets ( ) include plural forms or synonyms.

Square brackets [ ] include cognate topics listed elsewhere in the Index.